Advances in Minimally Invasive Liver Resection for Cancer Therapies

Yutaro Kato, Atsushi Sugioka, Masayuki Kojima, Satoshi Mii, Yuichiro Uchida and Hideaki Iwama et al.
Minimally Invasive Anatomic Liver Resection for Hepatocellular Carcinoma Using the Extrahepatic Glissonian Approach: Surgical Techniques and Comparison of Outcomes with the Open Approach and between the Laparoscopic and Robotic Approaches
Reprinted from: *Cancers* **2023**, *15*, 2219, doi:10.3390/cancers15082219 113

Luigi Cioffi, Giulio Belli, Francesco Izzo, Corrado Fantini, Alberto D'Agostino and Gianluca Russo et al.
Minimally Invasive ALPPS Procedure: A Review of Feasibility and Short-Term Outcomes
Reprinted from: *Cancers* **2023**, *15*, 1700, doi:10.3390/cancers15061700 133

Tijs J. Hoogteijling, Jasper P. Sijberden, John N. Primrose, Victoria Morrison-Jones, Sachin Modi and Giuseppe Zimmitti et al.
Laparoscopic Right Hemihepatectomy after Future Liver Remnant Modulation: A Single Surgeon's Experience
Reprinted from: *Cancers* **2023**, *15*, 2851, doi:10.3390/cancers15102851 144

Alexandra Nassar, Stylianos Tzedakis, Alix Dhote, Marie Strigalev, Romain Coriat and Mehdi Karoui et al.
Multiple Laparoscopic Liver Resection for Colorectal Liver Metastases
Reprinted from: *Cancers* **2023**, *15*, 435, doi:10.3390/cancers15020435 156

Takuya Minagawa, Osamu Itano, Minoru Kitago, Yuta Abe, Hiroshi Yagi and Taizo Hibi et al.
Surgical and Oncological Outcomes of Salvage Hepatectomy for Locally Recurrent Hepatocellular Carcinoma after Locoregional Therapy: A Single-Institution Experience
Reprinted from: *Cancers* **2023**, *15*, 2320, doi:10.3390/cancers15082320 168

Contents

About the Editor vii

Preface ix

Zenichi Morise
Editorial (Preface) for the Special Issue on Advances in Minimally Invasive Liver Resection for Cancer Therapies
Reprinted from: Cancers 2023, 15, 3520, doi:10.3390/cancers15133520 1

Gianluca Cassese, Ho-Seong Han, Boram Lee, Hae Won Lee, Jai Young Cho and Roberto Troisi
Leaping the Boundaries in Laparoscopic Liver Surgery for Hepatocellular Carcinoma
Reprinted from: Cancers 2022, 14, 2012, doi:10.3390/cancers14082012 5

Winifred M. Lo, Samer T. Tohme and David A. Geller
Recent Advances in Minimally Invasive Liver Resection for Colorectal Cancer Liver Metastases—A Review
Reprinted from: Cancers 2022, 15, 142, doi:10.3390/cancers15010142 19

Yoshiki Fujiyama, Taiga Wakabayashi, Kohei Mishima, Malek A. Al-Omari, Marco Colella and Go Wakabayashi
Latest Findings on Minimally Invasive Anatomical Liver Resection
Reprinted from: Cancers 2023, 15, 2218, doi:10.3390/cancers15082218 34

Federica Cipriani, Francesca Ratti, Gianluca Fornoni, Rebecca Marino, Antonella Tudisco and Marco Catena et al.
Conversion of Minimally Invasive Liver Resection for HCC in Advanced Cirrhosis: Clinical Impact and Role of Difficulty Scoring Systems
Reprinted from: Cancers 2023, 15, 1432, doi:10.3390/cancers15051432 43

Giammauro Berardi, Edoardo Maria Muttillo, Marco Colasanti, Germano Mariano, Roberto Luca Meniconi and Stefano Ferretti et al.
Challenging Scenarios and Debated Indications for Laparoscopic Liver Resections for Hepatocellular Carcinoma
Reprinted from: Cancers 2023, 15, 1493, doi:10.3390/cancers15051493 58

Shogo Tanaka, Shoji Kubo and Takeaki Ishizawa
Positioning of Minimally Invasive Liver Surgery for Hepatocellular Carcinoma: From Laparoscopic to Robot-Assisted Liver Resection
Reprinted from: Cancers 2023, 15, 488, doi:10.3390/cancers15020488 75

Zenichi Morise, Luca Aldrighetti, Giulio Belli, Francesca Ratti, Tan To Cheung and Chung Mau Lo et al.
An International Retrospective Observational Study of Liver Functional Deterioration after Repeat Liver Resection for Patients with Hepatocellular Carcinoma
Reprinted from: Cancers 2022, 14, 2598, doi:10.3390/cancers14112598 88

Hirokatsu Katagiri, Hiroyuki Nitta, Syoji Kanno, Akira Umemura, Daiki Takeda and Taro Ando et al.
Safety and Feasibility of Laparoscopic Parenchymal-Sparing Hepatectomy for Lesions with Proximity to Major Vessels in Posterosuperior Liver Segments 7 and 8
Reprinted from: Cancers 2023, 15, 2078, doi:10.3390/cancers15072078 98

Editor
Zenichi Morise
Department of Surgery
Fujita Health University
School of Medicine
Okazaki, Aichi
Japan

Editorial Office
MDPI
St. Alban-Anlage 66
4052 Basel, Switzerland

This is a reprint of articles from the Special Issue published online in the open access journal *Cancers* (ISSN 2072-6694) (available at: www.mdpi.com/journal/cancers/special_issues/advances_in_LRCT).

For citation purposes, cite each article independently as indicated on the article page online and as indicated below:

Lastname, A.A.; Lastname, B.B. Article Title. *Journal Name* **Year**, *Volume Number*, Page Range.

ISBN 978-3-0365-8685-4 (Hbk)
ISBN 978-3-0365-8684-7 (PDF)
doi.org/10.3390/books978-3-0365-8684-7

© 2023 by the authors. Articles in this book are Open Access and distributed under the Creative Commons Attribution (CC BY) license. The book as a whole is distributed by MDPI under the terms and conditions of the Creative Commons Attribution-NonCommercial-NoDerivs (CC BY-NC-ND) license.

Advances in Minimally Invasive Liver Resection for Cancer Therapies

Editor

Zenichi Morise

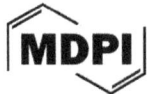

Basel • Beijing • Wuhan • Barcelona • Belgrade • Novi Sad • Cluj • Manchester

About the Editor

Zenichi Morise

Zenichi Morise is a Professor/Chairman of the department (Surgery) in Fujita Health University School of Medicine Okazaki Medical Center. He was born in 1962 at Kurume-city Fukuoka Japan and graduated Keio University in 1987. He is the founding past director of Fujita Health University Okazaki Medical Center. In the role, he developed the university hospital from scratch and ran until it became well-functioning and profitable. As well as this, he conducted the project of accommodating and caring for 128 COVID-19-positive patients from the cruise ship just before the openings both of the pandemic in Japan and the hospital (Feb-Mar 2020) [N Engl J Med. 2020; 383:885-886. doi:10.1056/NEJMc2013020].

He has been working on hepato-pancreato-biliary, mainly liver, surgeries. Currently, his research interest is minimally invasive liver surgery, especially for HCC. He published the world-first paper describing the novel concept of "Caudal approach" in laparoscopic liver surgery in 2013. The concept was defined as a main conceptual change of laparoscopic liver resection in the 2nd International Consensus Conference and followed by many papers, including his own works. He has been doing research about the advantages of minimally invasive liver surgery, such as for patients with impaired liver function and repeat liver resection. He conducted several ILLS (International laparoscopic liver society)-related projects and published the papers, including laparoscopic repeat liver resection.

Preface

To all friends and colleagues of ILLS.

World-famous prominent teams of surgeons and researchers wrote papers for this topic.

This Special Issue, "Advances in Minimally Invasive Liver Resection for Cancer Therapies", is dedicated to the further steps that should be taken towards implementing minimally invasive liver resection as a standard surgical practice of cancer therapy.

Zenichi Morise
Editor

Editorial

Editorial (Preface) for the Special Issue on Advances in Minimally Invasive Liver Resection for Cancer Therapies

Zenichi Morise

Department of Surgery, School of Medicine, Fujita Health University Okazaki Medical Center, 1 Gotanda Harisakicho, Okazaki 444-0827, Aichi, Japan; zmorise@fujita-hu.ac.jp; Tel.: +81-564-64-8800; Fax: +81-564-64-8135

After the initial reports of laparoscopic liver resection (LLR) in the early 1990s, minimally invasive liver resection has been rapidly developing based on technical and instrumental improvements [1] during its first 30 years, with two international consensus conferences [2,3] and three world congresses of the International Laparoscopic Liver Society [4]. Resections in the anterolateral segments and left lateral sectionectomy were established as common surgical procedures. Laparoscopic hemi-hepatectomies and sectionectomies (excluding left lateral sectionectomy), handling straightforward caudal–cranial transection planes suitable for the laparoscopic approach, followed them [1,3]. Partial resections and segmentectomies in posterosuperior segments (segments 1, 4a, 7, and 8), repeat LLR, and various untypical anatomical resections (such as extended anatomical resections, combinations of small anatomical resections, and hepatic-vein-guided resections, with or without preoperative simulations and intraoperative navigations) are now on their way to being established as generalized practices that many centers can adapt. Many attempts to conquer its specific disadvantages, such as the lack of a 3D view, movement restriction, little tactile sensation, and difficulty to obtain a good overview for the whole operative field, were performed. Thereafter, almost all styles of LLR without vessel reconstruction can be currently performed in many centers. However, the difficulty leading to open conversion and morbidity/mortality is different in each specific case. It not only depends on the resection style but also tumor condition (size/number/location/proximity to major vessels) as well as a patient's general condition (performance status, comorbidities, etc.) and liver condition (such as background chronic liver diseases (CLDs) in hepatocellular carcinoma (HCC) patients and post-chemotherapy liver damage in patients with colorectal liver metastasis (CRCLM)). For these situations, several difficulty scoring systems (DSSs) have been developed for patient selection and the safe dissemination of procedures based on a learning curve.

During these developments, not only the feasibility after conquering disadvantages but also specific advantages were discussed. Less intraoperative blood loss, less morbidity, and shorter hospital stays with comparable long-term outcomes have been generally reported for HCC and CRCLM [5–7]. We reported the novel concept of a "caudal approach to LLR" in 2013 [8], which was defined as a main conceptual change from open liver resection to LLR in the statement of the 2nd International Consensus Conference on LLR [3]. We reported that this LLR-specific approach can cause the benefits of LLR for CLD patients who sometimes develop postoperative liver failure and often need repeated treatments for multifocal and metachronous HCC [5,9]. The basic approach of LLR, the "caudal approach", can make minimum manipulation (damage) of the residual liver and surrounding structures (such as collateral vessels in CLD patients) possible, and leads to less liver-related morbidity/mortality plus less deterioration of liver function after liver resection. Similarly, repeat liver resection can be performed with minimum adhesiolysis in the approach, with the benefits of less blood loss, less morbidity, and shorter hospital stays with comparable operation times and long-term outcomes [10] (Figure 1).

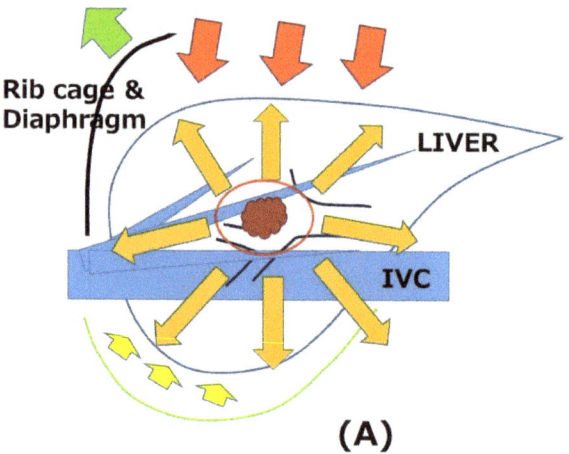

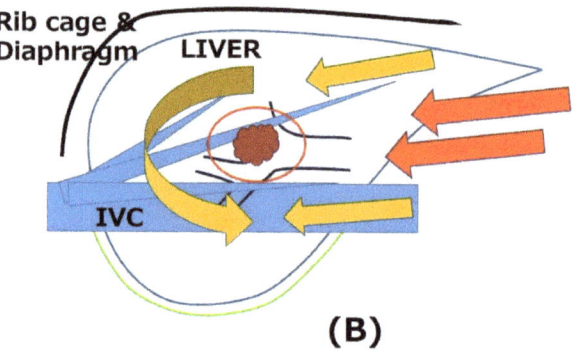

Figure 1. Open (**A**) and laparoscopic "caudal approach" (**B**) repeat liver resections [11]. Liver resection is a procedure in which the liver protected inside a subphrenic "rib cage" is handled and resected. The directions of view and manipulation in each approach are indicated with red arrows. (**A**) In open liver resection, the cage is opened with a big subcostal incision followed by lifting of the costal arch, and the mobilized liver is picked up from the retroperitoneum. (**B**) In the laparoscopic approach, the instruments were introduced into the cage from the caudal direction and the surgery was performed with minimal damage to the associated structures.

This field is still developing. LLR for cancers has been mainly applied for the patients with HCC and CRCLM as curative-intent resection [12]. LR for each disease has its own specificity based on disease characteristics and background liver condition. HCC patients mostly with a CLD background often develop postoperative liver failure and multifocal metachronous HCCs that need repeated treatment of liver resection in combination with (sometimes as a salvage therapy for) RFA/TACE during their long-term treatment histories. For those patients, LLR is now applied for its advantages. Anatomical resection is recommended for the disease due to its feature of spreading through the portal vein system. Precise anatomical LLR using ICG staining, etc., is developing. CRCLM patients often have postchemotherapy liver injury and multiple tumors. LLR could be used for fragile and congestive livers, with its merit of less bleeding. Multiple tumors need intraoperative precise tumor-localization as well as pre- and intraoperative precise planning for the extent of resections. The localization of tumors by using ICG fluorescence in LLR is spreading. In order to expand the indication of liver resection for multiple CRCLM, two-stage hepatectomy, future remnant liver hypertrophy with portal vein embolization, and associated liver partition with portal vein ligation for staged hepatectomy have been introduced. Multiple parenchymal-sparing resections are also performed. For liver resections with these procedures, reports of LLR application are increasing. Furthermore, the early introduction of adjuvant chemotherapy after LLR with early recovery may lead to better long-term outcomes. It is an important topic.

Biliary tract carcinoma (BTC) is also one of the candidates for LLR application [12]. However, the surgery for BTC needs lymph node dissection and bile duct resection plus reconstruction. Although there are reports of LLR for peripheral intrahepatic cholangiocarcinoma, which is often treated like HCC, and gall bladder carcinoma without the need of bile duct resection, the surgeries for the other BTCs with the needs of liver resection plus lymph node dissection/bile duct resection are currently in their developing stage. Recently emerging robot-assisted LLR could work with advantages in those cases, besides complicated resections for other tumors.

Based on the above-mentioned current status, world-famous prominent teams of researchers and surgeons wrote papers on topics in which they are interested. This Special Issue, "Advances in Minimally Invasive Liver Resection for Cancer Therapies", is dedicated to the further steps that should be taken toward implementing minimally invasive liver resection as a standard surgical practice of cancer therapy.

Conflicts of Interest: The authors declare no conflict of interest.

References

1. Morise, Z.; Wakabayashi, G. First quarter century of laparoscopic liver resection. *World J. Gastroenterol.* **2017**, *23*, 3581–3588. [CrossRef] [PubMed]
2. Buell, J.F.; Cherqui, D.; Geller, D.A.; O'Rourke, N.; Iannitti, D.; Dagher, I.; Koffron, A.J.; Thomas, M.; Gayet, B.; Han, H.S.; et al. The international position on laparoscopic liver surgery: The Louisville Statement, 2008. *Ann. Surg.* **2009**, *250*, 825–830. [CrossRef] [PubMed]
3. Wakabayashi, G.; Cherqui, D.; Geller, D.A.; Buell, J.F.; Kaneko, H.; Han, H.S.; Asbun, H.; O'Rourke, N.; Tanabe, M.; Koffron, A.J.; et al. Recommendations for laparoscopic liver resection: A report from the second international consensus conference held in Morioka. *Ann. Surg.* **2015**, *261*, 619–629. [PubMed]
4. Cherqui, D.; Wakabayashi, G.; Geller, D.A.; Buell, J.F.; Han, H.S.; Soubrane, O.; O'Rourke, N. International Laparoscopic Liver Society. The need for organization of laparoscopic liver resection. *J. Hepatobiliary Pancreat. Sci.* **2016**, *23*, 665–667. [CrossRef] [PubMed]
5. Morise, Z.; Ciria, R.; Cherqui, D.; Chen, K.H.; Belli, G.; Wakabayashi, G. Can we expand the indications for laparoscopic liver resection? A systematic review and meta-analysis of laparoscopic liver resection for patients with hepatocellular carcinoma and chronic liver disease. *J. Hepatobiliary Pancreat. Sci.* **2015**, *22*, 342–352. [CrossRef] [PubMed]
6. Takahara, T.; Wakabayashi, G.; Beppu, T.; Aihara, A.; Hasegawa, K.; Gotohda, N.; Hatano, E.; Tanahashi, Y.; Mizuguchi, T.; Kamiyama, T.; et al. Long-term and perioperative outcomes of laparoscopic versus open liver resection for hepatocellular carcinoma with propensity score matching: A multi-institutional Japanese study. *J. Hepatobiliary Pancreat. Sci.* **2015**, *22*, 721–727. [CrossRef] [PubMed]
7. Beppu, T.; Wakabayashi, G.; Hasegawa, K.; Gotohda, N.; Mizuguchi, T.; Takahashi, Y.; Hirokawa, F.; Taniai, N.; Watanabe, M.; Katou, M.; et al. Long-term and perioperative outcomes of laparoscopic versus open liver resection for colorectal liver metastases with propensity score matching: A multi-institutional Japanese study. *J. Hepatobiliary Pancreat. Sci.* **2015**, *22*, 711–720. [CrossRef] [PubMed]
8. Tomishige, H.; Morise, Z.; Kawabe, N.; Nagata, H.; Ohshima, H.; Kawase, J.; Arakawa, S.; Yoshida, R.; Isetani, M. Caudal approach to pure laparoscopic posterior sectionectomy under the laparoscopy-specific view. *World J. Gastrointest. Surg.* **2013**, *5*, 173–177. [CrossRef] [PubMed]
9. Berardi, G.; Morise, Z.; Sposito, C.; Igarashi, K.; Panetta, V.; Simonelli, I.; Kim, S.; Goh, B.K.P.; Kubo, S.; Tanaka, S.; et al. Development of a nomogram to predict outcome after liver resection for hepatocellular carcinoma in Child-Pugh B cirrhosis. *J. Hepatol.* **2020**, *72*, 75–84. [CrossRef] [PubMed]
10. Morise, Z.; Aldrighetti, L.; Belli, G.; Ratti, F.; Belli, A.; Cherqui, D.; Tanabe, M.; Wakabayashi, G.; ILLS-Tokyo Collaborator group. Laparoscopic repeat liver resection for hepatocellular carcinoma: A multicentre propensity score-based study. *Br. J. Surg.* **2020**, *107*, 889–895. [CrossRef] [PubMed]

11. Morise, Z.; Katsuno, H.; Kikuchi, K.; Endo, T.; Matsuo, K.; Asano, Y.; Horiguchi, A. Laparoscopic Repeat Liver Resection—Selecting the Best Approach for Repeat Liver Resection. *Cancers* **2023**, *15*, 421. [CrossRef] [PubMed]
12. Morise, Z. Current status of minimally invasive liver surgery for cancers. *World J. Gastroenterol.* **2022**, *28*, 6090–6098. [CrossRef] [PubMed]

Disclaimer/Publisher's Note: The statements, opinions and data contained in all publications are solely those of the individual author(s) and contributor(s) and not of MDPI and/or the editor(s). MDPI and/or the editor(s) disclaim responsibility for any injury to people or property resulting from any ideas, methods, instructions or products referred to in the content.

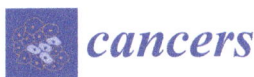 *cancers*

Review

Leaping the Boundaries in Laparoscopic Liver Surgery for Hepatocellular Carcinoma

Gianluca Cassese [1,2], Ho-Seong Han [1,*], Boram Lee [1], Hae Won Lee [1], Jai Young Cho [1] and Roberto Troisi [2]

1. Department of HPB Surgery, Seoul National University Bundang Hospital, Seongnam 13620, Korea; gianluca.cassese@unina.it (G.C.); boramlee0827@snubh.org (B.L.); lansh@hanmail.net (H.W.L.); jycho@snubh.org (J.Y.C.)
2. Minimally Invasive and Robotic HPB Surgery Unit, Department of Clinical Medicine and Surgery, Federico II University, 80131 Naples, Italy; roberto.troisi@unina.it
* Correspondence: hanhs@snubh.org; Tel.: +82-31-787-7091

Simple Summary: Recent advances in surgical techniques and perioperative management lead to a redefinition of the actual frontiers of Laparoscopic Liver Resection (LLR) by including patients with more advanced disease. Nonetheless, because of both underlying liver conditions and technical difficulty, LLR for Hepatocellular Carcinoma (HCC) is still considered as a challenging procedure. Specific concerns exist about LLR in cirrhotic patients, posterosuperior segments, giant and multiple tumors, as well as repeat resections. This review focuses on the specific limits of this approach in HCC patients in order to put into practice all the pre- and intra-operative precautions to overcome their boundaries, making this technique the standard of care within high-volume hepatobiliary centers.

Abstract: The minimally invasive approach for hepatocellular carcinoma (HCC) had a slower diffusion compared to other surgical fields, mainly due to inherent peculiarities regarding the risks of uncontrollable bleeding, oncological inadequacy, and the need for both laparoscopic and liver major skills. Recently, laparoscopic liver resection (LLR) has been associated with an improved postoperative course, including reduced postoperative decompensation, intraoperative blood losses, length of hospitalization, and unaltered oncological outcomes, leading to its adoption within international guidelines. However, LLR for HCC still faces several limitations, mainly linked to the impaired function of underlying parenchyma, tumor size and numbers, and difficult tumor position. The aim of this review is to highlight the state of the art and future perspectives of LLR for HCC, focusing on key points for overcoming currents limitations and pushing the boundaries in minimally invasive liver surgery (MILS).

Keywords: laparoscopic liver resection; hepatocellular carcinoma; overcoming the limits; minimally invasive liver surgery

Citation: Cassese, G.; Han, H.-S.; Lee, B.; Lee, H.W.; Cho, J.Y.; Troisi, R. Leaping the Boundaries in Laparoscopic Liver Surgery for Hepatocellular Carcinoma. *Cancers* **2022**, *14*, 2012. https://doi.org/10.3390/cancers14082012

Academic Editor: Adam E. Frampton

Received: 1 March 2022
Accepted: 12 April 2022
Published: 15 April 2022

Publisher's Note: MDPI stays neutral with regard to jurisdictional claims in published maps and institutional affiliations.

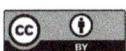

Copyright: © 2022 by the authors. Licensee MDPI, Basel, Switzerland. This article is an open access article distributed under the terms and conditions of the Creative Commons Attribution (CC BY) license (https://creativecommons.org/licenses/by/4.0/).

1. Introduction

Liver cancer is the fifth-most-common cancer in the world and the fourth-most-common cause of cancer-related death [1]. With an estimated incidence from 500,000 to 1 million per year, hepatocellular carcinoma (HCC) accounts for about 90% of liver cancers and is still associated with a poor prognosis [2]. When it is diagnosed in the early stages, 5-year overall survival (OS) reaches 50–70%, thanks to the advances in both surgical and medical therapy [2]. Surgical treatments include liver transplantation (LT) and liver resections, with a recurrence rate as high as 20% after LT and 70% after liver resection [3]. LT is the best curative treatment in cirrhotic patients, but due to organ shortages and the long waiting times associated with the consequent risk of dropout for tumor progression, it should be reserved for patients who are not candidates for LR or RFA due to uncompensated cirrhosis, patients with bad prognostic factors on pathological examination after resection, and those with recurrent HCC in transplantable patients [4]. Accordingly, liver resection is still considered the first-line treatment for HCC in patients with compensated cirrhosis [5]. Thermal ablation is considered to be effective only for lesions smaller than 3 cm when technically feasible. On the other side, for non-resectable liver disease, trans-arterial chemoembolization (TACE) represents the treatment of choice if the patient has a suitable performance status. Medical therapy is reserved for cases with disseminated disease or when other therapies are not feasible. To date, it is mainly based on the use of sorafenib, a kinase inhibitor, but thanks to an improved understanding of molecular pathways of HCC carcinogenesis, other immunotherapy drugs are licensed in some countries or currently in an advanced phase of clinical trials [6,7].

Since the first laparoscopic liver resection (LLR) was reported by Reich and colleagues in 1991 [8], its spreading has been slower when compared to other surgical specialties. This has been due to different reasons, including the technical complexity of parenchymal transection and hilar dissection, the risk for massive bleeding, the oncological concerns about resection margins (limited by the initial unavailability of intraoperative ultrasounds), and the consideration of cirrhotic patients as too fragile and complex for a minimally invasive approach. Slowly, more and more papers focusing on LLR have been published, indicating that minimally invasive liver surgery (MILS) is a viable option for both primary and secondary liver diseases [9].

In the setting of hepatocellular carcinoma (HCC) treatment, international guidelines have officially approved the use of laparoscopy in the treatment of early-stage disease [10,11]. Indeed, different authors have proposed that MILS could decrease the risk for postoperative decompensation of HCC patients, and in everyday practice, high-volume centers routinely perform LLR also for challenging cases in fragile cirrhotic patients [12,13].

However, several limitations to the universal adoption of LLR for HCC still exist. Firstly, the minimally invasive liver surgeon must be confident with both laparoscopy and open liver surgery. Secondly, there is the need for performing more complex procedures than for other liver pathologies, which includes anatomical resections (AR), thanks to the theoretical advantage of excising the entire primary tumor along with adjacent liver parenchyma containing micro-metastases, even if survival advantages are still debated [14,15]. Finally, other challenges are represented by tumor location, tumor size, the proximity of the tumor to large vessels, and underlying liver function. All these aspects are not considered a contraindication per se but can be limiting with regard to the laparoscopic approach.

In this review, we will first summarize the current indications and limitations for LLR for HCC, and then we will focus on the strategies for overcoming the current challenges.

2. Current Indications and Limitations of LLR for HCC

Several advantages have been proven in patients undergoing minimally invasive surgery in other surgical fields, including reduced length of hospital stay, postoperative pain, bleedings, complication rates related to surgical incision, and improved postoperative quality of life. However, after 30 years since the first reported LLR, a randomized trial testing the efficacy and safety of a laparoscopic approach for HCC treatment still does not exist. To date, only one randomized controlled trial investigating LLR has been published, the OSLO-COMET, focused on patients with colorectal liver metastases undergoing parenchymal-sparing liver surgery, therefore including mainly atypical resections in non-cirrhotic patients, showing reduced postoperative complications and hospital stay in the laparoscopic group [16].

Even in the absence of randomized trials, recommendations for implementation and adoption of LLR in HCC were proposed by expert consensus conferences, then followed by recent guidelines based on non-randomized studies. The first international expert consensus was held in Louisville in 2008 [17]. This conference defined univocal terminology about laparoscopic procedures (pure, hand-assisted laparoscopy, and hybrid techniques). It was highlighted that major laparoscopic liver resections had been performed with safety and efficacy equaling open surgery in highly specialized centers, however underlining the potentially unsafe and rapid dissemination of such difficult procedures in the absence of structured training and renown certification.

The Southampton Consensus Guidelines (2018) can be considered the actual clinical practices guidelines, aiming to guide "the safe development and progression of laparoscopic liver surgery" [18]. These guidelines underlined that the majority of the evidence was published from surgeons experienced in both laparoscopic techniques and liver surgery, working in high-volume centers, and recognized that in expert hands, major LLR is associated with reduced hospital stay and blood loss, while oncological outcomes are comparable to open liver resection (OLR) [18]. There is a specific section involving HCC, stating that the available data from literature strongly suggested that LLR for HCC treatment is associated with reduced blood loss, transfusion rate, postoperative ascites, liver failure, and hospital stay with comparable operation time, disease-free margin, and recurrence rates [19,20]. Furthermore, in a propensity score-matched study focused on minor resections, a laparoscopic approach was found to be the only independent factor to reduce the complication rate in resections for HCC [21].

Thus, the adoption of LLR for HCC should now be recommended in each high-volume HPB center. During the initial phases, clinical practice should follow a step-wise approach, starting from minor liver resection in anterolateral segments, followed by major liver resections and resections of lesions located in posterosuperior segments, which are the most difficult due to the orientation of the transection planes. To guide this approach, several difficulty scores and classification systems have been described. Unfortunately, to date, most of the available scores consider only some aspects, and there is not a score able to predict all the different possible outcomes.

Even after the consensus statements, the role of LLR in some situations is still debated, such as for difficultly located HCC and for multiple or giant lesions.

3. Perioperative Management of HCC Patients Undergoing LLR

In the near-zero mortality era, with all technological advances available in surgical, anesthesiologic, radiological, and hepatological fields, attention must be focused not only on intraoperative aspects but also pre- and postoperative assessments. Meticulous preparation of the patient, with attention to every aspect concerning the different phases of management, is the key to finally overcoming different limits in the treatment of HCC patients.

3.1. Tumor Anatomical Modeling and Surgical Planning

One of the most important differences from other surgeries is that liver resections need a wide preoperative evaluation with very tailored surgical planning. A precise study of our patient's anatomy, as well as the exact location of the lesion within the liver and its relationship to vascular structures, is essential to correctly plan LLR. Anatomical and positional aspects seem to be even more important in HCC surgery, given the importance of performing anatomical resections, which implies the removal of the entire portal territory nourishing the tumor, which could be associated with better short-term oncological results [14,22]. Therefore, different imaging modalities have been improved, such as 3D reconstructions for a more accurate study of exact lesion positioning with regard to vascular and biliary structures [23].

When dealing with large resections, especially in the case of cirrhotic liver, multiple tumors, or large-sized lesions, the risk for post-hepatectomy liver failure (PHLF) is still an important cause of mortality [24]. The preoperative evaluation should also be aimed to identify all the possible preoperative risk factors for PHLF in order to mitigate them and prevent fearsome postoperative complications as much as possible [25]. While the biggest part of these risk factors cannot be modified, we can act on the volume of the liver remnant. Thus, a precise volume analysis must always be carried out before a major hepatectomy. Vauthey et al. introduced a formula for a precise evaluation based on a correlation of liver volume with body surface area (eTLV: = $-794.41 + 1267.28 \times$ body surface area) [26]. As widely validated in literature, the estimated FRL can be calculated by the ratio of

FRL volume and eTLV ($FRL_{Standard} = LRV/TLV_{Standard} \times 100\%$) [27]. It is considered safe an FRL of $\geq 20\%$ of volume in case of normal liver, $\geq 30\%$ after chemotherapy, 40% for steatotic and cholestatic liver, and $\geq 50\%$ in case of cirrhosis [28].

3.2. Evaluation of Liver Function

Stratification in cirrhotic patients always has to be assessed using the Child–Turcot–Pugh (CTP) and the Model for End-Stage Liver Disease (MELD) score, as recommended in international guidelines [10,11]. In particular, the Barcelona Clinic Liver Cancer (BCLC) staging system is the most widely adopted, and it takes into account simultaneously the liver function evaluation with CTP score, patient performance status, and tumor characteristics, allowing a prognostic stratification and guiding treatment allocation [7,10]. However, both scoring systems present some weak points. They are not useful in non-cirrhotic patients, and they cannot accurately identify patients at risk for postoperative liver failure [29]. In particular, an impaired CTP can hide a wide range of cirrhosis severity (the "ceiling effect"), as well as a suitable CTP, cannot show different underlying conditions ("floor effect") [30]. Similarly, newer scores have been proposed, such as ALBI and ABIC scores, but they cannot be used in all settings of patients, and they are not universally adopted [31]. Thus, other liver function tests should be used in addition.

The measurement of indocyanine green (ICG) clearance is widely performed in Asia, as well as in high-volume Western HPB centers. It is a dynamic method that evaluates the hepatic clearance of indocyanine green 15 min after its intravenous administration (ICG-R15), and it is usually delayed in cases of liver disease [32]. A decisional algorithm with excellent results in cirrhotic patients was developed by Makuuchi et al., according to which major resections should only be performed in patients with ICG-R15 lower than 10–20%, while neither minor resections when ICG-R15 is higher than 40% [33]. As a weak point, we can underline that it can evaluate only global liver function without specific information about the remnant. Furthermore, the use of ICG is impaired by hyperbilirubinemia since the uptake is mediated by common hepatic transporters.

Hepatobiliary scintigraphy with 99mTc-mebrofenin (HBS) is the most widely used nuclear medicine imaging technique to assess liver function. The 99mTc-mebrofenin extraction rate is correlated to underlying parenchymal status and to ICG clearance (sharing the same OATPB1/B3 transporters) [34]. In addition, it allows an evaluation of regional and segmental repartitions by the calculation of the 99mTc-mebrofenin extraction rate in the volume of interest, such as our FRL. At the segmental level, the FRL function appears to better predict the risk of PHLF than volumetric-based parameters [35]. Sadly, it is cost- and facilities-demanding, and it is impaired by hyperbilirubinemia.

3.3. Augmentation Volume Procedures

When needed, different strategies can be used to induce compensatory hypertrophy of FRL to reduce the risk of PHLF. To date, portal vein embolization (PVE) is considered the standard of care procedure for the FRL augmentation, with indications that include HCC on the cirrhotic liver. Up to 85% of patients can undergo liver resection after 4–6 weeks, which means that there is almost a 20% of failure rate due to both insufficient FLR or tumor progression in the waiting time [36]. To prevent tumor growth between PVE and LR, the addition of sequential preoperative trans-arterial chemoembolization (TACE) has been proposed, also obtaining a higher degree of hypertrophy [37]. However, the association of these procedures can lead to a worse inflammation of the hepatic pedicle, making the consequent surgical resection more difficult from the technical point of view.

Guiu et al. proposed the liver venous deprivation (LVD) technique, based on the simultaneous embolization of the hepatic vein ($\pm$ the median) and the ipsilateral portal vein, with an amplatzer plug positioned at about 10 mm from the ostium [38]. Preliminary results from a study with HBS showed +66% FLR function at day 7 after LVD when compared with PVE, an increase in the kinetic growth factor of 75%, as well as encouraging perioperative and oncological outcomes [39]. Such results must be validated by further randomized studies, and its role in cirrhotic patients is debated [40].

Associated liver partition with portal vein ligation for stage hepatectomy (ALPPS) is a two-staged hepatectomy (TSH) firstly described by Schnitzbauer et al. in 2012, with the main advantage of sensitively reducing the delay among first and second procedures [41]. The main issue for ALPPS is an increased risk of postoperative morbidity and mortality, especially for cirrhotic patients. Actually, the best setting for ALPPS is represented by patients treated for colorectal liver metastasis with an age inferior to 60 years old, reaching a mortality among 5% [42], even if cases of successful ALPPS have also been reported for advanced HCC with portal vein thrombosis [43].

3.4. Evaluation of Portal Hypertension

According to different international guidelines, preoperative portal hypertension should be assessed in cirrhotic patients undergoing liver resections [10,44]. The gold-standard technique is HVPG measurement, but it is not routinely performed because of technical and logistical issues. Thus, other methods have been proposed. In cirrhotic patients, a liver stiffness of <20 kPa and a platelet count of >150,000/dL are associated with a very low risk of clinically significant portal hypertension (CSPH) [45]. Recently, spleen stiffness has been suggested as a new non-invasive tool to predict CSPH and post-surgical morbidity and mortality [46]. Even if very promising, further prospective studies are needed before its routine use in the treatment algorithm for cirrhotic patients.

Furthermore, even if liver resections in patients with portal hypertension have traditionally shown high morbidity, thanks to ongoing improvements in surgical technique and intensive care management, they are considered feasible in selected patients in high-volume centers, leading to suitable long-term results, especially after LLR [47,48]. Azoulay et al. showed 79 patients with acceptable mortality, morbidity, and liver decompensation rates for HCC patients with CSPH. Furthermore, the laparoscopic approach was the sole predictor of a textbook outcome [49].

3.5. Intraoperative Management

Thanks to developments in surgical and anesthetic techniques, high-volume centers have reported operative mortality for LLR of less than 5% [50]. However, LLR for HCC has to face specific risks that must be well managed by both the surgeon and anesthetist by using a standardized perioperative protocol.

LLR carries an important risk of blood loss for the dissection of the hepatic vein, inferior vein cava, portal vein, and the transection of a highly vascularized parenchyma. Increased blood loss and perioperative blood transfusions are associated with worse perioperative morbidity and mortality [51]. Both surgeons and anesthesiologists must contribute to decreasing intraoperative blood loss. Surgeons can use vascular clamps intraoperatively, with more or less important hemodynamic implications: even if some small resections on a normal liver can be avoided, in order to not cause an ischemic injury to the remaining liver and intestinal congestion, a Pringle maneuver (selective or not) should be prepared when performing major resections, as recently shown in a propensity-matched analysis on 209 patients [52]. Anesthesiologists can reduce central venous pressure (CVP) during the parenchymal transection: randomized trials have shown how a low CVP during parenchymal transection results in decreased blood loss and transfusion requirements [53]. A problem with this procedure could be the possibility of renal injury, especially in cirrhotic patients, but to date, there is no evidence of such improved risk.

Air embolism is another known intraoperative complication of LLR that can result from the use of pneumoperitoneum, with various precautions that have been proposed to reduce this risk. However, more recent evidence showed no increased risk of air embolism during LLR compared with OLR, neither depending on patient positioning [53].

4. Overcoming old limits

4.1. LLR in Cirrhotic Liver

HCC develops in a cirrhotic liver in approximately 80–90% of cases, and the incidence of cirrhosis is expected to increase worldwide due to the prevalence of obesity, fatty liver disease, and alcoholic steato-hepatitis [54]. After an initial phase in which the presence of cirrhosis was considered a contraindication to laparoscopy, several studies investigated the outcomes of LLR in cirrhotic patients. These patients often present a risk of postoperative hepatic decompensation and failure, as well as low platelets and impaired coagulation. A metanalysis of 11 studies comprising 1618 patients indicated a 16–26% reduction in the hazard ratio of death for patients with HCC and cirrhosis who underwent LLR [55]. In addition, LLR was associated with reduced blood loss, reduced major complications, and shorter length of hospital stay.

When considering liver resection in patients with liver cirrhosis, it is important to consider not only the oncological outcomes but also the surgical stress on both the patient and the liver. An important consequent advantage of LLR in cirrhotic patients is the lower incidence of postoperative liver failure and ascites, given the reduced interruption of portosystemic shunts and the avoidance of electrolyte imbalances as a result of the exposure of the abdominal content to the air [12]. Furthermore, the reduced invasiveness of laparoscopy, which minimizes liver manipulation, preserves collateral vessels and the abdominal musculature, and can be a key factor in expanding the classic limitations of liver surgery [56]. In fact, the advantages of LLR have been confirmed even in advanced Child-B cirrhotic patients: a propensity score-matched study involving international high-volume centers showed reduced blood loss, morbidity, and major complications in the LLR group in this setting [57].

4.2. Giant Tumors

In the first years of the spread of LLR, huge-volume tumors were considered a contraindication due to both technical and oncological issues. The last decades saw an extension of tumor burden-related indications for LR. Currently, the EASL guidelines recommend LR in cases of a resectable lesion regardless of its size, while the AASLD guidelines advocate LR in patients with Child–Pugh A cirrhosis and resectable HCC with a diameter less than 5 cm. Meanwhile, according to APASL, all tumors without extrahepatic metastases are potentially resectable regardless number and size of lesions [10,11,44]. However, expert centers published several experiences involving LLR for giant tumors, and, as the technical challenges become easier to face with widespread minimally invasive experience, the fear for oncological results and PHLF still exists.

Recently, Hong et al. published suitable long-term outcomes from a nationwide cohort of 466 patients with large HCC, suggesting a worse prognosis in subgroups with low platelets and tumors >10 cm [58]. Similarly, suitable long-term outcomes for giant HCC were shown by Thng et al., who found the presence of satellite nodules and blood transfusions as the only negative predictors of worse prognosis [59]. The safety of LLR for large malignant tumors was previously reported by different authors, with a recent international multicenter matched cohort study with regression discontinuity analyses that also concluded that the safety of MILS also for tumors larger than 10 cm, even if technically demanding [60,61]. Accordingly, the size of the tumor is taken into account in the Iwate difficulty score so that tumors larger than 3 cm are considered of increased difficulty [62].

Giant tumors indeed are extremely demanding to operate on, where limits of what is considered technically feasible can easily be reached. The placement of trocars, the mobilization of a liver lobe, and the accidental tumor perforation by shear forces are examples of possible intraoperative difficulties. Further arguments against the laparoscopic procedure for giant tumors include that conventional recovery bags are too small, and a comparatively long incision is required to retrieve the specimen. In this respect, the question of feasibility depends primarily on whether the resection can be performed safely, and, if technically feasible, well-known advantages of LLR have also been confirmed in the literature for giant tumors [63].

Therefore, the decision whether to operate laparoscopically or rather conventionally open should be based on the findings and, again, on the own learning curve and personal experiences made. In our experience, the trocars' positioning is fundamental, and it depends on both the experience of the surgeon of the center, as well as on the segment to be resected. The manipulation of the liver must be performed with caution, using protections under the hepatic retractors so as not to damage the tumor capsule. The mobilization of the liver can also be performed laparoscopically in the case of large tumors, in which case the correct trocar positioning and the experience of both the surgeon and the operator that holds the rotating camera are once again important.

4.3. Multiple Tumors

Besides giant tumors, the role of LLR in the case of multiple HCCs is also debated. From an oncological point of view, in Western countries, the best candidates have always been defined as those with a single tumor, and the treatment of multifocal non-metastatic HCC consisted of LT, within Milan criteria, or ablation/chemoembolization for the remaining patients [10]. As early as 2014, Eastern countries did not consider the presence of multiple HCCs as a contraindication, and a recent Japanese national series reported better results in Child A patients than radiofrequency or TACE in terms of OS, albeit at the cost of greater morbidity [64]. A definitive green light came from a randomized trial confirming that LR provided better OS for patients with multiple HCC outside of Milan criteria than TACE [65], even if the number of tumors was an independent risk factor. Recently a propensity score-matched analysis including multiple HCC within Milan criteria finally confirmed the safety of the laparoscopic approach [66].

Obviously, published data come from the long experience of high-volume centers for complex LLR. In our experience, an expert ultrasonography-guided parenchymal dissection is indispensable [67]. Three-dimensional laparoscopy should be mentioned as an additional supportive visual tool, as well as the use of ICG that can further help to both detect superficial lesions and guide difficult parenchymal dissection [32]. Further technological research is supposed to help surgeons in this scenario, such as the application of virtual realities, which could also be beneficial in this context [68].

In conclusion, LLR should be considered in multinodular HCCs, but more robust studies are needed to support clinical practice. A personalized strategy can also be proposed, combining both laparoscopic ablation and resection when technically demanding, and the size and position of the lesions can benefit from it [69].

4.4. Difficult Positions

The technical difficulty associated with LLR is linked to different aspects, such as parenchymal transection, hemostasis at the transection plane, and limited ability to explore deep and posterior regions of the liver. Therefore, LLR was initially reserved for superficial or left-sided lesions. The successive improvements in laparoscopic techniques and the introduction of new technologies mean that LLR is technically feasible in postero-superior (PS) segments (I, IVa, VII, VIII), too [70] (Figures 1 and 2). LLR of PS segments are considered major liver resections, according to the most recent international consensus [18], since they have shown a significantly longer operative time, length of hospital stay, rate of open conversion, and estimated blood loss when compared to antero-lateral resections [71].

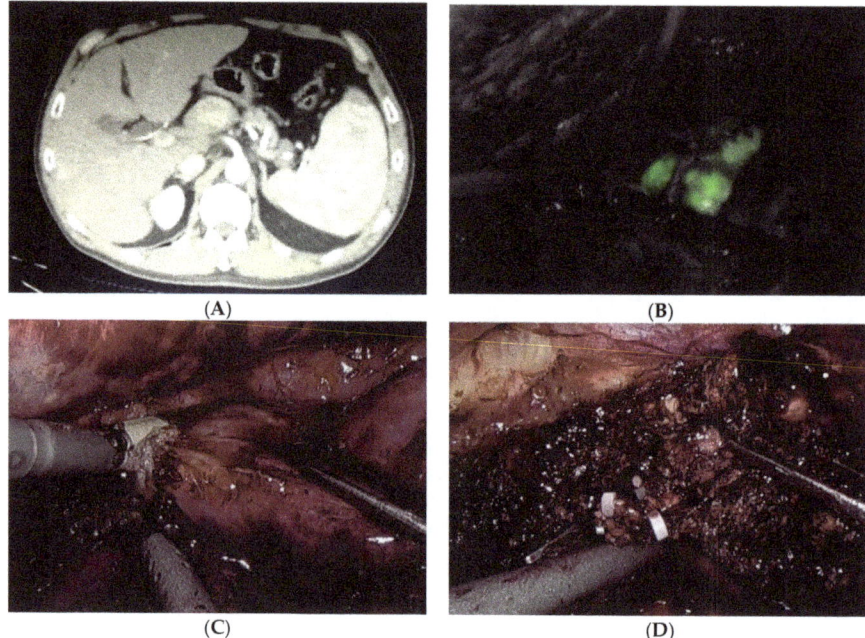

Figure 1. Laparoscopic resection of caudate lobe for hepatocellular carcinoma. (**A**) CT scan with arterial wash-in. (**B**) ICG enhancement of the lesion, assuring negative resection margins. (**C**) Parenchymal transection. (**D**) Securing spigelian vessels.

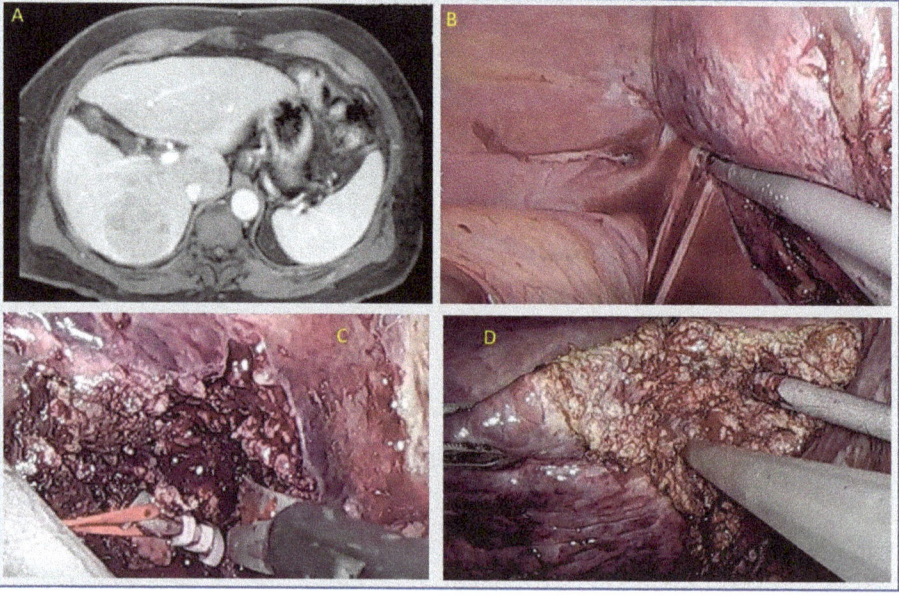

Figure 2. Laparoscopic right posterior sectionectomy. (**A**) CT scan with portal wash-out. (**B**) Mobilization of right lobe. (**C**) Selective ligation of right posterior portal branch. (**D**) Parenchymal transection by using ultrasonic cavitron.

At the same time, improved laparoscopic techniques, better visualization of the operative field using a flexible laparoscope, and routine use of an ultrasonic cavitron for transecting the deeper portion of the liver parenchyma have allowed to reach excellent outcomes for LLR for HCC located in the PS segments, resulting in reduced blood loss, fewer complications, and shorter postoperative hospital stay compared with OLR tor the same segments in retrospective studies [72,73]. An international multicenter randomized trial for LLR in PS segments (orange segments trial) is still ongoing, and it will allow obtaining a definitive confirmation.

Segments 7 and 8 are the more posterior ones, rated as 5 on the Iwate score, because of unfavorable working angles and a poor operating view, especially with the classic trocar positioning, from caudal to cranial. Thus, different approaches have been proposed: Morise proposed a left lateral position for posterior sectionectomy and the semi-prone position S7 segmentectomy, with or without an intercostal placement or a lateral positioning of the trocars [74]. Newer dissection strategies have also been proposed, such as the diamond technique, allowing safe LLR in PS segments, even in cirrhotic patients [75].

In our experience, it is the surgeon's ability to master both hepatic anatomy and laparoscopic liver surgery that makes the difference, with the need to know how to deal with any dangerous bleeding from the hepatic veins and probably know when to convert to prevent them happen. The approaches described in the literature can probably all be used indifferently but consistently with the experience of the surgeon and the center. Finally, also for the resections of the PS segments, and perhaps above all, technology can once again come to our aid for the resections of patients with HCC. In fact, the use of the ICG allows obtaining both a positive and a negative counter-staining, facilitating the transection line in the Glissonian approach for anatomical resections, as originally described by Takasaki, useful specifically for HCC treatment [32,76]. At the same time, 3D modeling or virtual reality could help to clarify the difficult relationships of the lesions with the hepatic veins, even if their real role needs to be proved [77].

4.5. Repeat Resection

As already mentioned, HCC has a high risk of recurrence after both LT and liver resection. Thus, repeat laparoscopic liver resection (RLLR) has increased thanks to the progressive wide adoption of LLR. Furthermore, LLR reduces the risk of further adhesions. Kanazawa et al. showed that the operation time for RLLR after previous LLR was significantly shorter than after OLR [78]. Belli et al. reported fewer postoperative complications, lower bleedings, and shorter hospital stay after RLLR than repeat OLR [79]. Recently, the feasibility of a laparoscopic approach for repeat resection after LT was also reported, pushing the limits of MILS even further [80].

Finally, Morise et al. recently published an international multi-institutional propensity score-based study of RLLR for HCC, showing less blood loss and hospital stay for the laparoscopic group, even if the LLR was preferred for patients with favorable tumor characteristics [81].

4.6. Robotic Liver Resection

Since the first series of robotic liver resections (RLR) reported by Giulianotti et al. in 2003, different advantages of this approach have been proposed: from the ability to articulate the instruments and the magnified three-dimensional vision to ergonomic advantages for the surgeon [82,83]. Several studies have investigated the safety and effectiveness of RLR in different situations, leading to the first international consensus statement on RLR in 2018 [84,85].

Safe and effective RLR for tumors located in the PS segment has been reported by several authors [86]. Similarly, robotic hemi-hepatectomies were associated with less intraoperative blood loss and a shorter operation time than LLR. Hu et al. published a meta-analysis including 487 RLR and 902 LLR showing fewer bleedings for RLR, with longer operation time than LLR [87]. There was no significant difference in hospital stay, conversion rate, R0 resection rate, and total complication rate between the two groups.

The high cost of treatment, as well as logistic and organizational aspects, may be the biggest shortcomings in the development of robotic surgery.

4.7. MILS and Liver Transplantation

Since the first laparoscopic hepatectomy (LDH) for a living donor LT (LDLT) was performed for a pediatric recipient by Cherqui in 2002, many transplant centers worldwide have adopted this approach, even if some concerns about donor safety still exist [88]. Hong et al. in 2021 published results from a Korean multicenter study on more than 500 LDH, showing similar outcomes to the open approach in terms of safety, with a decreasing operation time [89]. Recently, two meta-analyses involving more than 1000 patients concluded the safety of LDH while showing some advantages in terms of lower blood loss and shorter hospital stay [90,91].

Similarly, the first robotic donor hepatectomy was a right hepatectomy reported by Giulianotti et al. in 2012, with the aim of applying the supposed advantages of the robotic approach also in the field of LT [92]. The first series published by Chen et al. showed comparable results for complication rates, blood loss, and recovery of donor liver function when compared to open hepatectomy, with a shorter length of stay and less postoperative pain, without open conversions; the robotic group had longer operation time [93]. Recent systematic reviews support the safety of the robotic approach, suggesting technical advantages regarding hilar dissection, with no major difference in terms of ischemic time or cosmesis [94]. Therefore, robotic donor hepatectomy has been proposed as a viable option for experienced surgeons in the latest recommendations on robotic liver surgery [85].

Finally, what seemed to be the major limitation for laparoscopic liver surgery, namely the implantation of the liver graft in the recipient, was also overcome in 2021, a historic event for LT. The operation carried out by Suh et coll. lasted 960 min, including pure laparoscopic total hepatectomy and pure laparoscopic implantation, through a suprapubic incision, and was shown to be safe, without postoperative complications [95]. Further prospective studies on larger sample sizes will have the task of clarifying the benefits of such an incredible procedure.

5. Conclusions

In conclusion, with the advances in surgical techniques and perioperative management experienced in the recent two decades, indications for LLR in HCC patients have tremendously improved and become technically practicable for the biggest part of lesions. Current advances in both surgical and medical treatment for HCC will probably redefine the actual frontiers of LLR by including patients with more advanced disease. With the exponential growth of LLRs performed around the world, it is important to know the specific limits of this approach in HCC patients in order to put into practice all the pre-, intra-, and postoperative precautions to overcome them, making this technique the standard of care within high-volume hepatobiliary centers. Expertise and learning curve should remain the mainstay, and the selection of appropriate candidates with meticulous preparation are the key points to ensure the success of the approach.

Funding: None.

Conflicts of Interest: The authors declare no conflict of interest.

References

1. Ferlay, J.; Soerjomataram, I.; Dikshit, R.; Eser, S.; Mathers, C.; Rebelo, M.; Parkin, D.M.; Forman, D.; Bray, F. Cancer incidence and mortality worldwide: Sources, methods and major patterns in GLOBOCAN 2012. *Int. J. Cancer* **2015**, *136*, E359–E386. [CrossRef] [PubMed]
2. Marrero, J.A.; Kulik, L.M.; Sirlin, C.B.; Zhu, A.X.; Finn, R.S.; Abecassis, M.M.; Roberts, L.R.; Heimbach, J.K. Diagnosis, Staging, and Management of Hepatocellular Carcinoma: 2018 Practice Guidance by the American Association for the Study of Liver Diseases. *Hepatol. Baltim. Md.* **2018**, *68*, 723–750. [CrossRef] [PubMed]
3. Llovet, J.M.; Kelley, R.K.; Villanueva, A.; Singal, A.G.; Pikarsky, E.; Roayaie, S.; Lencioni, R.; Koike, K.; Zucman-Rossi, J.; Finn, R.S. Hepatocellular carcinoma. *Nat. Rev. Dis. Primer* **2021**, *7*, 6. [CrossRef] [PubMed]
4. Tribillon, E.; Barbier, L.; Goumard, C.; Irtan, S.; Perdigao-Cotta, F.; Durand, F.; Paradis, V.; Belghiti, J.; Scatton, O.; Soubrane, O. When Should We Propose Liver Transplant After Resection of Hepatocellular Carcinoma? A Comparison of Salvage and De Principe Strategies. *J. Gastrointest. Surg. Off. J. Soc. Surg. Aliment. Tract.* **2016**, *20*, 66–76. [CrossRef] [PubMed]
5. Graf, D.; Vallböhmer, D.; Knoefel, W.T.; Kröpil, P.; Antoch, G.; Sagir, A.; Häussinger, D. Multimodal treatment of hepatocellular carcinoma. *Eur. J. Intern. Med.* **2014**, *25*, 430–437. [CrossRef]
6. Nakano, S.; Eso, Y.; Okada, H.; Takai, A.; Takahashi, K.; Seno, H. Recent Advances in Immunotherapy for Hepatocellular Carcinoma. *Cancers* **2020**, *12*, 775. [CrossRef]
7. Bruix, J.; Chan, S.L.; Galle, P.R.; Rimassa, L.; Sangro, B. Systemic treatment of hepatocellular carcinoma: An EASL position paper. *J. Hepatol.* **2021**, *75*, 960–974. [CrossRef]
8. Reich, H.; McGlynn, F.; DeCaprio, J.; Budin, R. Laparoscopic excision of benign liver lesions. *Obstet. Gynecol.* **1991**, *78*, 956–958.
9. Nguyen, K.T.; Gamblin, T.C.; Geller, D.A. World review of laparoscopic liver resection-2,804 patients. *Ann. Surg.* **2009**, *250*, 831–841. [CrossRef]
10. European Association for the Study of the Liver. European Association for the Study of the Liver EASL Clinical Practice Guidelines: Management of hepatocellular carcinoma. *J. Hepatol.* **2018**, *69*, 182–236. [CrossRef]
11. Omata, M.; Cheng, A.-L.; Kokudo, N.; Kudo, M.; Lee, J.M.; Jia, J.; Tateishi, R.; Han, K.-H.; Chawla, Y.K.; Shiina, S.; et al. Asia-Pacific clinical practice guidelines on the management of hepatocellular carcinoma: A 2017 update. *Hepatol. Int.* **2017**, *11*, 317–370. [CrossRef] [PubMed]
12. Morise, Z. Laparoscopic liver resection for the patients with hepatocellular carcinoma and chronic liver disease. *Transl. Gastroenterol. Hepatol.* **2018**, *3*, 41. [CrossRef] [PubMed]
13. Molina, V.; Sampson-Dávila, J.; Ferrer, J.; Fondevila, C.; Díaz Del Gobbo, R.; Calatayud, D.; Bruix, J.; García-Valdecasas, J.C.; Fuster, J. Benefits of laparoscopic liver resection in patients with hepatocellular carcinoma and portal hypertension: A case-matched study. *Surg. Endosc.* **2018**, *32*, 2345–2354. [CrossRef] [PubMed]
14. Famularo, S.; Di Sandro, S.; Giani, A.; Lauterio, A.; Sandini, M.; De Carlis, R.; Buscemi, V.; Romano, F.; Gianotti, L.; De Carlis, L. Long-term oncologic results of anatomic vs. parenchyma-sparing resection for hepatocellular carcinoma. A propensity score-matching analysis. *Eur. J. Surg. Oncol.* **2018**, *44*, 1580–1587. [CrossRef]
15. Liu, H.; Hu, F.-J.; Li, H.; Lan, T.; Wu, H. Anatomical vs nonanatomical liver resection for solitary hepatocellular carcinoma: A systematic review and meta-analysis. *World J. Gastrointest. Oncol.* **2021**, *13*, 1833–1846. [CrossRef]
16. Chan, A.K.C.; Jamdar, S.; Sheen, A.J.; Siriwardena, A.K. The OSLO-COMET randomized controlled trial of laparoscopic versus open resection for colorectal liver metastases. *Ann. Surg.* **2018**, *267*, 199–207. [CrossRef]
17. Buell, J.F.; Cherqui, D.; Geller, D.A.; O'Rourke, N.; Iannitti, D.; Dagher, I.; Koffron, A.J.; Thomas, M.; Gayet, B.; Han, H.S.; et al. The international position on laparoscopic liver surgery: The Louisville Statement, 2008. *Ann. Surg.* **2009**, *250*, 825–830. [CrossRef]
18. Abu Hilal, M.; Aldrighetti, L.; Dagher, I.; Edwin, B.; Troisi, R.I.; Alikhanov, R.; Aroori, S.; Belli, G.; Besselink, M.; Briceno, J.; et al. The Southampton Consensus Guidelines for Laparoscopic Liver Surgery: From Indication to Implementation. *Ann. Surg.* **2018**, *268*, 11–18. [CrossRef]
19. Jiang, B.; Yan, X.-F.; Zhang, J.-H. Meta-analysis of laparoscopic versus open liver resection for hepatocellular carcinoma. *Hepatol. Res.* **2018**, *48*, 635–663. [CrossRef]
20. Xiong, J.-J.; Altaf, K.; Javed, M.A.; Huang, W.; Mukherjee, R.; Mai, G.; Sutton, R.; Liu, X.-B.; Hu, W.-M. Meta-analysis of laparoscopic vs open liver resection for hepatocellular carcinoma. *World J. Gastroenterol. WJG* **2012**, *18*, 6657–6668. [CrossRef]
21. Sposito, C.; Battiston, C.; Facciorusso, A.; Mazzola, M.; Muscarà, C.; Scotti, M.; Romito, R.; Mariani, L.; Mazzaferro, V. Propensity score analysis of outcomes following laparoscopic or open liver resection for hepatocellular carcinoma. *Br. J. Surg.* **2016**, *103*, 871–880. [CrossRef] [PubMed]
22. Hidaka, M.; Eguchi, S.; Okuda, K.; Beppu, T.; Shirabe, K.; Kondo, K.; Takami, Y.; Ohta, M.; Shiraishi, M.; Ueno, S.; et al. Impact of Anatomical Resection for Hepatocellular Carcinoma With Microportal Invasion (vp1): A Multi-institutional Study by the Kyushu Study Group of Liver Surgery. *Ann. Surg.* **2020**, *271*, 339–346. [CrossRef] [PubMed]
23. Yeo, C.T.; MacDonald, A.; Ungi, T.; Lasso, A.; Jalink, D.; Zevin, B.; Fichtinger, G.; Nanji, S. Utility of 3D Reconstruction of 2D Liver Computed Tomography/Magnetic Resonance Images as a Surgical Planning Tool for Residents in Liver Resection Surgery. *J. Surg. Educ.* **2018**, *75*, 792–797. [CrossRef] [PubMed]
24. Ocak, İ.; Topaglu, S.; Acarli, K. Posthepatectomy liver failure. *Turk. J. Med. Sci.* **2020**, *50*, 1491–1503. [CrossRef] [PubMed]

25. Longbotham, D.; Young, A.; Nana, G.; Feltbower, R.; Hidalgo, E.; Toogood, G.; Lodge, P.A.; Attia, M.; Rajendra Prasad, K. The impact of age on post-operative liver function following right hepatectomy: A retrospective, single centre experience. *HPB* **2020**, *22*, 151–160. [CrossRef]
26. Vauthey, J.-N.; Abdalla, E.K.; Doherty, D.A.; Gertsch, P.; Fenstermacher, M.J.; Loyer, E.M.; Lerut, J.; Materne, R.; Wang, X.; Encarnacion, A.; et al. Body surface area and body weight predict total liver volume in Western adults. *Liver Transplant. Off. Publ. Am. Assoc. Study Liver Dis. Int. Liver Transplant Soc.* **2002**, *8*, 233–240. [CrossRef]
27. Small, B.G.; Wendt, B.; Jamei, M.; Johnson, T.N. Prediction of liver volume - a population-based approach to meta-analysis of paediatric, adult and geriatric populations—An update. *Biopharm. Drug Dispos.* **2017**, *38*, 290–300. [CrossRef]
28. Clavien, P.-A.; Petrowsky, H.; DeOliveira, M.L.; Graf, R. Strategies for safer liver surgery and partial liver transplantation. *N. Engl. J. Med.* **2007**, *356*, 1545–1559. [CrossRef]
29. Northup, P.G.; Wanamaker, R.C.; Lee, V.D.; Adams, R.B.; Berg, C.L. Model for End-Stage Liver Disease (MELD) predicts nontransplant surgical mortality in patients with cirrhosis. *Ann. Surg.* **2005**, *242*, 244–251. [CrossRef]
30. Cassese, G.; Han, H.-S.; Al Farai, A.; Guiu, B.; Troisi, R.I.; Panaro, F. Future remnant Liver optimization: Preoperative assessment, volume augmentation procedures and management of PVE failure. *Minerva Surg.* Epub ahead of print. **2022**. [CrossRef]
31. Dominguez, M.; Rincón, D.; Abraldes, J.G.; Miquel, R.; Colmenero, J.; Bellot, P.; García-Pagán, J.-C.; Fernández, R.; Moreno, M.; Bañares, R.; et al. A new scoring system for prognostic stratification of patients with alcoholic hepatitis. *Am. J. Gastroenterol.* **2008**, *103*, 2747–2756. [CrossRef] [PubMed]
32. Cassese, G.; Troisi, R.I. Indocyanine green applications in hepato-biliary surgery. *Minerva Surg.* **2021**, *76*, 199–201. [CrossRef] [PubMed]
33. Miyagawa, S.; Makuuchi, M.; Kawasaki, S.; Kakazu, T. Criteria for safe hepatic resection. *Am. J. Surg.* **1995**, *169*, 589–594. [CrossRef]
34. Hoekstra, L.T.; de Graaf, W.; Nibourg, G.A.A.; Heger, M.; Bennink, R.J.; Stieger, B.; van Gulik, T.M. Physiological and biochemical basis of clinical liver function tests: A review. *Ann. Surg.* **2013**, *257*, 27–36. [CrossRef] [PubMed]
35. Rassam, F.; Olthof, P.B.; Richardson, H.; van Gulik, T.M.; Bennink, R.J. Practical guidelines for the use of technetium-99m mebrofenin hepatobiliary scintigraphy in the quantitative assessment of liver function. *Nucl. Med. Commun.* **2019**, *40*, 297–307. [CrossRef] [PubMed]
36. Alvarez, F.A.; Castaing, D.; Figueroa, R.; Allard, M.A.; Golse, N.; Pittau, G.; Ciacio, O.; Sa Cunha, A.; Cherqui, D.; Azoulay, D.; et al. Natural history of portal vein embolization before liver resection: A 23-year analysis of intention-to-treat results. *Surgery* **2018**, *163*, 1257–1263. [CrossRef]
37. Esposito, F.; Lim, C.; Lahat, E.; Shwaartz, C.; Eshkenazy, R.; Salloum, C.; Azoulay, D. Combined hepatic and portal vein embolization as preparation for major hepatectomy: A systematic review. *HPB* **2019**, *21*, 1099–1106. [CrossRef]
38. Guiu, B.; Chevallier, P.; Denys, A.; Delhom, E.; Pierredon-Foulongne, M.-A.; Rouanet, P.; Fabre, J.-M.; Quenet, F.; Herrero, A.; Panaro, F.; et al. Simultaneous trans-hepatic portal and hepatic vein embolization before major hepatectomy: The liver venous deprivation technique. *Eur. Radiol.* **2016**, *26*, 4259–4267. [CrossRef]
39. Khayat, S.; Cassese, G.; Quenet, F.; Cassinotto, C.; Assenat, E.; Navarro, F.; Guiu, B.; Panaro, F. Oncological Outcomes after Liver Venous Deprivation for Colorectal Liver Metastases: A Single Center Experience. *Cancers* **2021**, *13*, 200. [CrossRef]
40. Guiu, B.; Herrero, A.; Panaro, F. Liver venous deprivation: A bright future for liver metastases—but what about hepatocellular carcinoma? *Hepatobiliary Surg. Nutr.* **2021**, *10*, 270–272. [CrossRef]
41. Schnitzbauer, A.A.; Lang, S.A.; Goessmann, H.; Nadalin, S.; Baumgart, J.; Farkas, S.A.; Fichtner-Feigl, S.; Lorf, T.; Goralcyk, A.; Hörbelt, R.; et al. Right portal vein ligation combined with in situ splitting induces rapid left lateral liver lobe hypertrophy enabling 2-staged extended right hepatic resection in small-for-size settings. *Ann. Surg.* **2012**, *255*, 405–414. [CrossRef] [PubMed]
42. Lang, H.; Baumgart, J.; Mittler, J. Associated Liver Partition and Portal Vein Ligation for Staged Hepatectomy (ALPPS) Registry: What Have We Learned? *Gut Liver* **2020**, *14*, 699–706. [CrossRef] [PubMed]
43. Di Benedetto, F.; Assirati, G.; Magistri, P. Full robotic ALPPS for HCC with intrahepatic portal vein thrombosis. *Int. J. Med. Robot. Comput. Assist. Surg. MRCAS* **2020**, *16*, e2087. [CrossRef] [PubMed]
44. Heimbach, J.K.; Kulik, L.M.; Finn, R.S.; Sirlin, C.B.; Abecassis, M.M.; Roberts, L.R.; Zhu, A.X.; Murad, M.H.; Marrero, J.A. AASLD guidelines for the treatment of hepatocellular carcinoma. *Hepatol. Baltim. Md* **2018**, *67*, 358–380. [CrossRef]
45. De Franchis, R.; Bosch, J.; Garcia-Tsao, G.; Reiberger, T.; Ripoll, C. Baveno VII Faculty Baveno VII—Renewing consensus in portal hypertension. *J. Hepatol.* **2021**, *76*, 959–975. [CrossRef]
46. Marasco, G.; Colecchia, A.; Colli, A.; Ravaioli, F.; Casazza, G.; Bacchi Reggiani, M.L.; Cucchetti, A.; Cescon, M.; Festi, D. Role of liver and spleen stiffness in predicting the recurrence of hepatocellular carcinoma after resection. *J. Hepatol.* **2019**, *70*, 440–448. [CrossRef]
47. Hackl, C.; Schlitt, H.J.; Renner, P.; Lang, S.A. Liver surgery in cirrhosis and portal hypertension. *World J. Gastroenterol.* **2016**, *22*, 2725–2735. [CrossRef]
48. Belli, A.; Cioffi, L.; Russo, G.; Belli, G. Liver resection for hepatocellular carcinoma in patients with portal hypertension: The role of laparoscopy. *Hepatobiliary Surg. Nutr.* **2015**, *4*, 417–421. [CrossRef]
49. Azoulay, D.; Ramos, E.; Casellas-Robert, M.; Salloum, C.; Lladó, L.; Nadler, R.; Busquets, J.; Caula-Freixa, C.; Mils, K.; Lopez-Ben, S.; et al. Liver resection for hepatocellular carcinoma in patients with clinically significant portal hypertension. *JHEP Rep. Innov. Hepatol.* **2021**, *3*, 100190. [CrossRef]

50. Srinivasa, S.; Hughes, M.; Azodo, I.A.; Adair, A.; Ravindran, R.; Harrison, E.; Wigmore, S.J. Laparoscopic liver resection in cirrhotics: Feasibility and short-term outcomes compared to non-cirrhotics. *ANZ J. Surg.* **2020**, *90*, 1104–1107. [CrossRef]
51. De Boer, M.T.; Molenaar, I.Q.; Porte, R.J. Impact of blood loss on outcome after liver resection. *Dig. Surg.* **2007**, *24*, 259–264. [CrossRef] [PubMed]
52. Al-Saeedi, M.; Ghamarnejad, O.; Khajeh, E.; Shafiei, S.; Salehpour, R.; Golriz, M.; Mieth, M.; Weiss, K.H.; Longerich, T.; Hoffmann, K.; et al. Pringle Maneuver in Extended Liver Resection: A propensity score analysis. *Sci. Rep.* **2020**, *10*, 8847. [CrossRef] [PubMed]
53. Otsuka, Y.; Katagiri, T.; Ishii, J.; Maeda, T.; Kubota, Y.; Tamura, A.; Tsuchiya, M.; Kaneko, H. Gas embolism in laparoscopic hepatectomy: What is the optimal pneumoperitoneal pressure for laparoscopic major hepatectomy? *J. Hepato-Biliary-Pancreat. Sci.* **2013**, *20*, 137–140. [CrossRef] [PubMed]
54. Kabir, T.; Tan, Z.Z.; Syn, N.L.; Wu, E.; Lin, J.D.; Zhao, J.J.; Tan, A.Y.H.; Hui, Y.; Kam, J.H.; Goh, B.K.P. Laparoscopic versus open resection of hepatocellular carcinoma in patients with cirrhosis: A meta-analysis. *Br. J. Surg.* **2021**, *109*, 21–29. [CrossRef] [PubMed]
55. Guro, H.; Cho, J.Y.; Han, H.-S.; Yoon, Y.-S.; Choi, Y.; Periyasamy, M. Current status of laparoscopic liver resection for hepatocellular carcinoma. *Clin. Mol. Hepatol.* **2016**, *22*, 212–218. [CrossRef] [PubMed]
56. Troisi, R.I.; Berardi, G.; Morise, Z.; Cipriani, F.; Ariizumi, S.; Sposito, C.; Panetta, V.; Simonelli, I.; Kim, S.; Goh, B.K.P.; et al. Laparoscopic and open liver resection for hepatocellular carcinoma with Child-Pugh B cirrhosis: Multicentre propensity score-matched study. *Br. J. Surg.* **2021**, *108*, 196–204. [CrossRef]
57. Hong, S.K.; Lee, K.-W.; Hong, S.Y.; Suh, S.; Hong, K.; Han, E.S.; Lee, J.-M.; Choi, Y.; Yi, N.-J.; Suh, K.-S. Efficacy of Liver Resection for Single Large Hepatocellular Carcinoma in Child-Pugh A Cirrhosis: Analysis of a Nationwide Cancer Registry Database. *Front. Oncol.* **2021**, *11*, 674603. [CrossRef]
58. Thng, Y.; Tan, J.K.H.; Shridhar, I.G.; Chang, S.K.Y.; Madhavan, K.; Kow, A.W.C. Outcomes of resection of giant hepatocellular carcinoma in a tertiary institution: Does size matter? *HPB* **2015**, *17*, 988–993. [CrossRef]
59. Shelat, V.G.; Cipriani, F.; Basseres, T.; Armstrong, T.H.; Takhar, A.S.; Pearce, N.W.; AbuHilal, M. Pure laparoscopic liver resection for large malignant tumors: Does size matter? *Ann. Surg. Oncol.* **2015**, *22*, 1288–1293. [CrossRef]
60. Cheung, T.-T.; Wang, X.; Efanov, M.; Liu, R.; Fuks, D.; Choi, G.-H.; Syn, N.L.; Chong, C.C.; Sucandy, I.; Chiow, A.K.H.; et al. Minimally invasive liver resection for huge ($\geq$10 cm) tumors: An international multicenter matched cohort study with regression discontinuity analyses. *Hepatobiliary Surg. Nutr.* **2021**, *10*, 587–597. [CrossRef]
61. Barron, J.O.; Orabi, D.; Moro, A.; Quintini, C.; Berber, E.; Aucejo, F.N.; Sasaki, K.; Kwon, C.-H.D. Validation of the IWATE criteria as a laparoscopic liver resection difficulty score in a single North American cohort. *Surg. Endosc.* **2021**, *36*, 3601–3609. [CrossRef] [PubMed]
62. Hu, M.; Chen, K.; Zhang, X.; Li, C.; Song, D.; Liu, R. Robotic, laparoscopic or open hemihepatectomy for giant liver haemangiomas over 10 cm in diameter. *BMC Surg.* **2020**, *20*, 93. [CrossRef] [PubMed]
63. Fukami, Y.; Kaneoka, Y.; Maeda, A.; Kumada, T.; Tanaka, J.; Akita, T.; Kubo, S.; Izumi, N.; Kadoya, M.; Sakamoto, M.; et al. Liver Resection for Multiple Hepatocellular Carcinomas: A Japanese Nationwide Survey. *Ann. Surg.* **2020**, *272*, 145–154. [CrossRef] [PubMed]
64. Yin, L.; Li, H.; Li, A.-J.; Lau, W.-Y.; Pan, Z.-Y.; Lai, E.C.H.; Wu, M.-C.; Zhou, W.-P. Partial hepatectomy vs. transcatheter arterial chemoembolization for resectable multiple hepatocellular carcinoma beyond Milan Criteria: A RCT. *J. Hepatol.* **2014**, *61*, 82–88. [CrossRef]
65. Peng, Y.; Liu, F.; Xu, H.; Lan, X.; Wei, Y.; Li, B. Outcomes of Laparoscopic Liver Resection for Patients with Multiple Hepatocellular Carcinomas Meeting the Milan Criteria: A Propensity Score-Matched Analysis. *J. Laparoendosc. Adv. Surg. Tech.* **2019**, *29*, 1144–1151. [CrossRef]
66. Ellebaek, S.B.; Fristrup, C.W.; Hovendal, C.; Qvist, N.; Bundgaard, L.; Salomon, S.; Støvring, J.; Mortensen, M.B. Randomized clinical trial of laparoscopic ultrasonography before laparoscopic colorectal cancer resection. *Br. J. Surg.* **2017**, *104*, 1462–1469. [CrossRef]
67. Sauer, I.M.; Queisner, M.; Tang, P.; Moosburner, S.; Hoepfner, O.; Horner, R.; Lohmann, R.; Pratschke, J. Mixed Reality in Visceral Surgery: Development of a Suitable Workflow and Evaluation of Intraoperative Use-cases. *Ann. Surg.* **2017**, *266*, 706–712. [CrossRef]
68. Herbold, T.; Wahba, R.; Bangard, C.; Demir, M.; Drebber, U.; Stippel, D.L. The laparoscopic approach for radiofrequency ablation of hepatocellular carcinoma–indication, technique and results. *Langenbecks Arch. Surg.* **2013**, *398*, 47–53. [CrossRef]
69. Cho, J.Y.; Han, H.-S.; Yoon, Y.-S.; Shin, S.-H. Feasibility of laparoscopic liver resection for tumors located in the posterosuperior segments of the liver, with a special reference to overcoming current limitations on tumor location. *Surgery* **2008**, *144*, 32–38. [CrossRef]
70. Yoon, Y.-S.; Han, H.-S.; Cho, J.Y.; Ahn, K.S. Total laparoscopic liver resection for hepatocellular carcinoma located in all segments of the liver. *Surg. Endosc.* **2010**, *24*, 1630–1637. [CrossRef]
71. Xiao, L.; Xiang, L.; Li, J.; Chen, J.; Fan, Y.; Zheng, S. Laparoscopic versus open liver resection for hepatocellular carcinoma in posterosuperior segments. *Surg. Endosc.* **2015**, *29*, 2994–3001. [CrossRef] [PubMed]

72. Haber, P.K.; Wabitsch, S.; Krenzien, F.; Benzing, C.; Andreou, A.; Schöning, W.; Öllinger, R.; Pratschke, J.; Schmelzle, M. Laparoscopic liver surgery in cirrhosis—Addressing lesions in posterosuperior segments. *Surg. Oncol.* **2019**, *28*, 140–144. [CrossRef] [PubMed]
73. Morise, Z. Laparoscopic liver resection for posterosuperior tumors using caudal approach and postural changes: A new technical approach. *World J. Gastroenterol.* **2016**, *22*, 10267–10274. [CrossRef] [PubMed]
74. Cipriani, F.; Shelat, V.G.; Rawashdeh, M.; Francone, E.; Aldrighetti, L.; Takhar, A.; Armstrong, T.; Pearce, N.W.; Abu Hilal, M. Laparoscopic Parenchymal-Sparing Resections for Nonperipheral Liver Lesions, the Diamond Technique: Technical Aspects, Clinical Outcomes, and Oncologic Efficiency. *J. Am. Coll. Surg.* **2015**, *221*, 265–272. [CrossRef] [PubMed]
75. Takasaki, K. Glissonean pedicle transection method for hepatic resection: A new concept of liver segmentation. *J. Hepatobiliary Pancreat. Surg.* **1998**, *5*, 286–291. [CrossRef] [PubMed]
76. Fang, C.; Zhang, P.; Qi, X. Digital and intelligent liver surgery in the new era: Prospects and dilemmas. *EBioMedicine* **2019**, *41*, 693–701. [CrossRef]
77. Kanazawa, A.; Tsukamoto, T.; Shimizu, S.; Kodai, S.; Yamamoto, S.; Yamazoe, S.; Ohira, G.; Nakajima, T. Laparoscopic liver resection for treating recurrent hepatocellular carcinoma. *J. Hepato-Biliary-Pancreat. Sci.* **2013**, *20*, 512–517. [CrossRef]
78. Belli, G.; Cioffi, L.; Fantini, C.; D'Agostino, A.; Russo, G.; Limongelli, P.; Belli, A. Laparoscopic redo surgery for recurrent hepatocellular carcinoma in cirrhotic patients: Feasibility, safety, and results. *Surg. Endosc.* **2009**, *23*, 1807–1811. [CrossRef]
79. Berardi, G.; Colasanti, M.; Ettorre, G.M. ASO Author Reflections: Pushing the Limits in Laparoscopic Liver Surgery for Hepatocellular Carcinoma. *Ann. Surg. Oncol.* **2022**. Epub ahead of print. [CrossRef]
80. Morise, Z.; Aldrighetti, L.; Belli, G.; Ratti, F.; Belli, A.; Cherqui, D.; Tanabe, M.; Wakabayashi, G. ILLS-Tokyo Collaborator group Laparoscopic repeat liver resection for hepatocellular carcinoma: A multicentre propensity score-based study. *Br. J. Surg.* **2020**, *107*, 889–895. [CrossRef]
81. Milone, L.; Daskalaki, D.; Fernandes, E.; Damoli, I.; Giulianotti, P.C. State of the art in robotic hepatobiliary surgery. *World J. Surg.* **2013**, *37*, 2747–2755. [CrossRef] [PubMed]
82. Zhang, C.-Z.; Li, N. Advances in minimally invasive surgery for hepatocellular carcinoma. *Hepatoma Res.* **2020**, *6*, 77. [CrossRef]
83. Giulianotti, P.C.; Coratti, A.; Angelini, M.; Sbrana, F.; Cecconi, S.; Balestracci, T.; Caravaglios, G. Robotics in general surgery: Personal experience in a large community hospital. *Arch. Surg.* **2003**, *138*, 777–784. [CrossRef] [PubMed]
84. Liu, R.; Wakabayashi, G.; Kim, H.-J.; Choi, G.-H.; Yiengpruksawan, A.; Fong, Y.; He, J.; Boggi, U.; Troisi, R.I.; Efanov, M.; et al. International consensus statement on robotic hepatectomy surgery in 2018. *World J. Gastroenterol.* **2019**, *25*, 1432–1444. [CrossRef] [PubMed]
85. Casciola, L.; Patriti, A.; Ceccarelli, G.; Bartoli, A.; Ceribelli, C.; Spaziani, A. Robot-assisted parenchymal-sparing liver surgery including lesions located in the posterosuperior segments. *Surg. Endosc.* **2011**, *25*, 3815–3824. [CrossRef] [PubMed]
86. Zhao, Z.-M.; Yin, Z.-Z.; Meng, Y.; Jiang, N.; Ma, Z.-G.; Pan, L.-C.; Tan, X.-L.; Chen, X.; Liu, R. Successful robotic radical resection of hepatic echinococcosis located in posterosuperior liver segments. *World J. Gastroenterol.* **2020**, *26*, 2831–2838. [CrossRef]
87. Hu, Y.; Guo, K.; Xu, J.; Xia, T.; Wang, T.; Liu, N.; Fu, Y. Robotic versus laparoscopic hepatectomy for malignancy: A systematic review and meta-analysis. *Asian J. Surg.* **2021**, *44*, 615–628. [CrossRef]
88. Cherqui, D.; Soubrane, O.; Husson, E.; Barshasz, E.; Vignaux, O.; Ghimouz, M.; Branchereau, S.; Chardot, C.; Gauthier, F.; Fagniez, P.L.; et al. Laparoscopic living donor hepatectomy for liver transplantation in children. *Lancet* **2002**, *359*, 392–396. [CrossRef]
89. Hong, S.K.; Choi, G.-S.; Han, J.; Cho, H.-D.; Kim, J.M.; Han, Y.S.; Cho, J.Y.; Kwon, C.H.D.; Kim, K.-H.; Lee, K.-W.; et al. Pure Laparoscopic Donor Hepatectomy: A Multicenter Experience. *Liver Transplant. Off. Publ. Am. Assoc. Study Liver Dis. Int. Liver Transplant. Soc.* **2021**, *27*, 67–76. [CrossRef]
90. Xu, J.; Hu, C.; Cao, H.-L.; Zhang, M.-L.; Ye, S.; Zheng, S.-S.; Wang, W.-L. Meta-Analysis of Laparoscopic versus Open Hepatectomy for Live Liver Donors. *PLoS ONE* **2016**, *11*, e0165319. [CrossRef]
91. Gao, Y.; Wu, W.; Liu, C.; Liu, T.; Xiao, H. Comparison of laparoscopic and open living donor hepatectomy. *Medicine* **2021**, *100*, e26708. [CrossRef] [PubMed]
92. Giulianotti, P.C.; Tzvetanov, I.; Jeon, H.; Bianco, F.; Spaggiari, M.; Oberholzer, J.; Benedetti, E. Robot-assisted right lobe donor hepatectomy. *Transpl. Int. Off. J. Eur. Soc. Organ Transplant* **2012**, *25*, e5–e9. [CrossRef] [PubMed]
93. Chen, P.-D.; Wu, C.-Y.; Hu, R.-H.; Ho, C.-M.; Lee, P.-H.; Lai, H.-S.; Lin, M.-T.; Wu, Y.-M. Robotic liver donor right hepatectomy: A pure, minimally invasive approach. *Liver Transplant Off. Publ. Am. Assoc. Study Liver Dis. Int. Liver Transplant. Soc.* **2016**, *22*, 1509–1518. [CrossRef] [PubMed]
94. Cho, H.-D.; Samstein, B.; Chaundry, S.; Kim, K.-H. Minimally invasive donor hepatectomy, systemic review. *Int. J. Surg. Lond. Engl.* **2020**, *82S*, 187–191. [CrossRef]
95. Suh, K.-S.; Hong, S.K.; Lee, S.; Hong, S.Y.; Suh, S.; Han, E.S.; Yang, S.-M.; Choi, Y.; Yi, N.-J.; Lee, K.-W. Pure laparoscopic living donor liver transplantation: Dreams come true. *Am. J. Transplant* **2022**, *22*, 260–265. [CrossRef]

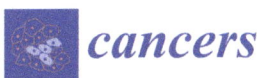

Review

Recent Advances in Minimally Invasive Liver Resection for Colorectal Cancer Liver Metastases—A Review

Winifred M. Lo, Samer T. Tohme and David A. Geller *

Division of Hepatobiliary and Pancreatic Surgery, University of Pittsburgh Medical Center, Pittsburgh, PA 15213, USA
* Correspondence: gellerda@upmc.edu; Tel.: +1-412-692-2001; Fax: +1-412-602-2002

Simple Summary: Minimally invasive surgery has been slowly incorporated into liver resection for metastatic colorectal cancer. Here, we review the perioperative safety and efficacy for laparoscopic and robotic approaches for patients with liver colorectal metastases. Laparoscopic liver resection (LLR) is associated with shorter hospital stays and similar post-operative complications to open techniques. This approach does not compromise oncologic outcomes or long-term overall survival. LLR allows for the earlier initiation of adjuvant chemotherapy. Studies also show that laparoscopic simultaneous resection of both colorectal and liver tumors can be safe in highly-selected patients. Early research on robotic liver resection has demonstrated a comparable safety profile to LLR and may improve the rate of R0 resection. Minimally invasive liver surgery is a safe and effective alternative for resection colorectal liver metastases in appropriately selected patients. It should be strongly considered in patients with one or two small, unilobar, and anterolateral tumors.

Abstract: Minimally invasive surgical (MIS) approaches to liver resection have been increasingly adopted into use for surgery on colorectal cancer liver metastases. The purpose of this review is to evaluate the outcomes when comparing laparoscopic liver resection (LLR), robotic liver resection (RLR), and open liver resection (OLR) for colorectal cancer liver metastases (CRLM) in 39 studies (2009–2022) that include a case-matched series, propensity score analyses, and three randomized clinical trials. LLR is associated with less intraoperative blood loss and shorter hospital stay compared with OLR. LLR can be performed with comparable operative time. LLR has similar rates of perioperative complications and mortality as OLR. There were no significant differences in 5-year overall or disease-free survival between approaches. Robotic liver resection (RLR) has comparable perioperative safety to LLR and may improve rates of R0 resection in certain patients. Finally, MIS approaches to the hepatic resection of CRLM reduce the time from liver resection to initiation of adjuvant chemotherapy. Thus, MIS liver surgery should be considered in the array of options for patients with CRLM, though thoughtful patient selection and surgeon experience should be part of that decision.

Keywords: minimally invasive surgery; laparoscopic liver resection; laparoscopic hepatectomy; colorectal cancer liver metastases; colon cancer; metastatic colorectal cancer; liver surgery

1. Introduction

Minimally invasive surgery (MIS) has advanced the field of complex surgical oncology over the last decade. Laparoscopic liver resection (LLR) surgery has been shown to provide clinical benefits without compromising oncologic outcomes [1–7]. In patients with colorectal cancer liver metastases (CRLM), a case-matched series, propensity score analyses, meta-analyses, and three randomized clinical trials have compared laparoscopic and open liver resection (OLR) for perioperative safety and efficacy. Recent advances include robotic liver resection (RLR) for CRLM, repeat LLR for CRLM, simultaneous MIS colon and liver resections, MIS approaches to posterior–superior segments, and associating liver partition

Citation: Lo, W.M.; Tohme, S.T.; Geller, D.A. Recent Advances in Minimally Invasive Liver Resection for Colorectal Cancer Liver Metastases—A Review. *Cancers* **2023**, *15*, 142. https://doi.org/10.3390/cancers15010142

Academic Editor: Massimo Rossi

Received: 12 October 2022
Revised: 29 November 2022
Accepted: 2 December 2022
Published: 26 December 2022

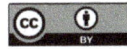

Copyright: © 2022 by the authors. Licensee MDPI, Basel, Switzerland. This article is an open access article distributed under the terms and conditions of the Creative Commons Attribution (CC BY) license (https://creativecommons.org/licenses/by/4.0/).

and portal vein ligation for the staged hepatectomy (ALPPS) approach for CRLM. Many of the recent findings have relied on single-center retrospective data, requiring careful interpretation of the data. This review examines the safety and efficacy of minimally invasive surgery (LLR and RLR) when compared with OLR for CRLM based on retrospective studies and randomized clinical trials in the last 13 years. It also reviews the limitations and remaining questions for future study.

2. Methods

A literature review was performed using PubMed, Web of Science, and Cochrane library using the search terms "laparoscopic surgery", "minimally invasive surgery", "robotic surgery", "colorectal cancer", and "liver resection". Papers published between January 2009 and March 2022 were evaluated for inclusion. Papers were excluded if they were not written in English, if their referenced procedures entailed only colon resection, if they reviewed liver surgery for other diagnoses, if they demonstrated outcomes not related to MIS, systematic reviews, case reports, case series regarding less than 10 patients, or if the full text could not be obtained. Conference abstracts were excluded. For papers that were review articles or meta-analyses, the reference list was manually reviewed for additional papers for inclusion. Thirty-nine papers were selected for in-depth review and inclusion (Figure 1). Data pulled from each paper included the numbers of patients, survival rates (disease-free, overall), complication rates, and mortality rates. This data was logged and reported in tables that are included for easier reference (Tables 1–5). If a study population performed propensity-score matching, the specific survival and perioperative safety data was extracted from that matched population.

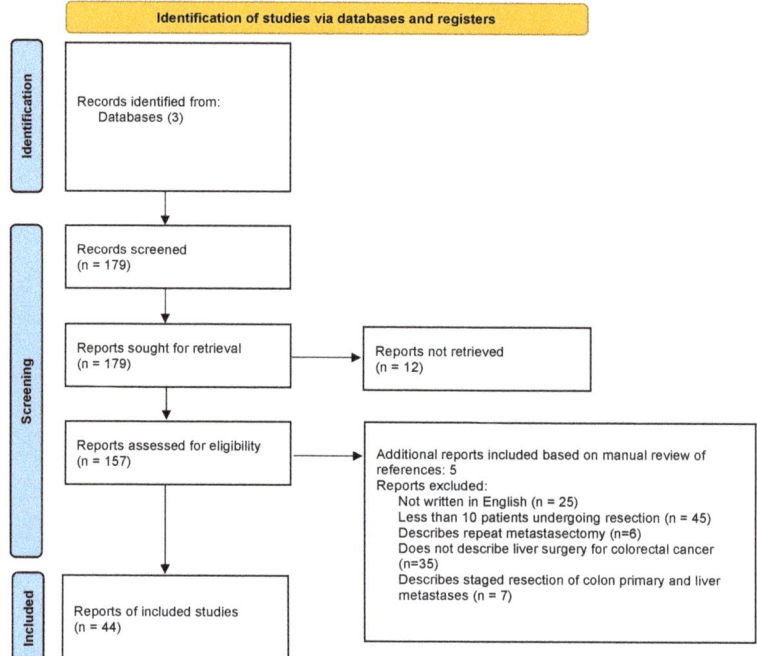

Figure 1. Flow diagram.

3. Results

3.1. Retrospective Case Series Comparing LLR with OLR

LLR has been evaluated extensively for safety and efficacy in several retrospective studies. These include both single-center and multi-center analyses with characterizations of LLR alone and LLR when compared with OLR in propensity- or case-matched analyses. In total, these include 3814 patients described in 39 studies published between 2009 and 2022 (Table 1) [8–27]. This number consisted of 1833 LLR and 1981 OLR patients. It should be noted that there is significant heterogeneity in patient selection, with limited information on tumor location within the liver, proximity to major vasculature (portal pedicle, hepatic vein), or objective assessment of intraoperative technical difficulty (i.e., Iwate score). Most patients represented oligometastatic disease with prior resection of the colon primary, although a proportion of patients undergoing open resection in one study had a significantly higher rate of simultaneous colon and liver resections [22]. LLR was associated with a similar median operative time to open procedures without any significant prolongation of operating time. Laparoscopic resection was associated with lower estimated blood loss (EBL) and a shorter length of hospital stay (LOS) (laparoscopic 3–12 days versus open resection 5–14 days). Pringle maneuver application and time were not consistently reported across studies. In general, these studies concluded that LLR could be safely performed without any significant increase in operating time and could be performed with less EBL and a shorter length of hospital stay versus OLR.

When evaluating for safety, most studies reported low mortality rates (0–3.9%). Additionally, when comparing perioperative mortality between surgical approaches, there was no significant difference between LLR and OLR (Table 1). Perioperative complication rates (all grades) ranged from 8.8–41%. Eight studies noted that LLR was associated with a significantly lower rate of perioperative complications. While this was not consistently seen across all studies, it is noteworthy that there were no reports of increased perioperative complication rates with LLR.

Table 1. Studies evaluating laparoscopic and open liver resections (2009–2022).

Author	Year	Nation	Multi-Center	Arm	N	5-y OS (%)	p-Value	5-y RFS (%)	p-Value	Complication Rate (%)	p-Value	Mortality Rate (%)	p-Value
Castaing [2]	2009	France	yes	OLR	60	56	0.32	27	0.32	33		1.7 *	
				LLR	60	64		35		30		1.7 *	
Nguyen [3]	2009	US	yes	LLR	109	50		43		11.9		0	
Sasaki [8]	2009	Japan	no	LLR	76	64		NR		3.7		0	
Bryant [9]	2009	France	no	LLR	22	64		47		NR		0	
Kazaryan [10]	2010	Norway		LLR	110	47		NR		14.3		0.8	
Topal [11]	2012	Belgium	no	OLR	193	59.5 $	0.63	30 $	NS	29	0.02	1	0.89
				LLR	81					13		0	
Cannon [12]	2012	US	no	OLR	140	42	0.82	15	0.35	50	0.07	1 **	0.96
				LLR	35	36		22		23		0 **	
Iwahashi [13]	2014	Japan	no	OLR	21	51	NS	25	NS	9.5	0.21	0	
				LLR	21	42		14		24		0	
Montalti [14]	2014	Belgium	no	OLR	57	65	0.36	38	0.24	32	0.03	0	
				LLR	57	60		29		16		0	
Beppu [15]	2015	Japan	yes	OLR	342	68	0.30	51	NR	12	0.63	0.6 *	
				LLR	171	70		53		14		0 *	
Allard [16]	2015	France	yes	OLR	153	75	0.72	36	0.60	32.7	0.0002	3.9	0.5
				LLR	153	78		32		12.4		2	
De'Angelis [17]	2015	France	no	OLR	52	62	0.51	21	0.71	17.9	0.23	3.8	0.49
				LLR	52	76		21		17.2		0	
Hasegawa [18]	2015	Japan	no	OLR	69	57	0.53	29	0.33	24.6	0.005	1.4	1
				LLR	102	49		40		8.8		0.98	
Lin [19]	2015	China	no	OLR	36	55	0.79	38	0.86	30.5	0.599	0	NR
				LLR	36	51		27		25		0	
Schiffman [20]	2015	International	yes	OLR	368	46	NS	26	NS	33.2	0.03	0.9	0.92
				LLR	242	51		32		20.3		0.5	
Cipriani [21]	2016	UK	no	OLR	133	63	NR	16	0.24	39.8	0.002	1.5 **	0.99
				LLR	133	64		16		23.3		0.8 **	

Table 1. Cont.

Author	Year	Nation	Multi-Center	Arm	N	5-y OS (%)	p-Value	5-y RFS (%)	p-Value	Complication Rate (%)	p-Value	Mortality Rate (%)	p-Value
Lewin [22]	2016	Australia	yes	OLR	138 ^	63	0.66	38	0.50	25	NR	1.4	
				LLR	146 ^	54		36		17		0	
Nomi [23]	2016	France	no	LLR	120	35.4 &		15 &		41.7	NR	0.8	
Maurette [24]	2017	Argentina	no	OLR	22	58.7 #	0.89	19 #	0.39	27	0.23	0	
				LLR	18	40 #		58 #		11		0	
Goumard [25]	2018	US	no	OLR	121	68	0.89	NR		59	0.001	0	
				LLR	43	81		NR		41		0	
Efanov [26]	2021	Russia	no	OLR	20	63	0.57	27	NR	10 ~	0.633	0	NR
				LLR	20	78		27		15 ~		0	
Nicolas [27]	2021	Argentina	no	OLR	56	77 ***	NS	20 ***	NS	16	0.3	1	NS
				LLR	26	75 ***		36 ***		2		0	

NR: not reported; NS: not significant; * 60-day mortality; ** 90-day mortality; *** 3-year results; ~ Grade 3+ complications; ^ reported as resections including multiple resections on same patient (specific breakdown not available in report); # 8-year survival; & large tumor cohort data included for reference; $: data reported for total study population only.

Oncologic outcomes are preserved with a laparoscopic approach. Five-year overall survival ranged from 36–81% in patients undergoing LLR and was not significantly different compared to patients undergoing OLR. Similarly, five-year recurrence-free or disease-free survival rates ranged from 14–53%, and were not significantly different from patients undergoing OLR (Table 1). While this is persuasive that LLR is a safe alternative to OLR, these conclusions needed to be tested in the context of a randomized control trial, leading to three studies that are described below.

3.2. Randomized Control Trials Comparing LLR vs. OLR

The randomized control trials comparing safety and efficacy in LLR versus OLR include ORANGE II, OSLO CoMET, and LapOpHuva (Table 2), which evaluated a total of 502 patients. Outcomes evaluated included perioperative safety, operating time, estimated blood loss or EBL, transfusion rate, hospital LOS, time to functional recovery, perioperative morbidity, perioperative mortality, resection margins, and survival.

3.2.1. ORANGE II

This study was one of the original randomized control trials evaluating safety and efficacy in LLR versus OLR [28]. This was a multi-center, double-blind randomized control trial comparing laparoscopic versus open left lateral sectionectomy. The primary outcome was the time to functional recovery. The secondary outcomes were postoperative LOS, readmission rate, total morbidity rate, and mortality. After four years of recruitment, only 29 patients were randomized. The trial was closed due to slow accrual rate, which is the primary limitation of interpreting this trial. While the patient cohorts were not powered to assess significant differences, the descriptive data suggested similar times to functional recovery, LOS, and overall morbidities. ORANGE II is important for demonstrating the feasibility and safety of performing LLR as an alternative to OLR and served as the groundwork for multiple subsequent trials.

Table 2. Randomized control trials comparing laparoscopic and open liver resection.

Author	Year	Nation	Study Type	Multi-Center	Arm	N	5-y OS (%)	p-Value	5-y RFS (%)	p-Value	Complications (%)	p-Value	Mortality (%)	p-Value
Wong [28]	2018	International	ORANGE II	yes	OLR	14	NR		NR		36	0.141	7.14	NR
					LLR	15	NR		NR		8		0	
Robles-Campos [29]	2019	Spain	LapOpHuva	no	OLR	97	47.4	0.82	23.9	0.23	23.7	0.025	1	NR
					LLR	96	49.3		22.7		11.5		1	
Aghayan [30,31]	2019	Netherlands	OSLO-CoMET	no	OLR	147	55	0.67	35.7	0.57	31	0.021	0.6	NR
					LLR	133	54		29.7		19		1	

NR: not reported.

3.2.2. LapOpHuva

This was a single-center RCT conducted in Spain [29]. Patients were randomized in a 1:1 format to either the LLR or OLR group after ensuring that they did not meet the exclusion criteria, which included a disseminated disease, large liver metastases, a tumor close to major vessels, or multiple bilobar tumors. If patients were safe and had no contraindications, they received adjuvant chemotherapy (specific regimen not reported). The primary end-point was 90-day post-operative morbidity. The secondary outcomes were the OS and disease-free survival (DFS), operating time, blood loss, transfusion rate, use of the Pringle maneuver, hospital length-of-stay, and 90-day mortality. After randomization, 193 patients were available for per-protocol analysis. For both population arms, similar numbers of patients presented with synchronous or bilobar liver metastases. Most patients had one–two tumors that were moderately sized (median diameter 3–4 cm). Similar proportions (27.2% vs. 33.3%, $p = 0.091$) received neoadjuvant therapy. There were no significant differences in the anatomic distributions of the tumors, with approximately 44% (OLR) and 41.7% (LLR) of patients presenting with tumor distributions in segments six–eight. There were similar rates of major liver resection between both arms (7.2 vs. 11.5%, $p = 0.434$), though the indices of technical difficulty could not be directly compared between both approaches. The Pringle maneuver was used more frequently in LLRs with longer occlusion times. There were no differences in operating times, EBL, or rates of blood transfusion between the OLR and LLR groups. Median hospital stay was shorter in LLR (4 vs. 6 days, $p < 0.001$). Post-op morbidity was significantly lower in LLR (11.5% vs. 23.7%, $p = 0.025$), though there were no differences in severe post-operative complications or post-operative mortality.

One advantage of the LapOpHuva trial is that the study included long-term oncologic outcomes. The median follow-up times were 36 (OLR) and 40 months (LLR). The five-year OS was 47.4% (OLR) and 49.3% (LLR, $p = 0.82$). Similarly, there were no differences in the 5-year DFS rates (23.9% vs. 22.7%, $p = 0.23$). Patients had similar rates of disease recurrence (71% vs. 67.7%, ns) between treatment groups, with no differences in distant or intrahepatic recurrences between technical approaches. At the time of data analysis, 46.4% (OLR) and 51% (LLR) of patients had died due to recurrent disease.

This trial was limited by having single-center, tertiary referral center design. By having two expert surgeons in each laparoscopic case and referencing at least 50 LLR cases prior to study initiation, the study represents a highly selected, expert surgeon population that would make these results less generalizable to the global population. Additionally, there is limited data on the number of patients successfully reaching adjuvant therapy—a common experience at many centers. Finally, a sizable proportion of patients underwent repeat resection (OLR 26, LLR 32), which confounds the estimation of OS benefit from the index resection.

3.2.3. OSLO CoMET

This trial was the first to directly compare laparoscopic versus open surgical approaches for CRLM [30]. In this single-center trial, the recruited patients had CRLM that could be resected with parenchyma-sparing (less than three consecutive segments) resection without requiring concomitant ablation, vascular or biliary reconstruction, or the synchronous resection of the primary tumor. Patients were randomized two weeks prior to surgery but not informed on which approach until the day of the procedure. The operating surgeon was scheduled based on departmental availability and procedure complexity, and could change from parenchyma-sparing resection to hemi-hepatectomy or ablation at their discretion. The primary outcome was the 30-day complication rate. The secondary outcomes included conversion to laparotomy, unfavorable intraoperative incidents, operating times, blood loss, transfusion rates, and lengths of hospital stay. Patient follow-ups were performed at 1 month and 4 months after procedure.

Two hundred and eighty patients were enrolled. When reviewing background characteristics, patients in both treatment arms had similar numbers of metastases, neoadjuvant chemotherapy, rates of prior liver surgery, Iwate complexity scores, and similar rates of tumor location in posterior liver segments. Patients who underwent LLR had a lower rate of significant post-op complication (19% vs. 31%, $p = 0.021$), with one death in the open-surgery group with an uncertain cause of death at autopsy. LLR patients had lower lengths of hospital stay (53 vs. 96 h, $p < 0.001$) and less narcotic requirements (52 vs. 170 mEQ, $p < 0.001$) than OLR patients. Additionally, there were no differences in operating time, EBL, unfavorable perioperative incidents, or rates of transfusion. There was also no difference in 30-day readmission or reoperation. LLR patients had comparable oncologic outcomes, including no difference in R0 resection, R1 resection, or missed lesions. Cost-analysis was performed comparing both treatment strategies and demonstrated LLR was associated with more upfront OR costs ($5472 vs. $4762, $p = 0.00$), but did not contribute to an increased cost of initial hospital stay or additional necessary treatments at 1 or 4 months. The initial cost-savings of OLR were abrogated by costs from inpatient hospital stay, leading to no difference in short-term cost analysis for the perioperative period. Thus, LLR seemed to offer comparable immediate perioperative and cost-efficacy outcomes to OLR without compromising oncologic results. Quality of life was reported separately and evaluated physical functioning, physical role, bodily pain, overall health, emotional health, mental health, and social functioning [31]. Patients who underwent LLR had better functions in physical roles, bodily pain, and social functioning compared with patients undergoing OLR at 1 month. By four months, patients who underwent OLR still reported decreased physicality, although all other metrics were similar with LLR patients.

The long-term outcomes from the OSLO CoMET trial were released in 2021 after a minimum of 46 months follow-up [31]. In the intention-to-treat analysis, the median OSs were 80 months vs. 70 months (LLR vs. OLR, HR 0.93, CI 0.67 to 1.30, $p = 0.67$). The five-year OS rates were also similar (LLR 54% vs. OLR 55%, CI -11.3 to 12.3, $p > 0.05$). Predictors of poor OS included a poor ECOG status, lymph node involvement with the rectal primary tumor, the size of the largest liver metastasis, and the presence of extrahepatic disease at time of liver surgery. Operative approach was not a predictor of OS. The median RFSs were reported on the per-protocol analysis only and were 17 months (LLR) and 16 months (OLR). Five-year recurrence-free survival rates were 30% (LLR) versus 36% (OLR, HR 1.09, 95% CI 0.80–1.49, $p = 0.57$). The disease recurred in 62–67% of patients in both cohorts, with the most common sites of recurrence being the liver, lungs, and peritoneum. The predictors of poor RFS included lymph node involvement on the colorectal primary tumor and extrahepatic disease at diagnosis. The operative approach was not a predictor of RFS. These findings support the theory that LLR can offer a safe and oncologically sound alternative to OLR with expedited healing and improved quality of life in the immediate post-operative period. This study notably evaluated for the receipt of neoadjuvant chemotherapy, location of tumor, perceived difficulty (Iwate score) with resection, and number of lesions–features which are not consistently reported in other studies. Its limitations include the single-center and non-blinded trial design, which would make it difficult to extrapolate these results to a less-experienced center with a lower volume. As a result, additional multi-center trials evaluating whether these outcomes can be recapitulated at other centers would be very helpful to the field. For example, the ORANGE II PLUS is a multicenter trial in patients undergoing planned hemi-hepatectomy randomized to either LLR or OLR in 16 European centers. The results from this trial have not yet been published.

3.2.4. Reflections on the Data—ORANGE II, OSLO CoMET, and LapOpHuva

The study investigators should be congratulated for conducting these trials which are challenging to accomplish and add critical information to the field. The most crucial element throughout these studies is the impact of patient selection. The single-institution RCTs favored patients with unilobar disease, single, smaller (<5 cm) metastases located in anterolateral segments, and who were amenable to parenchymal-sparing surgery. These patients were fortunate enough to have little disease burden, tumors away from major vessels or bile ducts, and were amenable to parenchyma-sparing surgery, which limits broader extrapolation to all patients with CRLM.

One complicating factor is the use of perioperative therapy. The use of systemic therapy, the type of regimen, the number of completed cycles, and the rates of completing all planned systemic therapy were unevenly reported between studies. Approximately 30% of LapOpHuva patients received systemic therapy, compared with 60–69% of patients in OSLO CoMET. Of note, neoadjuvant and adjuvant chemotherapy are often given to patients with resectable CRLM, although EORTC 40983 did not show any significant 5-yr OS benefit with use of 3 months neoadjuvant and 3 months adjuvant FOLFOX compared with surgery alone [32,33]. The use of neoadjuvant/adjuvant chemotherapy may be a significant confounding factor that was not accounted for throughout these surgical trials.

Finally, these studies were based at tertiary referral centers with high volumes in liver surgery, allowing for learning and expertise in laparoscopic approaches. Thus, safety and efficacy can be estimated for high-volume referral centers, but may not be reproducible when applied in the less-experienced centers. Collectively, these studies provide valuable information that can be extrapolated to similarly selected patients. LLR can be technically feasible, safe, and oncologically comparable to OLR for CRLM resection, and should be considered in patients who meet the selection criteria of the published RCTs.

3.3. Robotic vs. Laparoscopic Liver Resection Surgery

Robotic liver resection (RLR) has been evaluated for differences in feasibility, perioperative safety, and oncologic outcomes. Kingham and colleagues initially compared robotic liver resection to open resection in a single-institution, case-matched series [34]. Sixty-five patients underwent RLR between 2002 and 2014. Selection criteria included patients with resectable liver lesions that did not require procedures more extensive than a hemihepatectomy, have an invasion of the IVC, have an invasion of the main, right, or left portal veins, or require vascular or biliary reconstruction. Patients between both cohorts had similar rates of malignant and benign lesions, and incidence of steatosis and hepatitis were similar between both groups. Patients undergoing RLR had shorter operating times (163 min vs. 210 min, $p = 0.017$), lower blood loss (100 vs. 300 mL, $p < 0.001$), and lower rates of Pringle maneuver use (9% vs. 75%, $p < 0.001$). This was despite a similar rate of wedge or segmentectomy resections between groups. There were no differences in R1 resection (1.6% vs. 15%, $p = 0.40$), major complication rates (5% vs. 6%, $p = 1.0$), or 90-day mortality rates (3% vs. 1.6%, $p = 1.0$) [34]. In this cohort, RLR was safe and offered comparable short-term oncologic outcomes to OLR in appropriately selected patients at experienced, tertiary-care referral centers.

RLR was subsequently compared to LLR for safety and efficacy. Five different retrospective cohort studies compared the robotic versus the laparoscopic approach for CRLM resection in 1869 patients total (Table 3) [35–39]. One of these studies was a multi-center retrospective study at an Italian center (59 study patients) [35], and may overlap with results published from the IGoMILS registry. The reported outcomes included perioperative safety, LOS, and survival. There were no differences in the estimated blood loss (EBL), transfusion rates, or perioperative morbidities between the LLR and RLR groups. No differences were noted in five-year disease-free (38 vs. 44%, ns) or overall survival (61 vs. 60%, $p > 0.05$) rates. There were conflicting reports regarding the operating times. Rahimli and colleagues found in their series that RLR (n = 12) was associated with a significantly longer operating time (342 vs. 200 min) but a higher tendency towards R0 resection (100% vs. 77%, $p > 0.05$) compared with LLR (n = 12) [37]. In their multi-center analysis, Masetti and colleagues found no differences in operating times between the RLR and LLR groups, and RLR was associated with lower rates of R1 resection (16.9 vs. 28.8%, ns) with greater distances in surgical margins than LLR [39]. Beard and colleagues reviewed the collective experience in six high-volume, tertiary referral centers in the U.S. and Belgium [36]. Propensity matching was performed to minimize the differences between the LLR and RLR patients. The total cohort comprised 629 patients, including 115 patients who underwent

RLR (2002–2017). Most procedures were parenchyma-sparing wedge resections. After matching for 115 LLR similar patients, there were no differences in reoperation rates (0.9% vs. 3.5%, ns), perioperative complications (27.8% vs. 31.3%, ns), perioperative mortality rates (1 LLR, 1 RLR from cardiac arrest), or margin statuses. After a median follow-up time of 2.8–3.1 years, there were no differences in the 5-year OSs or DFS. A separate meta-analysis evaluated seven retrospective cohort studies examining LLR vs. RLR in a cohort of 525 patients [38]. There were no differences in the perioperative complication rates, perioperative mortalities, rates of conversion to open procedure, R1 resections, blood transfusions, operating times, or lengths of hospital stay. No survival data could be extrapolated from the cohort studies.

Table 3. Studies comparing robotic and open liver resections.

Author	Year	Nation	Multi-Center	Arm		5-y OS (%)	p-Value	5-y RFS/DFS (%)	p-Value	Complications (%)	p-Value	Periop Mortality	p-Value
Guerra [35]	2018	Italy	yes	LLR	0							0	
				RLR	59	66		41.9		27		0	
Beard [36]	2019	US	yes	LLR	115	60	0.78	44	0.62	32	0.66	0.9	1
				RLR	115	61		38		36		0.9	
Rahimli [37]	2020	Germany	no	LLR	13	100 *	NS	54.9 *	NS	15.3	NS	0	NR
				RLR	12	44 *		33.3 *		25		0	
Ziogas [38]	2020	International	yes	LLR	300	NR		NR		28	0.13	0.3	0.75
				RLR	225	NR		NR		18		0	
Masetti [39]	2022	Italy	Yes	LLR	953	NR		NR		20	0.906	0.3	0.792
				RLR	77	NR		NR		19.5		0	

* denotes 3-year survival data; NR: not reported; NS: not significant.

When reviewed in total, there were no differences in perioperative complications or mortalities when comparing RLR to LLR across any of the five studies. In the two studies that reported on survival data, there were no differences in five-year RFSs or OSs between the RLR and LLR approaches. In conclusion, RLR appears to be feasible, safe, and may improve margin resections without compromising survival. It is not surprising that the difference in perioperative safety and transfusion is comparable between RLR and LLR for the general patient population undergoing resection for CRLM. Patients with large tumors with close proximities to hilar structures and major vessels are less likely to be incorporated in this patient population. Additional study is warranted for evaluating tumors in difficult locations, with predicted high Iwate scores for surgical complexity, and, with time, with tumors adjacent to major vessels. Furthermore, the long-term survival results have yet to mature and be reported in major study centers.

3.4. Laparoscopic vs. Open Simultaneous Liver and Colon Resections for Synchronous Disease

Select patients who present with CRLM at diagnosis may be eligible for synchronous resection. Advances in the laparoscopic technique, perioperative care, and the use of systemic therapy have made it possible to attempt synchronous resection in appropriately selected patients. Eleven single-center and multi-center retrospective cohort studies evaluated whether laparoscopic simultaneous resection could be safely performed for patients with synchronous stage IV CRLM disease (Table 4) [40–51]. Of note, all of these studies were performed outside of the United States (France, Spain, Israel, UK, Italy, South Korea, and multi-national), and evaluated a total of 490 study patients undergoing laparoscopic simultaneous resections. Procedures were performed at tertiary referral centers with extensive prior experience in laparoscopic and open liver surgeries. They evaluated feasibility, perioperative safety, and survival.

Table 4. Studies evaluating synchronous resections of colon primary and metastatic liver tumors.

Author	Year	Nation	Study Type	Arm	N	3-y OS	p-Value	3-y RFS	p-Value	Complications (%)	p-Value	Periop Mortality (%)	p-Value
Akiyoshi [40]	2009	Japan	Single-center, retrospective	Lap	10	NR		NR		10		0	
Polignano [41]	2012	UK	Single-center, retrospective	Lap	13			90		28		0	
Hatwell [42]	2012	France	Single-center, retrospective	Lap	51	NR		NR		55		0	
Ferretti [43]	2015	International	Multi-center, retrospective	Lap	142	71.9 *		63 *		31		2.1	
Muangkaew [44]	2015	South Korea	Single-center, retrospective	Lap	55					76		0	
Tranchart [45]	2015	International	Multi-center, retrospective	Lap	89	78	0.17	64	0.13	15	1	6	0.49
				Open	89	65		52		15		0	
Chen [46]	2018	Taiwan	Single-center, retrospective	Lap	16	73	0.99	35	0.14	25	0.06	0	NR
				Open	22	48		15		36		0	
Bizzoca [47]	2019	Italy	Single-center, retrospective	Lap	17					47		0	
van der Poel [48]	2019	International	Multi-center, retrospective	Lap	61	NR		NR		15	0.237	0	1
				Open	61	NR		NR		9		2	
Perfecto [50]	2021	Spain	Single-center, retrospective	Lap	15	92.3		24		26.6		0	
Sawaied [51]	2021	Israel	Multi-center, retrospective	Lap	21	87	0.64	48	0.92	33	0.15	0	0.48
				Open	42	57		40		52		2	

* denotes 5-year survival; NR: not reported.

The laparoscopic resection of the synchronous disease was as safe as open resection. There were no differences in blood loss or transfusion rates. Two studies noted slightly longer operating times, although these was not significantly different from open procedures. About 5–8% of laparoscopic procedures required conversion to an open procedure, which was consistent across multiple multi-center trials. The perioperative complication rates ranged from 10–76%, with approximately 20% constituting major complications. There were no differences in major or minor complications between the laparoscopic and open procedures. The perioperative mortality was quite low, with only four deaths reported across all studies (one from open surgery, one due to liver hemorrhage requiring reoperation, one from multi-organ system failure, and one from acute coronary syndrome). The hospital length-of-stay was inconsistently reported, but ranged from 6–16 days for both the laparoscopic and open surgery cohorts. The rates of anastomotic leaks and hospital readmissions were inconsistently reported across all studies.

Oncologic and survival outcomes were premature for the study cohorts, as most reports had median follow-up times of 24–26 months for both the open and laparoscopic surgery groups. OS and DFS were the most common oncologic outcomes reported, but varied in reporting style (i.e., 3-year versus 5-year follow-up, disease recurrence rates, etc.), making consistent comparisons across study groups challenging. Several studies did not report patient OS or DFS at all. In the five studies that reported a three-year OS, there were no differences between the laparoscopic and open surgery groups, with rates that ranged from 48–92.3% [43,45,47,50,51]. The three-year DFS ranged from 15–64%, and was also similar between both groups. These findings suggest that laparoscopic synchronous resection is at least comparable to open resection from the perioperative safety and short-term oncologic outcome perspectives in appropriately selected patients. However, it is worth nothing that many of the technical advantages associated with laparoscopic resection, such as decreased blood loss and decreased overall complication rates, are lost when applying these surgical approaches to synchronous colon and liver resections. Additionally, not all patients are appropriate for selection for laparoscopic synchronous resection. These studies favored anterolateral liver tumors over posterior tumors.

The findings for these studies are limited by the pragmatic limitations of appropriate patient selection. This warrants careful interpretation of the literature and extrapolation. For example, there was significant heterogeneity between patient cohorts with respect to the receipt of systemic therapy. For some studies, most patients did not receive neoadjuvant therapy, and in others, less patients in the open group received adjuvant chemotherapy. Additionally, the type of systemic chemotherapy and the use of biologic agents (i.e., cetuximab, bevacizumab) were not delineated in these studies, adding potential additional heterogeneity. Most studies selected for solitary liver tumors less than 3 cm in greatest diameter, and were amenable to non-anatomic resections. Some studies specifically selected for lesions in anterolateral segments only, and specifically avoided very-low-lying rectal lesions. While these are appropriate and key factors to consider in pre-operative patient selection, it is important to understand these study limitations, especially when applying to one's own practice. As such, there are limited evidence-based guidelines available for guidance on patient and tumor selection. One example, which nicely reviews expert consensus and evidence-based recommendations, is the Italian consensus on minimally invasive simultaneous resections [52].

3.5. MIS Approaches Are Associated with Shorter Times to Adjuvant Therapy

While MIS approaches to liver resection show comparable safety and efficacy to open resection, they are associated with earlier recovery and the initiation of systemic therapy. Three papers evaluated this question in retrospective cohort analyses (Table 5) [53–55]. Tohme and colleagues identified that patients undergoing MIS liver resection were able to start systemic therapy within 42 days after resection, as compared with 63 days in patients recovering from open resection ($p < 0.001$). These results were corroborated by Mbah and Kawai and colleagues as well. This may be because patients undergoing MIS resections experience lower rates of blood loss and perioperative complications and are more likely to have a short length of hospital stay [54,55]. Patients who experience even grade one or grade two complications may experience a delay in return to full functional capacity, thus contributing to a delay in initiating adjuvant therapy. Thus, there may be a potential advantage in using MIS approaches for liver resection to facilitate sooner recovery and the continuation of oncologic care.

Table 5. Studies evaluating time to adjuvant therapy after liver surgery for colorectal liver metastases.

Author	Year	Nation	N	Arm	5-y OS	p-Value	5-y RFS	Complications (%)	p-Value	Periop Mortality (%)	p-Value	Time to Chemo (days)	p-Value
Tohme [53]	2015	US	66	OLR	38	0.06	NR	38	0.19	0	1	63	0.001
			66	MIR	51		NR	26		0		42	
Mbah [54]	2017	US	44	OLR	NR		NR	36	0.03	1.6	1	39	0.0001
			76	LLR	NR		NR	14		1.1		24	
Kawai [55]	2018	France	87	OLR	NR		NR	28	0.61	0	NR	53	0.01
			30	LLR	NR		NR	33		0		45	

NR: not reported.

3.6. Limitations

The limitations of specific RCTs and surgical approaches were reviewed within the respective sections. However, there are some overarching limitations with our review. First, most of the published papers entailed single-center, retrospective studies from high-volume centers over extended periods of time. These inherently reflect bias from surgeons with extensive experience in laparoscopic (and robotic) colon and liver surgery and patient and tumor selection. Even within study groups, there was heterogeneity in reporting the number of lesions, the sizes of the greatest liver lesions, the unilobar versus bilobar distributions, the individual tumor locations, the anticipated technical difficulties, and whether the tumors had been treated with neoadjuvant chemotherapy. The types and numbers of cycles of systemic therapy were not universally reported, nor were the common mutational profiles (i.e., KRAS, BRAF, MSI) that are typically reviewed in patients with a systemic disease today. These reporting characteristics have significant influences on perioperative morbidity and long-term oncologic results. These data points should be considered for inclusion in prospective trials for future studies aiming to evaluate perioperative safety and oncologic outcomes.

Furthermore, several of the studies have not yet reported more-updated results for long-term survival outcomes. While OSLO-COMET and LapOpHuva reported median follow-ups of at least 40+ months, some of the retrospective cohort studies only have mature data for 3-year survival (RFS, OS). These are important to reassess as we proceed with recommending RLR and laparoscopic simultaneous resections for appropriately selected patients.

The data reported from high-volume referral centers do not imply endorsement for broad integration. Surgeons need to reflect upon their own case volume and technical competence with liver surgery, laparoscopic surgery, and robotic surgery when considering embarking on these approaches for their own patients.

Finally, there are inherent limitations to the nature of a review. The papers we identified for inclusion were selected based on search terms, identification through our selected search engines, and availability in English and in full text. Our determined exclusion criteria may have excluded reports with smaller cohorts.

4. Conclusions

Minimally invasive approaches to hepatobiliary surgery have made significant advances in the last 15 years. The recent literature has demonstrated that LLR and RLR can be performed with acceptable perioperative safety without adversely affecting overall survival. MIS approaches can be associated with lower blood loss, shorter hospital stays, and lower rates of perioperative complications. Furthermore, advances in laparoscopic techniques and expertise may facilitate the synchronous resection of colorectal and liver tumors in patients who present with a synchronous stage-four disease. Another benefit to LLR for CRLM is the earlier initiation of adjuvant systemic chemotherapy. The current data represents the outcomes of careful patient selection and experience in advanced laparoscopic and robotic liver surgery techniques at tertiary referral centers. As MIS liver resection continues to diffuse globally, it is hoped that additional studies will provide more data on the benefits and outcomes of laparoscopic and robotic liver resections.

Author Contributions: Conceptualization, literature review, analysis, and manuscript writing—W.M.L., S.T.T. and D.A.G. All authors have read and agreed to the published version of the manuscript.

Funding: This research received no external funding.

Conflicts of Interest: The authors declare no conflict of interest.

References

1. Nguyen, K.T.; Gamblin, T.C.; Geller, D.A. World Review of Laparoscopic Liver Resection—2,804 Patients. *Ann. Surg.* **2009**, *250*, 831–841. [CrossRef] [PubMed]
2. Castaing, D.; Vibert, E.; Ricca, L.; Azoulay, D.; Adam, R.; Gayet, B. Oncologic Results of Laparoscopic Versus Open Hepatectomy for Colorectal Liver Metastases in Two Specialized Centers. *Ann. Surg.* **2009**, *250*, 849–855. [CrossRef] [PubMed]
3. Nguyen, K.T.; Marsh, J.W.; Tsung, A.; Steel, J.J.L.; Gamblin, T.C.; Geller, D.A. Comparative Benefits of Laparoscopic vs Open Hepatic Resection: A 2. critical appraisal. *Arch. Surg.* **2011**, *146*, 348–356. [CrossRef] [PubMed]
4. Nguyen, K.T.; Laurent, A.; Dagher, I.; Geller, D.A.; Steel, J.; Thomas, M.T.; Marvin, M.; Ravindra, K.V.; Mejia, A.; Lainas, P.; et al. Minimally Invasive Liver Resection for Metastatic Colorectal Cancer: A multi-institutional, international report of safety, feasibility, and early outcomes. *Ann. Surg.* **2009**, *250*, 842–848. [CrossRef]
5. Ratti, F.; Fiorentini, G.; Cipriani, F.; Catena, M.; Paganelli, M.; Aldrighetti, L. Laparoscopic vs Open Surgery for Colorectal Liver Metastases. *JAMA Surg.* **2018**, *153*, 1028. [CrossRef]
6. Ciria, R.; Cherqui, D.; Geller, D.A.; Briceno, J.; Wakabayashi, G. Comparative Short-term Benefits of Laparoscopic Liver Resection: 9000 cases and climbing. *Ann. Surg.* **2016**, *263*, 761–777. [CrossRef]
7. Fretland, Å.A.; Dagenborg, V.J.; Bjørnelv, G.M.W.; Kazaryan, A.M.; Kristiansen, R.; Fagerland, M.W.; Hausken, J.; Tønnessen, T.I.; Abildgaard, A.; Barkhatov, L.; et al. Laparoscopic Versus Open Resection for Colorectal Liver Metastases. *Ann. Surg.* **2018**, *267*, 199–207. [CrossRef]
8. Sasaki, K.; Nair, A.; Moro, A.; Augustin, T.; Quintini, C.; Berber, E.; Aucejo, F.N.; Kwon, C.H.D. A chronological review of 500 minimally invasive liver resections in a North American institution: Overcoming stagnation and toward consolidation. *Surg. Endosc.* **2022**, *36*, 6144–6152. [CrossRef]
9. Bryant, R.; Laurent, A.; Tayar, C.; Cherqui, D. Laparoscopic liver resection – understanding its role in current practice: The Henri Mondor Hospital experience. *Ann. Surg.* **2009**, *250*, 103–111. [CrossRef]
10. Kazaryan, A.M.; Marangos, I.P.; Røsok, B.I.; Rosseland, A.R.; Villanger, O.; Fosse, E.; Mathisen, O.; Edwin, B. Laparoscopic Resection of Colorectal Liver Metastases: Surgical and long-term oncologic outcome. *Ann. Surg.* **2010**, *252*, 1005–1012. [CrossRef]
11. Topal, H.; Tiek, J.; Aerts, R.; Topal, B. Outcome of laparoscopic major liver resection for colorectal metastases. *Surg. Endosc.* **2012**, *26*, 2451–2455. [CrossRef] [PubMed]
12. Cannon, R.M.; Scoggins, C.R.; Callender, G.G.; McMasters, K.M.; Martin, R.C. Laparoscopic versus open resection of hepatic colorectal metastases. *Surgery* **2012**, *152*, 567–574. [CrossRef] [PubMed]
13. Iwahashi, S.; Shimada, M.; Utsunomiya, T.; Imura, S.; Morine, Y.; Ikemoto, T.; Arakawa, Y.; Mori, H.; Kanamoto, M.; Yamada, S. Laparoscopic hepatic resection for metastatic liver tumor of colorectal cancer: Comparative analysis of short- and long-term results. *Surg. Endosc.* **2013**, *28*, 80–84. [CrossRef] [PubMed]
14. Montalti, R.; Berardi, G.; Laurent, S.; Sebastiani, S.; Ferdinande, L.; Libbrecht, L.; Smeets, P.; Brescia, A.; Rogiers, X.; de Hemptinne, B.; et al. Laparoscopic liver resection compared to open approach in patients with colorectal liver metastases improves further resectability: Oncological outcomes of a case-control matched-pairs analysis. *Eur. J. Surg. Oncol. (EJSO)* **2014**, *40*, 536–544. [CrossRef] [PubMed]
15. Beppu, T.; Wakabayashi, G.; Hasegawa, K.; Gotohda, N.; Mizuguchi, T.; Takahashi, Y.; Hirokawa, F.; Taniai, N.; Watanabe, M.; Katou, M.; et al. Long-term and perioperative outcomes of laparoscopic versus open liver resection for colorectal liver metastases with propensity score matching: A multi-institutional Japanese study. *J. Hepato-Biliary-Pancreat. Sci.* **2015**, *22*, 711–720. [CrossRef]
16. Allard, M.-A.; Cunha, A.S.; Gayet, B.; Adam, R.; Goere, D.; Bachellier, P.; Azoulay, D.; Ayav, A.; Navarro, F.; Pessaux, P. Early and Long-term Oncological Outcomes After Laparoscopic Resection for Colorectal Liver Metastases. *Ann. Surg.* **2015**, *262*, 794–802. [CrossRef]
17. De'Angelis, N.; Eshkenazy, R.; Brunetti, F.; Valente, R.; Costa, M.; Disabato, M.; Salloum, C.; Compagnon, P.; Laurent, A.; Azoulay, D. Laparoscopic Versus Open Resection for Colorectal Liver Metastases: A Single-Center Study with Propensity Score Analysis. *J. Laparoendosc. Adv. Surg. Tech.* **2015**, *25*, 12–20. [CrossRef]

18. Hasegawa, Y.; Kitago, M.; Abe, Y.; Kitagawa, Y. Does laparoscopic resection for colorectal cancer liver metastasis have a long-term oncologic advantage? *Hepatobiliary Surg. Nutr.* **2021**, *10*, 246–248. [CrossRef]
19. Lin, Q.; Ye, Q.; Zhu, D.; Wei, Y.; Ren, L.; Zheng, P.; Xu, P.; Ye, L.; Lv, M.; Fan, J.; et al. Comparison of minimally invasive and open colorectal resections for patients undergoing simultaneous R0 resection for liver metastases: A propensity score analysis. *Int. J. Color. Dis.* **2014**, *30*, 385–395. [CrossRef]
20. Schiffman, S.C.; Kim, K.H.; Tsung, A.; Marsh, J.W.; Geller, D.A. Laparoscopic versus open liver resection for metastatic colorectal cancer: A metaanalysis of 610 patients. *Surgery* **2015**, *157*, 211–222. [CrossRef]
21. Cipriani, F.; Rawashdeh, M.; Stanton, L.; Armstrong, T.; Takhar, A.; Pearce, N.W.; Primrose, J.; Abu Hilal, M. Propensity score-based analysis of outcomes of laparoscopic *versus* open liver resection for colorectal metastases. *Br. J. Surg.* **2016**, *103*, 1504–1512. [CrossRef]
22. Lewin, J.W.; O'Rourke, N.A.; Chiow, A.K.H.; Bryant, R.; Martin, I.; Nathanson, L.K.; Cavallucci, D.J. Long-term survival in laparoscopic vs open resection for colorectal liver metas-tases: Inverse probability of treatment weighting using propensity scores. *HPB* **2016**, *18*, 183–191. [CrossRef] [PubMed]
23. Nomi, T.; Fuks, D.; Louvet, C.; Nakajima, Y.; Gayet, B. Outcomes of Laparoscopic Liver Resection for Patients with Large Colorectal Liver Metastases: A Case-Matched Analysis. *World J. Surg.* **2016**, *40*, 1702–1708. [CrossRef]
24. Maurette, R.J.; Ejarque, M.G.; Mihura, M.; Bregante, M.; Bogetti, D.; Pirchi, D. Laparoscopic liver resection in metastatic colorectal cancer treatment: Comparison with long-term results using the conventional approach. *Ecancermedicalscience* **2017**, *11*, 775. [CrossRef] [PubMed]
25. Goumard, C.; You, Y.N.; Okuno, M.; Kutlu, O.; Chen, H.-C.; Simoneau, E.; Vega, E.A.; Chun, Y.-S.; Tzeng, C.D.; Eng, C.; et al. Minimally invasive management of the entire treatment sequence in patients with stage IV colorectal cancer: A propensity-score weighting analysis. *HPB* **2018**, *20*, 1150–1156. [CrossRef]
26. Efanov, M.; Granov, D.; Alikhanov, R.; Rutkin, I.; Tsvirkun, V.; Kazakov, I.; Vankovich, A.; Koroleva, A.; Kovalenko, D. Expanding indications for laparoscopic parenchyma-sparing resection of posterosuperior liver segments in patients with colorectal metastases: Comparison with open hepatectomy for immediate and long-term outcomes. *Surg. Endosc.* **2020**, *35*, 96–103. [CrossRef] [PubMed]
27. Nicolás, M.; Czerwonko, M.; Ardiles, V.; Claria, R.S.; Mazza, O.; de Santibañes, E.; Pekolj, J.; de Santibañes, M. Laparoscopic vs open liver resection for metastatic colorectal cancer: Analysis of surgical margin status and survival. *Langenbeck's Arch. Surg.* **2022**, *407*, 1113–1119. [CrossRef]
28. Wong-Lun-Hing, E.M.; van Dam, R.M.; van Breukelen, G.J.P.; Tanis, P.J.; Ratti, F.; van Hillegersberg, R.; Slooter, G.D.; de Wilt, J.H.W.; Liem, M.S.L.; de Boer, M.T.; et al. Randomized clinical trial of open versus laparoscopic left lateral hepatic sectionectomy within an enhanced recovery after surgery programme (ORANGE II study). *Br. J. Surg.* **2017**, *104*, 525–535. [CrossRef]
29. Robles-Campos, R.; Lopez-Lopez, V.; Brusadin, R.; Lopez-Conesa, A.; Gil-Vazquez, P.J.; Navarro-Barrios, Á.; Parrilla, P. Open versus minimally invasive liver surgery for colorectal liver metastases (LapOpHuva): A prospective randomized controlled trial. *Surg. Endosc.* **2019**, *33*, 3926–3936. [CrossRef]
30. Aghayan, D.L.; Kazaryan, A.M.; Dagenborg, V.J.; Røsok, B.I.; Fagerland, M.M.W.; Bjørnelv, M.G.M.W.; Kristiansen, B.R.; Flatmark, K.; Fretland, A.; Edwin, B. Long-Term Oncologic Outcomes After Laparoscopic Versus Open Resection for Colorectal Liver Metastases: A randomized trial. *Ann. Intern. Med.* **2021**, *174*, 175–182. [CrossRef]
31. Fretland, Å.A.; Dagenborg, V.J.; Bjørnelv, G.M.W.; Aghayan, D.L.; Kazaryan, A.M.; Barkhatov, L.; Kristiansen, R.; Fagerland, M.W.; Edwin, B.; Andersen, M.H. Quality of life from a randomized trial of laparoscopic or open liver resection for colorectal liver metastases. *Br. J. Surg.* **2019**, *106*, 1372–1380. [CrossRef] [PubMed]
32. Nordlinger, B.; Sorbye, H.; Glimelius, B.; Poston, G.J.; Schlag, P.M.; Rougier, P.; Bechstein, W.O.; Primrose, J.N.; Walpole, E.T.; Finch-Jones, M.; et al. Perioperative FOLFOX4 chemotherapy and surgery versus surgery alone for resectable liver metastases from colorectal cancer (EORTC 40983): Long-term results of a randomised, controlled, phase 3 trial. *Lancet Oncol.* **2013**, *14*, 1208–1215. [CrossRef] [PubMed]
33. Nordlinger, B.; Sorbye, H.; Glimelius, B.; Poston, G.J.; Schlag, P.M.; Rougier, P.; Bechstein, W.O.; Primrose, J.N.; Walpole, E.T.; Finch-Jones, M.; et al. Perioperative chemotherapy with FOLFOX4 and surgery versus surgery alone for resectable liver metastases from colorectal cancer (EORTC Intergroup trial 40983): A randomised controlled trial. *Lancet* **2008**, *371*, 1007–1016. [CrossRef]
34. Kingham, T.P.; Leung, U.; Kuk, D.; Gönen, M.; D'Angelica, M.I.; Allen, P.J.; DeMatteo, R.P.; Laudone, V.P.; Jarnagin, W.R.; Fong, Y. Robotic Liver Resection: A Case-Matched Comparison. *World J. Surg.* **2016**, *40*, 1422–1428. [CrossRef]
35. Guerra, F.; Guadagni, S.; Pesi, B.; Furbetta, N.; Di Franco, G.; Palmeri, M.; Annecchiarico, M.; Eugeni, E.; Coratti, A.; Patriti, A.; et al. Outcomes of robotic liver resections for colorectal liver metastases. A multi-institutional analysis of minimally invasive ultrasound-guided robotic surgery. *Surg. Oncol.* **2018**, *28*, 14–18. [CrossRef] [PubMed]
36. Beard, R.E.; Khan, S.; Troisi, R.I.; Montalti, R.; Vanlander, A.; Fong, Y.; Kingham, T.P.; Boerner, T.; Berber, E.; Kahramangil, B.; et al. Long-Term and Oncologic Outcomes of Robotic Versus Laparoscopic Liver Resection for Metastatic Colorectal Cancer: A Multicenter, Propensity Score Matching Analysis. *World J. Surg.* **2019**, *44*, 887–895. [CrossRef] [PubMed]
37. Rahimli, M.; Perrakis, A.; Schellerer, V.; Gumbs, A.; Lorenz, E.; Franz, M.; Arend, J.; Negrini, V.-R.; Croner, R.S. Robotic and laparoscopic liver surgery for colorectal liver metastases: An experience from a German Academic Center. *World J. Surg. Oncol.* **2020**, *18*, 333. [CrossRef]

38. Ziogas, I.A.; Giannis, D.; Esagian, S.M.; Economopoulos, K.P.; Tohme, S.; Geller, D.A. Laparoscopic versus robotic major hepatectomy: A systematic review and meta-analysis. *Surg. Endosc.* **2020**, *35*, 524–535. [CrossRef]
39. Masetti, M.; Fallani, G.; Ratti, F.; Ferrero, A.; Giuliante, F.; Cillo, U.; Guglielmi, A.; Ettorre, G.M.; Torzilli, G.; Vincenti, L.; et al. Minimally invasive treatment of colorectal liver metastases: Does robotic surgery provide any technical advantages over laparoscopy? A multicenter analysis from the IGoMILS (Italian Group of Minimally Invasive Liver Surgery) registry. *Updat. Surg.* **2022**, *74*, 535–545. [CrossRef]
40. Akiyoshi, T.; Kuroyanagi, H.; Saiura, A.; Fujimoto, Y.; Koga, R.; Konishi, T.; Ueno, M.; Oya, M.; Seki, M.; Yamaguchi, T. Simultaneous Resection of Colorectal Cancer and Synchronous Liver Metastases: Initial Experience of Laparoscopy for Colorectal Cancer Resection. *Dig. Surg.* **2009**, *26*, 471–475. [CrossRef]
41. Polignano, F.M.; Quyn, A.J.; Sanjay, P.; Henderson, N.A.; Tait, I.S. Totally laparoscopic strategies for the management of colorectal cancer with synchronous liver metastasis. *Surg. Endosc.* **2012**, *26*, 2571–2578. [CrossRef] [PubMed]
42. Hatwell, C.; Bretagnol, F.; Farges, O.; Belghiti, J.; Panis, Y. Laparoscopic resection of colorectal cancer facilitates simultaneous surgery of synchronous liver metastases. *Color. Dis.* **2012**, *15*, e21–e28. [CrossRef] [PubMed]
43. Ferretti, S.; Tranchart, H.; Buell, J.F.; Eretta, C.; Patriti, A.; Spampinato, M.G.; Huh, J.W.; Vigano, L.; Han, H.S.; Ettorre, G.M.; et al. Laparoscopic Simultaneous Resection of Colorectal Primary Tumor and Liver Metastases: Results of a Multicenter International Study. *World J. Surg.* **2015**, *39*, 2052–2060. [CrossRef]
44. Muangkaew, P.; Cho, J.Y.; Han, H.-S.; Yoon, Y.-S.; Choi, Y.; Jang, J.Y.; Choi, H.; Jang, J.S.; Kwon, S.U. Outcomes of Simultaneous Major Liver Resection and Colorectal Surgery for Colorectal Liver Metastases. *J. Gastrointest. Surg.* **2015**, *20*, 554–563. [CrossRef]
45. Tranchart, H.; Fuks, D.; Vigano, L.; Ferretti, S.; Paye, F.; Wakabayashi, G.; Ferrero, A.; Gayet, B.; Dagher, I. Laparoscopic simultaneous resection of colorectal primary tumor and liver metastases: A propensity score matching analysis. *Surg. Endosc.* **2015**, *30*, 1853–1862. [CrossRef]
46. Chen, Y.-W.; Huang, M.-T.; Chang, T.-C. Long term outcomes of simultaneous laparoscopic versus open resection for colorectal cancer with synchronous liver metastases. *Asian J. Surg.* **2018**, *42*, 217–223. [CrossRef] [PubMed]
47. Bizzoca, C.; DelVecchio, A.; Fedele, S.; Vincenti, L. Simultaneous Colon and Liver Laparoscopic Resection for Colorectal Cancer with Synchronous Liver Metastases: A Single Center Experience. *J. Laparoendosc. Adv. Surg. Tech.* **2019**, *29*, 934–942. [CrossRef]
48. Van der Poel, M.J.; Barkhatov, L.; Fuks, D.; Berardi, G.; Cipriani, F.; Aljaiuossi, A.; Lainas, P.; Dagher, I.; D'Hondt, M.; Rotellar, F.; et al. Multicentre propensity score-matched study of laparoscopic versus open repeat liver resection for colorectal liver metastases. *Br. J. Surg.* **2019**, *106*, 783–789. [CrossRef]
49. Van der Poel, M.J.; Tanis, P.J.; Marsman, H.A.; Rijken, A.M.; Gertsen, E.C.; Ovaere, S.; Gerhards, M.F.; Besselink, M.G.; D'Hondt, M.; Gobardhan, P.D. Laparoscopic combined resection of liver metastases and colorectal cancer: A multicenter, case-matched study using propensity scores. *Surg. Endosc.* **2018**, *33*, 1124–1130. [CrossRef]
50. Perfecto, A.; Gastaca, M.; Prieto, M.; Cervera, J.; Ruiz, P.; Ventoso, A.; Palomares, I.; García, J.M.; Valdivieso, A. Totally laparoscopic simultaneous resection of colorectal cancer and synchronous liver metastases: A single-center case series. *Surg. Endosc.* **2021**, *36*, 980–987. [CrossRef]
51. Sawaied, M.; Berger, Y.; Mahamid, A.; Abu-Zaydeh, O.; Verter, E.; Khoury, W.; Goldberg, N.; Sadot, E.; Haddad, R. Laparoscopic Versus Open Simultaneous Resection of Primary Colorectal Cancer and Associated Liver Metastases: A Comparative Retrospective Study. *Surg. Laparosc. Endosc. Percutaneous Tech.* **2021**, *32*, 73–78. [CrossRef] [PubMed]
52. Rocca, A.; Cipriani, F.; Belli, G.; Berti, S.; Boggi, U.; Bottino, V.; Cillo, U.; Cescon, M.; Cimino, M.; Corcione, F.; et al. The Italian Consensus on minimally invasive simultaneous resections for synchronous liver metastasis and primary colorectal cancer: A Delphi methodology. *Updat. Surg.* **2021**, *73*, 1247–1265. [CrossRef] [PubMed]
53. Tohme, S.; Goswami, J.; Han, K.; Chidi, A.P.; Geller, D.A.; Reddy, S.; Gleisner, A.; Tsung, A. Minimally Invasive Resection of Colorectal Cancer Liver Metastases Leads to an Earlier Initiation of Chemotherapy Compared to Open Surgery. *J. Gastrointest. Surg.* **2015**, *19*, 2199–2206. [CrossRef] [PubMed]
54. Mbah, N.; Agle, S.C.; Philips, P.; Egger, M.E.; Scoggins, C.R.; McMasters, K.M.; Martin, R.C. Laparoscopic hepatectomy significantly shortens the time to postoperative chemotherapy in patients undergoing major hepatectomies. *Am. J. Surg.* **2017**, *213*, 1060–1064. [CrossRef]
55. Kawai, T.; Goumard, C.; Jeune, F.; Savier, E.; Vaillant, J.-C.; Scatton, O. Laparoscopic liver resection for colorectal liver metastasis patients allows patients to start adjuvant chemotherapy without delay: A propensity score analysis. *Surg. Endosc.* **2018**, *32*, 3273–3281. [CrossRef]

Disclaimer/Publisher's Note: The statements, opinions and data contained in all publications are solely those of the individual author(s) and contributor(s) and not of MDPI and/or the editor(s). MDPI and/or the editor(s) disclaim responsibility for any injury to people or property resulting from any ideas, methods, instructions or products referred to in the content.

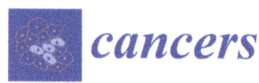

Communication

Latest Findings on Minimally Invasive Anatomical Liver Resection

Yoshiki Fujiyama [1,2,*], Taiga Wakabayashi [1,2], Kohei Mishima [1,2,3], Malek A. Al-Omari [1,2], Marco Colella [1,2] and Go Wakabayashi [1,2]

1. Department of Surgery, Ageo Central General Hospital, Saitama 362-8588, Japan; malekamo86@yahoo.com (M.A.A.-O.); mrccolella@gmail.com (M.C.); gowaka@ach.or.jp (G.W.)
2. Center for Advanced Treatment of Hepatobiliary and Pancreatic Diseases, Ageo Central General Hospital, Saitama 362-8588, Japan
3. Institute for Research against Digestive Cancer (IRCAD), 67091 Strasbourg, France
* Correspondence: fujiyama.yoshiki@kitasato-u.ac.jp; Tel.: +81-48-773-1111; Fax: +81-48-773-7122

Simple Summary: The safety of minimally invasive anatomical liver resection is a major concern for hepatobiliary surgeons. The Precision Anatomy for Minimally Invasive Hepato-Biliary-Pancreatic Surgery Expert Consensus Meeting was held in 2021. In this meeting, the importance of intraoperative staining of the dominant portal venous region was confirmed, with indocyanine green playing a central role. This article describes the latest findings on minimally invasive laparoscopic anatomical liver resection using the indocyanine green negative staining technique.

Abstract: Minimally invasive liver resection (MILR) is being widely utilized owing to recent advancements in laparoscopic and robot-assisted surgery. There are two main types of liver resection: anatomical (minimally invasive anatomical liver resection (MIALR)) and nonanatomical. MIALR is defined as a minimally invasive liver resection along the respective portal territory. Optimization of the safety and precision of MIALR is the next challenge for hepatobiliary surgeons, and intraoperative indocyanine green (ICG) staining is considered to be of considerable importance in this field. In this article, we present the latest findings on MIALR and laparoscopic anatomical liver resection using ICG at our hospital.

Keywords: MIALR; Tokyo 2020 terminology; ICG negative staining

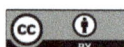

1. Introduction

With recent developments in minimally invasive surgeries, laparoscopic and robot-assisted procedures have become increasingly popular for hepatobiliary surgery [1–5]. Two international consensus conferences [6,7] and one international guideline conference [8] have been held to promote the safe use of minimally invasive liver resection (MILR). Safe and minimally invasive anatomical liver resection (MIALR) is the next keystone in hepatobiliary surgery [9–12]. To address the safety of MIALR, the Precision Anatomy for Minimally Invasive Hepato-Biliary-Pancreatic (HBP) Surgery Expert Consensus Meeting (PAM-consensus meeting) was held in Japan in 2021 [13,14]. Based on this meeting, the Tokyo 2020 Terminology of Liver Anatomy and Resections (Tokyo 2020 terminology) was recommended as an important guideline [15]. The Tokyo 2020 terminology defines anatomical liver resection more clearly, updating the Brisbane 2000 terminology of liver anatomy and resections [16–18]. The PAM consensus meeting and the Tokyo 2020 terminology addressed the importance of regional staining for safe MIALR. We believe that indocyanine green (ICG) plays a central role in MIALR, and that liver resection along the intersegmental plane with ICG negative staining is an acceptable basic technique for MIALR. This paper describes the latest findings on MIALR and our MIALR technique using ICG green-negative staining.

2. Latest Findings on the MIALR–PAM Consensus Meeting and Tokyo 2020 Terminology

MIALR has gradually become widely available worldwide following two international consensus conferences and one international guideline conference. However, the definition of MIALR and its associated surgical procedures have not been well formulated. An expert consensus meeting on the Precision Anatomy for Minimally Invasive HBP Surgery (the PAM consensus meeting) was held during the 32nd Annual Meeting of the Hepatobiliary and Pancreatic Surgery Society in February 2021. Hepatobiliary surgeons worldwide shared their opinions regarding the definition and safe surgical procedures for MIALR [9,19–21]. The main points of the PAM consensus meeting were published as the Tokyo 2020 Terminology of Liver Anatomy and Resections (Tokyo 2020 terminology). The Tokyo 2020 terminology is an important milestone in the field of liver surgery. The key points are listed below.

Key point 1: MIALR is defined as the complete resection of the liver parenchyma within the region of the respective portal vein.

Key point 2: Segmentectomy is defined as the complete resection of the third portal vein branch of the Couinaud classification. Subsegmentectomy is defined as the resection of the area beyond the third portal vein branch of the Couinaud classification, with each area defined as a "cone unit."

Key point 3: Two approaches to accessing the Glisson's sheath have been described: the Glissonean approach (GA), which secures Glisson's sheath in one piece, and the hilar approach (HA), which separates the artery, portal vein, and bile ducts individually. In MIALR, the GA is more suitable than the HA, particularly when approaching peripherally from secondary Glissonean branches.

Key point 4: The intersegmental/sectional plane (IP) is the boundary of each portal-dominant territory, and the vein passing through the IP is defined as the intersegmental/sectional vein (IV). Preoperative three-dimensional (3D) simulations are useful for visualizing the IPs and IVs. The dissection of the liver parenchyma along the correct IP is crucial for a precise anatomical liver resection.

Key point 5: To visualize the IPs in MIALR, negative staining with intravenous contrast after blocking the target Glisson or positive staining via direct injection into the portal vein is recommended.

3. Laparoscopic Anatomic Liver Resection at Ageo Central General Hospital (ACGH)

As of April 2016, all laparoscopic liver resections without biliary or vascular reconstruction are covered by health insurance in Japan. Thanks to this coverage, we performed 213 laparoscopic anatomical liver resections as of March 2022 (Table 1) [22–25]. In some cases, subsegmentectomy targeting the periphery beyond the third branch of Glisson's sheath was performed to achieve both anatomical resection and sparing of the liver parenchyma. All liver resections without biliary or vascular reconstruction were considered as indications for MIALR. Regarding the indications for anatomical resection, we performed anatomical resection for hepatocellular carcinoma, except in cases with a peripherally located tumor. For diseases other than hepatocellular carcinoma, we chose anatomical resection when the carcinoma-bearing Glisson was more central than the tertiary branch. This is because we believe that anatomical resection is a more physiological procedure that follows hepatic blood flow. The indications for the 213 patients and short-term outcomes are shown in Tables 1 and 2, respectively. As shown in the tables, our MIALR procedure was characterized by the anatomical resection of metastatic tumors (Table 1) and a large number of segmentectomy/subsegmentectomy cases (Table 2).

Table 1. Indications of 213 MIALR cases.

Disease	n (%)
Hepatocellular carcinoma	104 (48.4%)
Metastatic tumor	72 (33.8%)
Intrahepatic cholangiocarcinoma	16 (7.5%)
Benign liver disease	11 (5.2%)
Malignant lymphoma	3 (1.4%)
Others	7 (3.3%)

n = 213.

Table 2. Types of surgical procedure and surgical outcome.

	Case (%)	Procedure		Operation Time (min)	Blood Loss (mL)	Conversion to Open	Postoperative Complication (CD ≥ IIIa)	Postoperative Hospital Stay (Day)
Hr3	1 (0.5%)	Left trisectionectomy	1 (0.5%)	354	188	0 (0%)	1 (100%)	47
Hr2	40 (19.4%)	Left hepatectomy	20 (9.4%)	353 (216–540)	210 (15–2737)	0 (0%)	1 (5.0%)	8 (5–15)
		Right hepatectomy	14 (6.6%)	448 (305–798)	118 (10–925)	0 (0%)	1 (7.1%)	11.5 (6–53)
		Central bisectionectomy	6 (2.8%)	372 (281–542)	646 (80–1241)	0 (0%)	1 (16.7%)	13.5 (6–142)
Hr1	60 (27.8%)	Right anterior sectionectomy	20 (9.4%)	389 (214–552)	429 (47–1881)	0 (0%)	4 (20.0%)	11 (6–90)
		Right posterior sectionectomy	19 (8.9%)	405 (304–639)	456 (5–1523)	1 (5.3%)	0 (0%)	11 (5–21)
		Left medial sectionectomy	15 (7.0%)	331 (215–420)	190 (5–867)	0 (0%)	0 (0%)	9 (6–97)
		Left lateral sectionectomy	6 (2.8%)	267 (149–439)	293 (35–2367)	0 (0%)	1 (16.7%)	9 (5–15)
HrS	112 (54.4%)	Segmentectomy	88 (41.3%)	338 (110–850)	193 (10–5600)	0 (0%)	10 (11.4%)	9 (5–251)
HrSS		Subsegmentectomy	24 (11.3%)	335 (163–585)	173 (25–710)	0 (0%)	2 (8.3%)	8 (6–76)

The main points of our laparoscopic anatomical liver resections are as follows: (1) preoperative 3D simulation imaging based on the cone unit theory and intraoperative 3D monitoring, and (2) an intraoperative Glissonean approach to secure the target Glisson and dissection of the liver parenchyma along the intersegmental plane using indocyanine green (ICG) negative staining. The details of our surgical technique are presented below.

3.1. Preoperative 3D Simulation Imaging and Intraoperative 3D Monitor

In all cases, 3D simulation images were constructed based on the preoperative dynamic computed tomography (CT) data (Zaiostation2, Ziosoft Co., Tokyo, Japan). Deciding which Glisson should be divided and which should be preserved is crucial to this technique. Based on the division/preservation, a hepatic dissection plane can be constructed, and a surgical outline can be created (Figure 1a–c). Intraoperatively, a 3D monitor (Atrena, Amin Co., Tokyo, Japan) was routinely used to project preoperative 3D simulation images. The advantage of using the Atrena intraoperatively is that the actual Glissonean branching can be compared with the simulated 3D images. In addition, 3D information regarding the distance or direction from the hepatic hilum can be used to accurately identify tumor-bearing Glissonean pedicles. The Atrena can be operated on a touch panel in a clean surgical field; therefore, Glissonean branching can be assessed and discussed in real time (Figure 1d). In our study, the error rate between the predicted liver resection volume calculated using the preoperative simulation and the actual resection volume was within 10% in more than 80% of all cases. Thus, we believe that creating a preoperative 3D simulation is useful for a safe and precise laparoscopic liver resection.

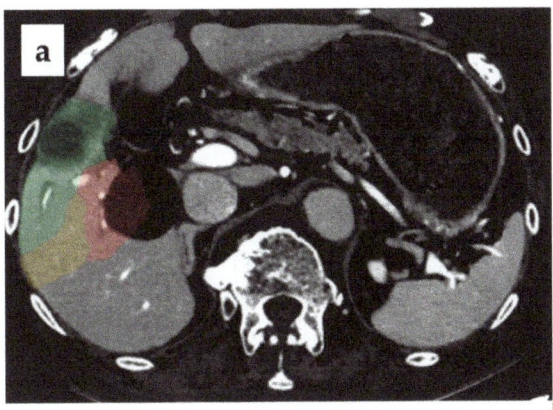
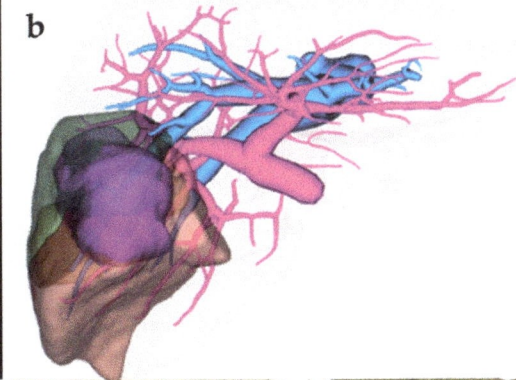

	Volume (cc)	%
Total liver	1422	100.0
S5-1 (red)	135	9.5
S5-2 (yellow)	28	2.0
S5-3 (green)	82	5.7
Residual liver	1184	82.8

Figure 1. Preoperative 3D simulation (S5 segmentectomy) and intraoperative 3D monitor. (**a**) Segment5 in this case consists of three cone units. (**b**) 3D-constructed image. (**c**) Liver volume calculation per cone unit. (**d**) 3D glasses were used during surgery, and simulated images were projected on a 3D monitor (center).

3.2. Liver Parenchyma Dissection with the Glissonean Approach and ICG Negative Staining

In our laparoscopic anatomical liver resections, the Glissonean approach was used to identify carcinoma-bearing Glissonean tumors by sequentially following them from the primary Glissonean branch to the periphery [26,27]. The target Glissonean pedicle was blocked with a bulldog clamp and ICG staining was performed using a basic technique [28,29]. The standard intravenous dose administration of ICG is 0.5 mg/body. When observed with an ICG camera (1688 AIM 4 K camera system, Stryker), a clear ICG demarcation between the fluorescent (preserved liver) and nonfluorescent (resected liver) areas appeared on the liver surface. Importantly, this ICG demarcation line was identified not only on the liver surface but also within the liver parenchyma, which is the dissecting plane of an anatomical liver resection IP. We believe that the risk of postoperative bile leakage is low if anatomical hepatic resection is performed along the correct IP because there are no transverse Glissonean sheaths across the IPs. Figures 2–4 show intraoperative images of left hepatectomy, posterior sectionectomy, and S3 subsegmentectomy.

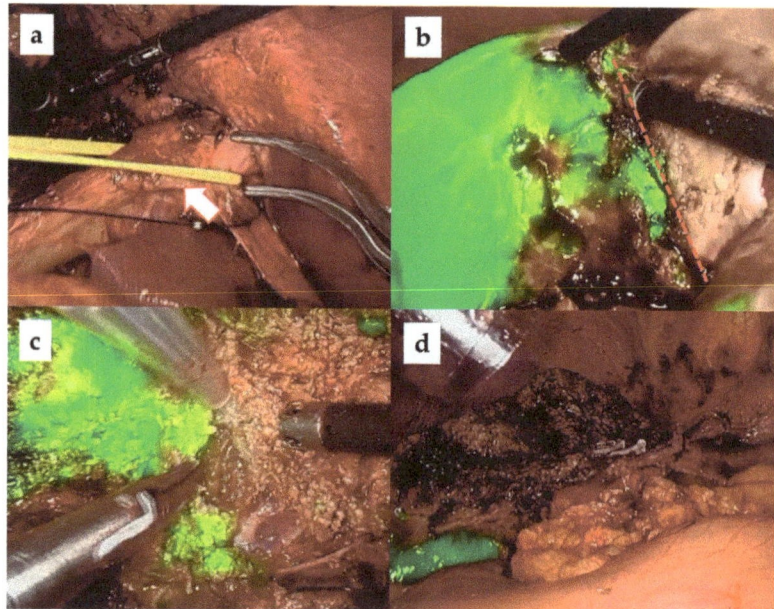

Figure 2. Laparoscopic left hepatectomy with ICG negative staining. (**a**) Securing and blocking the main trunk of the left branch of Glisson (arrow). (**b**) ICG demarcation line is observed in the center of the gallbladder bed (dotted line). (**c**) Liver parenchymal dissection along the intersegmental plane. (**d**) Liver cut surface.

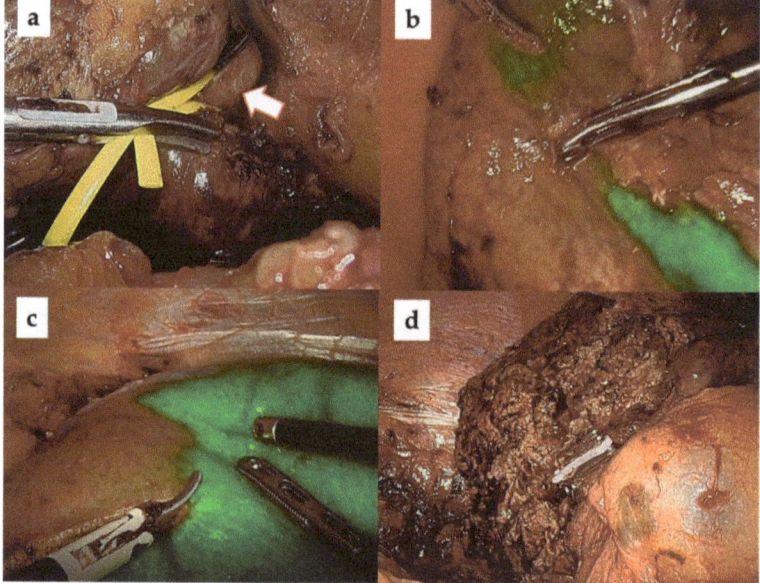

Figure 3. Laparoscopic right posterior sectionectomy with ICG negative staining. (**a**) Securing the main trunk of the right posterior branch of Glisson (arrow). (**b**) ICG demarcation line (dorsal). (**c**) ICG demarcation line (ventral). (**d**) Liver cut surface.

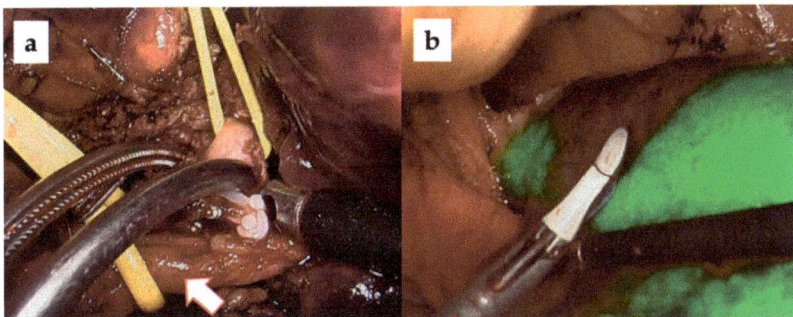

Figure 4. Laparoscopic subsegmentectomy (S3) with ICG negative staining (**a**) Securing and blocking the one of the branches of G3 (arrow: main trunk of G3). (**b**) ICG demarcation of subsegmentectomy of S3 (cone unit resection).

Robot-assisted hepatectomy has been covered by health insurance in Japan since April 2022. We performed robot-assisted hepatectomy using the same concepts as laparoscopic hepatectomy, namely, the Glissonean approach and ICG negative staining. We have performed 21 cases of robot-assisted liver resection as of March 2023. The multiarticulation unique to robotic surgery overcomes the limitations of the movement of surgical instruments restricted by laparoscopic ports. The articulation of robotic surgery facilitates the approach to vessels such as the Glisson and hepatic veins from any angle, which is a major advantage over laparoscopic surgery.

4. Discussion

One of the most significant technical differences between open and laparoscopic surgery is the angle of the surgical field of view; open surgery provides a cranial view, whereas laparoscopy provides a caudal view [30]. The hepatic-vein-guided approach (HVGA), a standard technique in open anatomical liver resections, is a vein-guided dissection of the liver parenchyma from the main hepatic vein to the periphery, which is a reasonable technique for open surgery in the cranial view. On the other hand, laparoscopic surgery, which provides a caudal view, is more suitable for the approach from the hepatic hilum as compared to open surgery. Therefore, the Glissonean approach (GA), which secures the Glissonean pedicles from the hepatic hilum, is a suitable surgical technique that takes advantage of laparoscopic surgery. Importantly, the HVGA and GA are not conflicting surgical approaches. The HVGA also plays an important role in MIALR by preventing disorientation during the liver parenchymal dissection, which is considered a pitfall of MIALR. Using the HVGA during MIALR has been advocated for by the PAM consensus/TOKYO 2020, and it is recommended that the tip of the device should be moved from the root to the periphery to prevent split bleeding [13]. Importantly, anatomical liver resection is not performed along the hepatic vein, but along the portal-vein-dominated area, based on Couinaud's definition. Therefore, exposing the major hepatic vein is not in itself the goal of anatomical liver resection, but is one of the techniques for safe liver resections. In our MIALR using the Glissonean approach and ICG negative staining, the dissection plane of the liver cut surface was not always flat, and the major hepatic vein was often not fully exposed.

At the PAM consensus meeting, visualization of the portal-dominant region using ICG during MIALR was recommended. However, whether negative or positive staining (PS) is the better technique for MIALR is a topic for future studies. In 2008, Aoki et al. reported the usefulness of positive staining in open anatomical liver resection [31]. In 2021, Felli et al. published a review paper on positive or negative staining, concluding that further case reports needed to be accumulated under standardized surgical conditions, including the dose and injection speed of ICG or observation devices. From our experience, PS seems to have greater technical difficulty and instability, but this may be due to a technical bias. The indications for PS and NS may differ depending on the tumor site, type of liver resection, and other factors. Subsegmentectomy for segment5, far from the hepatic hilum, may be a good indication for PS, whereas segmentectomy for segment7—in which it is technically difficult to puncture the target Glissons from the body surface and close to the hepatic hilum—may be a good indication for NS. The superiority of PS over NS is an important topic for future research.

The validity of anatomical hepatectomy for HCC has been widely reported, but is currently controversial for CRLM [32–34]. As shown in the results, we often performed anatomical resections for CRLMs. Anatomical hepatectomy for CRLM may seem contrary to the concept of parenchyma-sparing surgeries. However, in some cases, we believe that liver parenchymal preservation and anatomical hepatectomy are compatible with the selection of Glissons after the third bifurcation of Couinaud, which is defined as a subsegmentectomy in the Tokyo 2020 terminology. Hepatic parenchymal dissection along the cone unit should theoretically have no Glisson's transection and may be an ideal hepatic resection. We are in the process of accumulating cases of anatomic liver resection for CRLM for further reports.

There is a technical learning curve for liver resection using the Glissonean approach and ICG-NS. We believe that the key to safely overcoming the learning curve is the standardization of surgical procedures. When adopting these techniques for liver resection, standardization plays an important role in sharing surgical strategies with the surgical team. The main points of our standardized procedure are as follows: (1) Construct a preoperative 3D simulation image based on the concept of cone units. (2) Use an intraoperative 3D monitor. (3) Essentially, adapt the same patient position, port placement, and surgical instruments. (4) Encircle the responsible Glissonean pedicles using the GA. (5) Tape and clamp the target Glissonean pedicles. (6) Conduct intraoperative US with perflubutane to check if simulated ischemic boundaries can be observed in the liver parenchyma. (7) Carry out ICG NS (always 0.5 mg/body iv). (8) Perform liver parenchyma transection along the intersegmental plane. (9) Use antiadhesion agents in preparation for repeat hepatectomy.

The technological evolution of minimally invasive surgery has brought about a new phase in liver resection, namely, the widespread use of robotic-assisted hepatectomies. The articulating capabilities of robotic surgery are very useful for the dissection of dorsal aspects, such as the Glisson and hepatic veins. Moreover, the double-console system, which allows for a one-click changeover of surgeons from trainees to proctors, helps trainees to train in robotic surgery efficiently and safely. However, for hepatic parenchymal resection, we look forward to further improvements in the performance of ICG cameras and surgical devices for robotic-assisted hepatectomy. Currently, ICG cameras for robotic surgery do not have an overlay feature, which makes the background appear darker during anatomical liver resection. We believe that robotic-assisted anatomical liver resections with the GA and ICG-NS can be performed more safely as the scope of ICG and the devices in robotic surgery improve.

5. Conclusions

Intraoperative ICG staining plays a central role in MIALR. MIALR with the Glissonean approach and ICG negative staining, which is our standard technique, is a useful technique using ICG.

Author Contributions: Conceptualization, G.W.; formal analysis, Y.F.; data curation, T.W., M.A.A.-O., M.C. and K.M.; writing—original draft preparation, Y.F.; supervision, G.W. All authors have read and agreed to the published version of the manuscript.

Funding: This research received no external funding.

Institutional Review Board Statement: The study was conducted in accordance with the Declaration of Helsinki, and approved by the Institutional Review Board of ageo central general hospital (Approval No.965).

Informed Consent Statement: Informed consent was obtained from all patients involved in the study.

Data Availability Statement: Data available on request due to restrictions eg privacy or ethical.

Acknowledgments: The authors would like to thank Kazuma Nakanishi (radiological technologist) for the technical assistance.

Conflicts of Interest: The authors declare no conflict of interest.

References

1. Morise, Z. Current status of minimally invasive liver surgery for cancers. *World J. Gastroenterol.* **2022**, *28*, 6090–6098. [CrossRef] [PubMed]
2. Ciria, R.; Berardi, G.; Alconchel, F.; Briceño, J.; Choi, G.H.; Wu, Y.; Sugioka, A.; Troisi, R.I.; Salloum, C.; Soubrane, O.; et al. The impact of robotics in liver surgery: A worldwide systematic review and short-term outcomes meta-analysis on 2728 cases. *J. Hepato-Biliary-Pancreat. Sci.* **2020**, *29*, 181–197. [CrossRef] [PubMed]
3. Wakabayashi, G.; Tanabe, M. ILLS 2019 and the development of laparoscopic liver resection in Japan. *J. Hepato-Biliary-Pancreat. Sci.* **2019**, *27*, 1–2. [CrossRef]
4. Wakabayashi, G.; Kaneko, H. Can major laparoscopic liver and pancreas surgery become standard practices? *J. Hepato-Biliary-Pancreat. Sci.* **2016**, *23*, 89–91. [CrossRef] [PubMed]
5. Kaneko, H.; Otsuka, Y.; Kubota, Y.; Wakabayashi, G. Evolution and revolution of laparoscopic liver resection in Japan. *Ann. Gastroenterol. Surg.* **2017**, *1*, 33–43. [CrossRef]
6. Buell, J.F.; Cherqui, D.; Geller, D.A.; O'Rourke, N.; Iannitti, D.; Dagher, I.; Koffron, A.J.; Thomas, M.; Gayet, B.; Han, H.S.; et al. The International Position on Laparoscopic Liver Surgery: The Louisville Statement, 2008. *Ann. Surg.* **2009**, *250*, 825–830. [CrossRef] [PubMed]
7. Wakabayashi, G.; Cherqui, D.; Geller, D.A.; Buell, J.F.; Kaneko, H.; Han, H.S.; Asbun, H.; O'rourke, N.; Tanabe, M.; Koffron, A.J.; et al. Recommendations for laparoscopic liver resection: A report from the second international consensus conference held in Morioka. *Ann. Surg.* **2015**, *261*, 619–629. [CrossRef]
8. Abu Hilal, M.; Aldrighetti, L.; Dagher, I.; Edwin, B.; Troisi, R.I.; Alikhanov, R.; Aroori, S.; Belli, G.; Besselink, M.; Briceno, J.; et al. The Southampton Consensus Guidelines for Laparoscopic Liver Surgery: From indication to implementation. *Ann. Surg.* **2018**, *268*, 11–18. [CrossRef]
9. Morimoto, M.; Monden, K.; Wakabayashi, T.; Gotohda, N.; Abe, Y.; Honda, G.; Abu Hilal, M.; Aoki, T.; Asbun, H.J.; Berardi, G.; et al. Minimally invasive anatomic liver resection: Results of a survey of world experts. *J. Hepato-Biliary-Pancreat. Sci.* **2021**, *29*, 33–40. [CrossRef]
10. Sugioka, A.; Kato, Y.; Tanahashi, Y. Systematic extrahepatic Glissonean pedicle isolation for anatomical liver resection based on Laennec's capsule: Proposal of a novel comprehensive surgical anatomy of the liver. *J. Hepato-Biliary-Pancreat. Sci.* **2017**, *24*, 17–23. [CrossRef]
11. Felli, E.; Ishizawa, T.; Cherkaoui, Z.; Diana, M.; Tripon, S.; Baumert, T.F.; Schuster, C.; Pessaux, P. Laparoscopic anatomical liver resection for malignancies using positive or negative staining technique with intraoperative indocyanine green-fluorescence imaging. *HPB* **2021**, *23*, 1647–1655. [CrossRef]
12. Ciria, R.; Berardi, G.; Nishino, H.; Chan, A.C.; Chanwat, R.; Chen, K.; Chen, Y.; Cheung, T.T.; Fuks, D.; Geller, D.A.; et al. A snapshot of the 2020 conception of anatomic liver resections and their applicability on minimally invasive liver surgery. A preparatory survey for the Expert Consensus Meeting on Precision Anatomy for Minimally Invasive HBP Surgery. *J. Hepato-Biliary-Pancreat. Sci.* **2021**, *29*, 41–50. [CrossRef]
13. Gotohda, N.; Cherqui, D.; Geller, D.A.; Abu Hilal, M.; Berardi, G.; Ciria, R.; Abe, Y.; Aoki, T.; Asbun, H.J.; Chan, A.C.Y.; et al. Expert Consensus Guidelines: How to safely perform minimally invasive anatomic liver resection. *J. Hepato-Biliary-Pancreat. Sci.* **2021**, *29*, 16–32. [CrossRef] [PubMed]
14. Nagakawa, Y.; Nakata, K.; Nishino, H.; Ohtsuka, T.; Ban, D.; Asbun, H.J.; Boggi, U.; He, J.; Kendrick, M.L.; Palanivelu, C.; et al. International expert consensus on precision anatomy for minimally invasive pancreatoduodenectomy: PAM-HBP surgery project. *J. Hepato-Biliary-Pancreat. Sci.* **2021**, *29*, 124–135. [CrossRef]
15. Wakabayashi, G.; Cherqui, D.; Geller, D.A.; Abu Hilal, M.; Berardi, G.; Ciria, R.; Abe, Y.; Aoki, T.; Asbun, H.J.; Chan, A.C.Y.; et al. The Tokyo 2020 terminology of liver anatomy and resections: Updates of the Brisbane 2000 system. *J. Hepato-Biliary-Pancreat. Sci.* **2021**, *29*, 6–15. [CrossRef] [PubMed]
16. Strasberg, S.; Belghiti, J.; Clavien, P.-A.; Gadzijev, E.; Garden, J.; Lau, W.-Y.; Makuuchi, M.; Strong, R. The Brisbane 2000 Terminology of Liver Anatomy and Resections. *HPB* **2000**, *2*, 333–339. [CrossRef]
17. Strasberg, S.M.; Phillips, C. Use and Dissemination of the Brisbane 2000 Nomenclature of Liver Anatomy and Resections. *Ann. Surg.* **2013**, *257*, 377–382. [CrossRef]
18. Strasberg, S.M. Nomenclature of hepatic anatomy and resections: A review of the Brisbane 2000 system. *J. Hepato-Biliary-Pancreat. Surg.* **2005**, *12*, 351–355. [CrossRef]

19. Morimoto, M.; Tomassini, F.; Berardi, G.; Mori, Y.; Shirata, C.; Abu Hilal, M.; Asbun, H.J.; Cherqui, D.; Gotohda, N.; Han, H.; et al. Glissonean approach for hepatic inflow control in minimally invasive anatomic liver resection: A systematic review. *J. Hepato-Biliary-Pancreat. Sci.* **2021**, *29*, 51–65. [CrossRef]
20. Monden, K.; Alconchel, F.; Berardi, G.; Ciria, R.; Akahoshi, K.; Miyasaka, Y.; Urade, T.; Vázquez, A.G.; Hasegawa, K.; Honda, G.; et al. Landmarks and techniques to perform minimally invasive liver surgery: A systematic review with a focus on hepatic outflow. *J. Hepato-Biliary-Pancreat. Sci.* **2021**, *29*, 66–81. [CrossRef]
21. Wakabayashi, T.; Cacciaguerra, A.B.; Ciria, R.; Ariizumi, S.; Durán, M.; Golse, N.; Ogiso, S.; Abe, Y.; Aoki, T.; Hatano, E.; et al. Landmarks to identify segmental borders of the liver: A review prepared for PAM-HBP expert consensus meeting 2021. *J. Hepato-Biliary-Pancreat. Sci.* **2021**, *29*, 82–98. [CrossRef]
22. Berardi, G.; Colasanti, M.; Meniconi, R.L.; Ferretti, S.; Guglielmo, N.; Mariano, G.; Burocchi, M.; Campanelli, A.; Scotti, A.; Pecoraro, A.; et al. The Applications of 3D Imaging and Indocyanine Green Dye Fluorescence in Laparoscopic Liver Surgery. *Diagnostics* **2021**, *11*, 2169. [CrossRef]
23. Mishima, K.; Wakabayashi, T.; Fujiyama, Y.; Alomari, M.; Colella, M.; Wakabayashi, G. Resection margin status in laparoscopic liver resection for colorectal liver metastases: Literature review and future perspectives. *Minerva Surg.* **2022**, *77*, 428–432. [CrossRef] [PubMed]
24. Funamizu, N.; Ozaki, T.; Mishima, K.; Igarashi, K.; Omura, K.; Takada, Y.; Wakabayashi, G. Evaluation of accuracy of laparoscopic liver mono-segmentectomy using the Glissonian approach with indocyanine green fluorescence negative staining by comparing estimated and actual resection volumes: A single-center retrospective cohort study. *J. Hepato-Biliary-Pancreat. Sci.* **2021**, *28*, 1060–1068. [CrossRef] [PubMed]
25. Mori, S.M.; Mishima, K.; Ozaki, T.; Fujiyama, Y.; Wakabayashi, G.M. Short-term Outcomes and Difficulty of Repeat Laparoscopic Liver Resection. *Ann. Surg. Open* **2022**, *3*, e191. [CrossRef]
26. Monden, K.; Sadamori, H.; Hioki, M.; Ohno, S.; Takakura, N. Intrahepatic Glissonean Approach for Laparoscopic Bisegmentectomy 7 and 8 With Root-Side Hepatic Vein Exposure. *Ann. Surg. Oncol.* **2021**, *29*, 970–971. [CrossRef]
27. Takasaki, K. Glissonean pedicle transection method for hepatic resection: A new concept of liver segmentation. *J. Hepato-Biliary-Pancreat. Surg.* **1998**, *5*, 286–291. [CrossRef]
28. Wakabayashi, T.; Cacciaguerra, A.B.; Abe, Y.; Bona, E.D.; Nicolini, D.; Mocchegiani, F.; Kabeshima, Y.; Vivarelli, M.; Wakabayashi, G.; Kitagawa, Y. Indocyanine Green Fluorescence Navigation in Liver Surgery: A Systematic Review on Dose and Timing of Administration. *Ann. Surg.* **2022**, *275*, 1025–1034. [CrossRef] [PubMed]
29. Otsuka, Y.; Matsumoto, Y.; Ito, Y.; Okada, R.; Maeda, T.; Ishii, J.; Kajiwara, Y.; Okubo, K.; Funahashi, K.; Kaneko, H. Intraoperative guidance using ICG fluorescence imaging system for safe and precise laparoscopic liver resection. *Int. J. Clin. Rev.* **2021**, *76*, 211–219. [CrossRef]
30. Wakabayashi, G.; Cherqui, D.; Geller, D.A.; Han, H.-S.; Kaneko, H.; Buell, J.F. Laparoscopic hepatectomy is theoretically better than open hepatectomy: Preparing for the 2nd International Consensus Conference on Laparoscopic Liver Resection. *J. Hepato-Biliary-Pancreat. Sci.* **2014**, *21*, 723–731. [CrossRef]
31. Aoki, T.; Yasuda, D.; Shimizu, Y.; Odaira, M.; Niiya, T.; Kusano, T.; Mitamura, K.; Hayashi, K.; Murai, N.; Koizumi, T.; et al. Image-Guided Liver Mapping Using Fluorescence Navigation System with Indocyanine Green for Anatomical Hepatic Resection. *World J. Surg.* **2008**, *32*, 1763–1767. [CrossRef] [PubMed]
32. Cucchetti, A.; Cescon, M.; Ercolani, G.; Bigonzi, E.; Torzilli, G.; Pinna, A.D. A Comprehensive Meta-regression Analysis on Outcome of Anatomic Resection Versus Nonanatomic Resection for Hepatocellular Carcinoma. *Ann. Surg. Oncol.* **2012**, *19*, 3697–3705. [CrossRef] [PubMed]
33. Kwon, J.H.; Lee, J.-W.; Lee, J.W.; Lee, Y.J. Effects of Anatomical or Non-Anatomical Resection of Hepatocellular Carcinoma on Survival Outcome. *J. Clin. Med.* **2022**, *11*, 1369. [CrossRef] [PubMed]
34. Brown, K.M.; Albania, M.F.; Samra, J.S.; Kelly, P.J.; Hugh, T.J. Propensity score analysis of non-anatomical *versus* anatomical resection of colorectal liver metastases. *BJS Open* **2019**, *3*, 521–531. [CrossRef] [PubMed]

Disclaimer/Publisher's Note: The statements, opinions and data contained in all publications are solely those of the individual author(s) and contributor(s) and not of MDPI and/or the editor(s). MDPI and/or the editor(s) disclaim responsibility for any injury to people or property resulting from any ideas, methods, instructions or products referred to in the content.

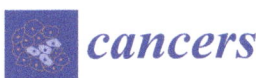

Article

Conversion of Minimally Invasive Liver Resection for HCC in Advanced Cirrhosis: Clinical Impact and Role of Difficulty Scoring Systems

Federica Cipriani [1,*], Francesca Ratti [1], Gianluca Fornoni [1], Rebecca Marino [1], Antonella Tudisco [1], Marco Catena [1] and Luca Aldrighetti [1,2]

[1] Hepatobiliary Surgery Division, IRCCS San Raffaele Scientific Institute, 20132 Milan, Italy
[2] Faculty of Medicine and Surgery, Vita-Salute San Raffaele University, 20132 Milan, Italy
* Correspondence: cipriani.federica@hsr.it

Simple Summary: It is essential to consider the specific impact that conversion can have in a context where MILR is so positively determinant, that is, hepatocellular carcinoma. It has not yet been specifically investigated what impact conversion may have in case of advanced cirrhosis, which is the central risk factor for specific postoperative complications and the context in which the loss of minimally invasive benefits can be particularly harmful. This study showed that conversion in the setting of advanced cirrhosis can be associated with non-inferior outcomes compared to compensated cirrhosis, provided careful patient selection is applied. Difficulty scoring systems may help in identifying the most appropriate candidates to maintain satisfactory outcomes, even in case of conversion, and become helpful in multidisciplinary treatment decisions.

Abstract: Background: Minimally invasive liver resections (MILRs) in cirrhosis are at risk of conversion since cirrhosis and complexity, which can be estimated by scoring systems, are both independent factors for. We aimed to investigate the consequence of conversion of MILR for hepatocellular carcinoma in advanced cirrhosis. Methods: After retrospective review, MILRs for HCC were divided into preserved liver function (Cohort-A) and advanced cirrhosis cohorts (Cohort-B). Completed and converted MILRs were compared (Compl-A vs. Conv-A and Compl-B vs. Conv-B); then, converted patients were compared (Conv-A vs. Conv-B) as whole cohorts and after stratification for MILR difficulty using Iwate criteria. Results: 637 MILRs were studied (474 Cohort-A, 163 Cohort-B). Conv-A MILRs had worse outcomes than Compl-A: more blood loss; higher incidence of transfusions, morbidity, grade 2 complications, ascites, liver failure and longer hospitalization. Conv-B MILRs exhibited the same worse perioperative outcomes than Compl-B and also higher incidence of grade 1 complications. Conv-A and Conv-B outcomes of low difficulty MILRs resulted in similar perioperative outcomes, whereas the comparison of more difficult converted MILRs (intermediate/advanced/expert) resulted in several worse perioperative outcomes for patients with advanced cirrhosis. However, Conv-A and Conv-B outcomes were not significantly different in the whole cohort where "advanced/expert" MILRs were 33.1% and 5.5% in Cohort A and B. Conclusions: Conversion in the setting of advanced cirrhosis can be associated with non-inferior outcomes compared to compensated cirrhosis, provided careful patient selection is applied (patients elected to low difficulty MILRs). Difficulty scoring systems may help in identifying the most appropriate candidates.

Keywords: laparoscopic liver resection; minimally invasive liver resection; conversion; cirrhosis; Child B; portal hypertension; difficulty score

Citation: Cipriani, F.; Ratti, F.; Fornoni, G.; Marino, R.; Tudisco, A.; Catena, M.; Aldrighetti, L. Conversion of Minimally Invasive Liver Resection for HCC in Advanced Cirrhosis: Clinical Impact and Role of Difficulty Scoring Systems. *Cancers* **2023**, *15*, 1432. https://doi.org/10.3390/cancers15051432

Academic Editor: Hiromitsu Hayashi

Received: 9 January 2023
Revised: 13 February 2023
Accepted: 22 February 2023
Published: 23 February 2023

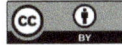

Copyright: © 2023 by the authors. Licensee MDPI, Basel, Switzerland. This article is an open access article distributed under the terms and conditions of the Creative Commons Attribution (CC BY) license (https://creativecommons.org/licenses/by/4.0/).

1. Introduction

Minimally invasive liver resections (MILRs) have seen a considerable diffusion as an alternative to the traditional open approach thanks to the evidence of positive effects, currently well known, for the postoperative course [1–5]. Since its onset, MILRs have been shown to be particularly beneficial for patients affected by hepatocellular carcinoma (HCC), being specifically associated with reduced postoperative ascites and hepatic insufficiency [6–13].

When approaching liver resection with minimally invasive techniques, it is known that conversion to laparotomy may be necessary to complete the operation safely [14–16]. Although this event should not necessarily be considered a complication or failure, it is well known that conversion actually has a non-negligible impact on results, being associated with inferior perioperative outcomes compared to both successfully completed MILRs and upfront open resections [17–21]. Consequently, it is recognized—and should be expected—that converted resections may at least lose some of the benefits of adopting a minimally invasive approach [22–25]. Therefore, it is essential to take into account the specific impact that conversion can have in a context where MILR is so positively determinant, that is, HCC.

It should also be considered that MILRs in cirrhosis are among the most complex minimally invasive liver surgeries and simultaneously exposed to a significant possibility of conversion given the reported role of cirrhosis as an independent factor for both conversion and MILR difficulty [26,27]. Furthermore, the MILR complexity itself should be considered a predisposing factor for conversion, which can be reliably estimated by existing complexity scoring systems [26,28].

Given the current trends to increasingly implement MILRs in cirrhosis and to consider minimally invasiveness as a potential means for an extension of HCC resective indications, the aim of this study was to investigate the consequence of conversion in the specific setting of advanced cirrhosis. In fact, it has not yet been investigated what impact conversion may have in the case of advanced cirrhosis, which represents the central risk factor for specific postoperative complications and the context in which the loss of minimally invasive benefits can be particularly harmful. The hypothesis was that advanced cirrhosis could adversely affect perioperative outcomes in case of conversion, with even inferior results compared to patients with compensated chronic liver disease. The ultimate purpose is to add useful knowledge helpful in the refinement of indications to resection for HCC and in line with technical and technological development, which is presently an ongoing process.

2. Materials and Methods

2.1. Study Design

Data of consecutive patients undergoing MILR at a single hepatobiliary center (January 2005–August 2022) were retrospectively reviewed for the purpose of this case series study. Patients affected by histologically proven HCC undergoing MILR were selected.

The study design is depicted in Figure 1.

Patients were separated into two cohorts according to the severity of chronic liver disease: cohort A including patients with preserved liver function (i.e., Child A without portal hypertension) and cohort B including patients with advanced liver disease (i.e., Child B/C cirrhosis or any Child stage associated with clinically significant portal hypertension defined as gastroesophageal varices on endoscopy or platelet count $< 100 \times 10^9/L$ in the presence of splenomegaly > 120 mm) [29,30].

Each cohort was further classified into a "minimally invasive completed" or "converted" group based on the occurrence of conversion to open during MILR. The two groups of converted patients (named Conv-A and Conv-B) were compared with minimally invasive completed patients (named Compl-A and Compl-B groups). To further enhance the analysis, liver resections were stratified in classes of increasing complexity using the Iwate criteria, a difficulty multiparametric scoring system specifically produced for MILR and already validated as the most reliable tool among difficulty scoring systems to predict conversion risk for HCC. Indeed, Lin and colleagues recently reported that, among existing difficulty scoring systems for MILR, only the Iwate criteria were able to predict conversion to laparotomy in the specific setting of HCC [26,28].

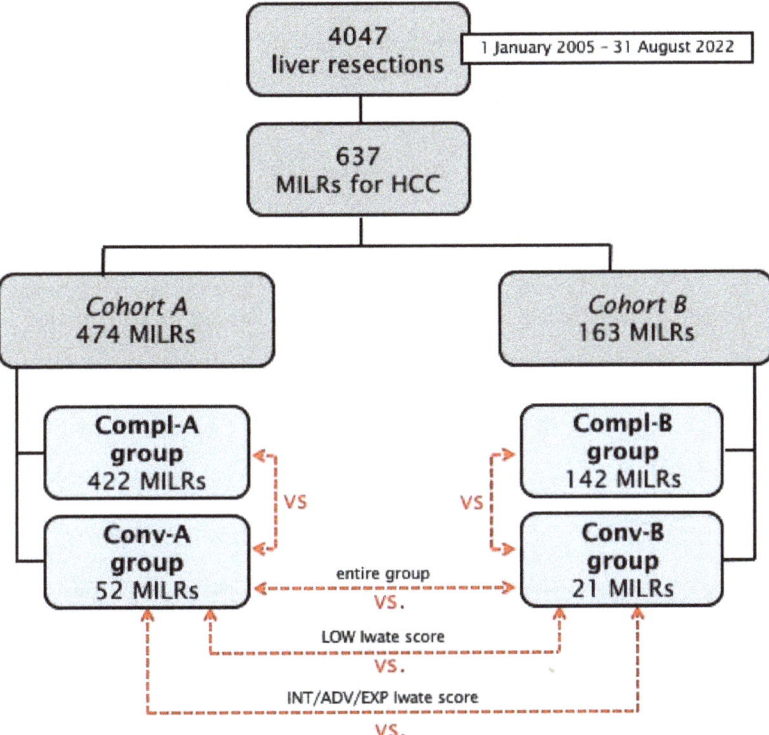

Figure 1. The study design. HCC stands for hepatocellular carcinoma. MILR stands for minimally invasive liver resection.

The analysis followed a three-step process:
1. Minimally invasive completed and converted patients in each cohort were compared (Compl-A vs. Conv-A and Compl-B vs. Conv-B) so as to test in our series the loss of advantage of conversion for any severity of chronic liver disease separately.
2. Converted patients of each cohort were compared (Conv-A vs. Conv-B) to test for differences in outcomes for converted patients with their severity of chronic liver disease.
3. Converted patients of each cohort were compared (Conv-A vs. Conv-B) selectively for low Iwate difficulty level and intermediate/expert/advanced Iwate difficulty level to test for differences in outcomes for converted patients with their severity of chronic liver disease in different settings of MILR complexity.

2.2. Outcome Measures

Data regarding the characteristics of patients, disease and perioperative course were collected. The analyzed baseline features included demographics, MELD score, ASA score, Charlson Comorbidity Index, background liver status, portal hypertension, baseline liver function, number of lesions, size of largest lesion (cm) and extent of resection.

Perioperative parameters were registered: operative time (minutes), estimated blood loss (mL), red blood cells and fresh frozen plasma transfusions, Pringle maneuver, completeness of resection (R0), conversion to open and reasons, mortality and both general and liver-specific morbidity, post-discharge readmission and length of stay (days).

2.3. Indications, Surgical Technique and Perioperative Management

The standard assessment of HCC patients included clinical examination and laboratory (liver function, serum tumor markers), endoscopic (esophagogastroduodenoscopy) and radiological tests (abdominal ultrasonography, thoracoabdominal contrast enhanced imaging) to assess liver function according to Child–Pugh score, signs of portal hypertension and tumor characteristics and staging. For all patients deemed eligible to liver resection, the treatment strategy was systematically evaluated at weekly multidisciplinary hepatobiliary meetings (inclusive of hepatobiliary surgeon, hepatologist and medical oncologist opinions) in order to validate the indication to surgery and technique.

Pure laparoscopic or robotic procedures were attempted in all patients, and no hybrid techniques were used. Our technique for MILR has been previously described [1,31–34]. Conversions were all performed directly to laparotomy, i.e., the standard, so as to protect the patient from complications related to late/emergency conversions [35].

Patients were managed with a perioperative fast-track protocol to enhance functional recovery. Functional recovery was considered achieved when all following criteria were met: adequate pain control with oral analgesics; independently mobile; tolerance of solid food; normal or improving blood tests; and no intravenous fluids. Patients are considered for discharge when both the functional recovery and patient's agreement are obtained. A specific analgesic and store red blood cells protocol is followed for pain management [36–38].

2.4. Definitions

Type of liver resections were classified according to the Brisbane 2000 Terminology of Liver Anatomy and Resections [39]. Postoperative morbidity, mortality and readmission were reviewed at 90 days after surgery and complications were graded according to the Clavien–Dindo classification of postoperative complications [40]. Liver-specific complications were liver failure (liver failure as an increased international normalized ratio and concomitant hyperbilirubinemia on or after postoperative day 5 [41]); ascitic decompensation (abdominal drainage above 10 mL/kg body weight/day after postoperative day 3 [42]); biliary leakage (bilirubin concentration in the drainage above three-fold of serum total bilirubin on or after pod 3) or the need for radiologic or operative intervention from a biliary collection or bile peritonitis [43].

2.5. Statistics

Data were expressed as median (with interquartile ranges) for continuous variables as their distribution was skewed (Shapiro-Wilk Test); categorical variables were expressed as absolute values and proportions. Continuous variables were compared using the nonparametric Mann–Whitney test; categorical variables were compared through the Fisher's exact or chi-square test. Statistical significance was set at $p < 0.05$. All analyses were performed using the statistical package SPSS 22.0 (SPSS, Chicago, IL, USA).

The work has been approved by the institutional Ethical Committee.

3. Results

The study population consisted of 637 MILRs for HCC (selected from a global pool of 4047 liver resections), divided into 474 pertaining to Cohort A and 163 to Cohort B (Figure 1).

The baseline characteristics of patients and operations included in Cohort A and B are depicted in Table 1.

Table 1. Baselines of MILRs for HCC in Child A and in advanced cirrhosis (Child B and Child A/B with portal hypertension) patients.

	Cohort A n = 474	Cohort B n = 163	p Value
Age, years	71 ± 5	73 ± 6	0.612
Gender [M/F], n (%)	208/266 (43.9/56.1%)	83/80 (50.9/49.1%)	0.845
MELD score, points	7	8	0.324
ASA score [1–2/3–4], n (%)	279/195 (58.8/41.2%)	79/84 (48.5/51.5%)	0.292
Charlson Comorbidity Index, points	9	12	0.478
Etiology of chronic liver disease, n (%)			0.658
Viral	73 (15.4%)	30 (18.4%)	
Alcoholic	106 (22.4%)	36 (22.1%)	
Metabolic	183 (38.6%)	41 (25.1%)	
Other/unknown	112 (23.6%)	56 (34.3%)	
Liver parenchyma, n (%)			0.020
Mild fibrosis (F0-1)	241 (50.8%)	65 (39.9%)	
Significant fibrosis (F2)	114 (24.0%)	49 (30.1%)	
Severe fibrosis (F3)	66 (13.9%)	37 (22.7%)	
Cirrhosis (F4)	53 (11.2%)	10 (6.1%)	
Tumor size, mm	51 ± 29	30 ± 11	0.031
Number of tumors [single/multiple], n (%)	350/124 (73.8/26.2%)	127/36 (77.9/22.1%)	0.541
Tumor location [anterolateral/posterosuperior], n (%)	262/212 (55.3/44.7%)	102/61 (62.6/37.4%)	0.040
Varices	0	61 (37.4%)	0.002
Ascites	0	22 (13.5%)	0.001
Platelet count < 80×10^9/L	0	67 (41.1%)	0.002
Previous liver resection, n (%)	75 (15.8%)	19 (11.6%)	0.429
Operation type			0.037
Wedge resection	94 (19.8%)	84 (51.5%)	
Anatomical segmentectomy	147 (31.0%)	32 (19.6%)	
Left lateral sectionectomy	64 (11.4%)	12 (7.4%)	
Hemihepatectomy	132 (27.8%)	27 (16.6%)	
Sectionectomy and other resection	37 (7.8%)	8 (4.9%)	
Iwate difficulty level			0.025
Low	152 (32.1%)	96 (58.9%)	
Intermediate	165 (34.8%)	58 (35.6%)	
Advanced/Expert	104/53 (21.9/11.2%)	9/0 (5.5/0%)	

There were no statistically significant differences in terms of age, gender, ASA score, Charlson Comorbidity Index, etiology of liver disease, MELD score, number of tumors and history of previous liver resection. Groups were well balanced between the approaches in terms of comorbidities, features of the liver parenchyma, etiology of liver disease and previous liver resection. Between Cohort A and B, the following parameters recorded a statistically significant difference: proportion of histological type of chronic liver disease, tumor locations, presence of varices, ascites or thrombocytopenia, tumor size, operation type and Iwate difficulty level. In particular, the proportion of MILRs classified as of "advanced/expert" difficulty was 33.1% in Cohort A and 5.5% in Cohort B (p = 0.025). Notably, there was no statistically significant difference in the median MELD score for both groups despite being higher in Cohort B; moreover, both groups were within 9 points, which is a value associated with acceptable risk liver surgery in terms of perioperative morbidity and mortality [44].

Cohort A resections were further classified into 422 Compl-A and 52 Conv-A (10.9% conversion rate) and Cohort B resections into 142 Compl-B and 21 Conv-B (12.9% conversion rate) (Figure 1). The cumulative conversion rate resulted in 11.4% (n = 73), and reasons of conversion had a comparable incidence among the two cohorts: the most frequent reason in both was bleeding or unsatisfactory hemostasis (40.4% and 52.4% of conversions, p = 0.475) followed by any concern of oncologic inadequacy (compromised margins or any doubt on radical resection), difficult adhesiolysis, unsatisfactory biliostasis and anesthesiological problems (Table 2).

Table 2. Conversions and reasons in MILRs for HCC in Child A and in advanced cirrhosis (Child B and Child A/B with portal hypertension) patients.

	Conv-A n = 52	Conv-B n = 21	p Value
Bleeding or unsatisfactory hemostasis, n (%)	21 (40.4)	11 (52.4)	0.475
Difficult adhesiolysis, n (%)	5 (9.6)	2 (9.5)	0.881
Concern of oncologic inadequacy, n (%)	20 (38.5)	6 (28.6)	0.639
Unsatisfactory Bili stasis, n (%)	4 (7.7)	1 (4.8)	0.129
Anesthesiological problems, n (%)	2 (3.8)	1 (4.8)	0.292

3.1. MILR in Patients with Preserved Liver Function: Completed versus Converted

Conv-A showed higher amount of blood loss (400 vs. 100 mL, $p = 0.009$) and incidence of fresh frozen plasma transfusions (21.1% vs. 3.3%, $p = 0.004$) than Compl-A. Moreover, global morbidity (23.1% vs. 11.8%, $p = 0.018$), grade 2 complications (13.4% vs. 6.4%, $p = 0.016$), ascites (17.3% vs. 5.0%, $p = 0.004$), postoperative liver failure (9.6% vs. 2.4%, $p = 0.018$) and pleural effusion (7.7% vs. 2.8%, $p = 0.015$) were more frequent in Conv-A group, as well as length of stay being longer (7 vs. 5 days, $p = 0.007$) and the readmission rate higher (7.7% vs. 1.9%, $p = 0.036$).

The rest of the parameters demonstrated nonsignificant differences (Table 3).

Table 3. Results of completed versus converted MILRs for HCC in Child A patients without portal hypertension.

	Compl-A n = 422	Conv-A n = 52	p Value
Operative time, minutes	210 (155–260)	190 (155–245)	0.488
Blood loss, mL	100 (50–160)	400 (150–570)	0.009
Red blood cell transfusion, n (%)	21 (4.9%)	3 (5.7%)	0.716
Fresh frozen plasma transfusion, n (%)	14 (3.3%)	11 (21.1%)	0.004
R0, n (%)	413 (97.8%)	50 (96.1%)	0.542
Use of Pringle maneuver, n (%)	358 (84.8%)	46 (88.5%)	0.671
Duration of Pringle maneuver, minutes	30 ± 20	40 ± 20	0.499
Total morbidity, n (%)	50 (11.8%)	12 (23.1%)	0.018
Grade 1	5 (1.2%)	2 (3.8%)	0.409
Grade 2	27 (6.4%)	7 (13.4%)	0.016
Grade 3	22 (5.2%)	3 (5.8%)	0.638
Grade 4	0	0	NC
Grade 5	0	0	NC
90-days mortality, n (%)	0	0	NC
Bleeding	8 (1.9%)	2 (3.8%)	0.841
Bile leak	17 (4.0%)	3 (5.7%)	0.778
Ascites	21 (5.0%)	9 (17.3%)	0.004
Postoperative liver failure	10 (2.4%)	5 (9.6%)	0.018
Collection	10 (2.4%)	2 (3.8%)	0.183
Chest infection	5 (1.2%)	1 (1.9%)	0.205
Pleural effusion	12 (2.8%)	4 (7.7%)	0.015
Length of stay, days	5 (3–6)	7 (5–10)	0.007
Readmissions, n (%)	8 (1.9%)	4 (7.7%)	0.036

NC: Not calculated.

3.2. MILR in Patients with Advanced Chronic Liver Disease: Completed versus Converted

As with cohort B, the parameters associated with a statistically significant difference in cohort A showed less favorable results for converted than completed MILRs: amount of blood loss (550 vs. 250 mL, $p = 0.007$), fresh frozen plasma transfusions (28.6% vs. 6.3%, $p = 0.003$), global morbidity (28.6% vs. 12.7%, $p = 0.002$), grade 2 complications (14.3% vs. 7.0%, $p = 0.021$), ascites (19.0% vs. 4.9%, $p = 0.008$), postoperative liver failure (9.5% vs. 2.8%, $p = 0.034$), pleural effusion (9.5% vs. 4.2%, $p = 0.039$), length of stay (8 vs. 5 days, $p = 0.005$) and readmission rate (9.5% vs. 3.5%, $p = 0.024$). In addition, Conv-B also showed a higher incidence of grade 1 complications (14.3% vs. 4.2%, $p = 0.032$).

The rest of the parameters demonstrated nonsignificant differences (Table 4).

Table 4. Results of completed versus converted MILRs for HCC in advanced cirrhosis patients (Child B and Child A/B with portal hypertension).

	Compl-B n = 142	Conv-B n = 21	p Value
Operative time, minutes	200 (160–280)	230 (180–290)	0.746
Blood loss, mL	250 (280–360)	550 (370–700)	0.007
Red blood cell transfusion, n (%)	5 (3.5%)	1 (4.7%)	0.655
Fresh frozen plasma transfusion, n (%)	9 (6.3%)	6 (28.6%)	0.003
R0, n (%)	138 (97.2%)	20 (95.2%)	0.903
Use of Pringle maneuver, n (%)	108 (76.0%)	17 (80.9%)	0.549
Duration of Pringle maneuver, minutes	35 ± 10	30 ± 15	0.336
Total morbidity, n (%)	18 (12.7%)	6 (28.6%)	0.002
Grade 1	6 (4.2%)	3 (14.3%)	0.032
Grade 2	10 (7.0%)	3 (14.3%)	0.021
Grade 3	2 (1.4%)	0	0199
Grade 4	0	0	NC
Grade 5	0	0	NC
90-days mortality, n (%)	0	0	NC
Bleeding	5 (3.5%)	1 (4.7%)	0.971
Bile leak	6 (4.2%)	1 (4.7%)	0.843
Ascites	7 (4.9%)	4 (19.0%)	0.008
Postoperative liver failure	4 (2.8%)	2 (9.5%)	0.034
Collection	3 (2.1%)	1 (4.8%)	0.437
Chest infection	2 (1.4%)	0	0.588
Pleural effusion	6 (4.2%)	2 (9.5%)	0.039
Length of stay, days	5 (3–7)	8 (4–10)	0.005
Readmissions, n (%)	5 (3.5%)	2 (9.5%)	0.024

NC: Not calculated.

3.3. Converted MILR: Patients with Preserved Liver Function versus Patients with Advanced Chronic Liver Disease (Whole Cohorts)

Conv-A and Conv-B groups showed similar perioperative outcomes as a statistically significant difference was recorded only for Grade 1 complications, which were higher for Conv-B patients (14.3% vs. 3.8%, $p = 0.030$). Indeed, all the other parameters showed comparable results between the two groups (Table 5).

Table 5. Results of converted MILRs for HCC: Child A versus converted MILRs in advanced cirrhosis (Child B and Child A/B with portal hypertension) patients.

	Conv-A n = 52	Conv-B n = 21	p Value
Operative time, minutes	190 (155–245)	230 (180–290)	0.574
Blood loss, mL	400 (150–570)	550 (370–700)	0.089
Red blood cell transfusion, n (%)	3 (5.7%)	1 (4.7%)	0.208
Fresh frozen plasma transfusion, n (%)	11 (21.1%)	6 (28.6%)	0.091
R0, n (%)	50 (96.1%)	20 (95.2%)	0.998
Use of Pringle maneuver, n (%)	46 (88.5%)	17 (80.9%)	0.991
Duration of Pringle maneuver, minutes	40 ± 20	30 ± 15	0.804
Total morbidity, n (%)	12 (23.1%)	6 (28.6%)	0.503
Grade 1	2 (3.8%)	3 (14.3%)	0.030
Grade 2	7 (13.4%)	3 (14.3%)	0.215
Grade 3	3 (5.8%)	0	0.622
Grade 4	0	0	NC
Grade 5	0	0	NC
90-days mortality, n (%)	0	0	NC
Bleeding	2 (3.8%)	1 (4.7%)	0.856
Bile leak	3 (5.7%)	1 (4.7%)	0.446
Ascites	9 (17.3%)	4 (19.0%)	0.101
Postoperative liver failure	5 (9.6%)	2 (9.5%)	0.923
Collection	2 (3.8%)	1 (4.8%)	0.748
Chest infection	1 (1.9%)	0	0.937
Pleural effusion	4 (7.7%)	2 (9.5%)	0.131
Length of stay, days	7 (5–10)	8 (4–10)	0.529
Readmissions, n (%)	4 (7.7%)	2 (9.5%)	0.785

NC: Not calculated.

3.4. Converted MILR: Patients with Preserved Liver Function versus Patients with Advanced Chronic Liver Disease (Low Iwate Difficulty Level)

Conv-A and Conv-B groups showed similar perioperative outcomes as a statistically significant difference was recorded only for Grade 1 complications, which were higher for Conv-B patients (12.5% vs. 6.6 %, p = 0.024). Indeed, all the other parameters showed comparable results between the two groups (Table 6).

Table 6. Results of converted MILRs for HCC: Child A versus converted MILRs in advanced cirrhosis (Child B and Child A/B with portal hypertension) patients for low Iwate difficulty level MILRs.

	Conv-A n = 15	Conv-B n = 8	p Value
Operative time, minutes	150 (130–210)	190 (150–230)	0.665
Blood loss, mL	300 (150–450)	450 (350–550)	0.183
Red blood cell transfusion, n (%)	1 (6.7%)	0	NC
Fresh frozen plasma transfusion, n (%)	2 (13.3%)	1 (12.5%)	0.912
R0, n (%)	14 (93.3%)	8 (100%)	0.832
Use of Pringle maneuver, n (%)	12 (80%)	6 (75%)	0.304
Duration of Pringle maneuver, minutes	30 ± 15	20 ± 15	0.628
Total morbidity, n (%)	3 (20%)	1 (12.5%)	0.078
Grade 1	1 (6.6%)	1 (12.5%)	0.024
Grade 2	2 (13.3%)	0	NC
Grade 3	0	0	NC
Grade 4	0	0	NC
Grade 5	0	0	NC
90-days mortality, n (%)	0	0	NC
Bleeding	1 (6.6%)	0	NC
Bile leak	0	1 (4.7%)	NC
Ascites	1 (6.6%)	0	NC
Postoperative liver failure	0	0	NC
Collection	1 (6.6%)	0	NC
Chest infection	0	0	NC
Pleural effusion	0	0	NC
Length of stay, days	6 (5–11)	7 (5–11)	0.779
Readmissions, n (%)	1 (6.6%)	1 (4.7%)	0.625

3.5. Converted MILR: Patients with Preserved Liver Function versus Patients with Advanced Chronic Liver Disease (Intermediate/Expert/Advanced Iwate Difficulty Level)

Conv-B showed a higher amount of blood loss (700 vs. 400 mL, $p = 0.029$), incidence of red blood cell transfusions (7.7% vs. 5.4%, $p = 0.034$) and fresh frozen plasma transfusions (38.5% vs. 24.3%, $p = 0.007$) than Conv-A. Moreover, global morbidity (38.5% vs. 24.3%, $p = 0.038$), grade 2 complications (23.1% vs. 13.5%, $p = 0.031$), ascites (30.8% vs. 21.6%, $p = 0.025$), collection (7.7% vs. 2.7%, $p = 0.034$) and pleural effusion (15.4% vs. 10.8%, $p = 0.037$) were more frequent in Conv-B group, as well as length of stay being longer (9 vs. 6 days, $p = 0.022$).

The rest of the parameters demonstrated nonsignificant differences (Table 7).

Table 7. Results of converted MILRs for HCC: Child A versus converted MILRs in advanced cirrhosis (Child B and Child A/B with portal hypertension) patients for intermediate/expert/advanced Iwate difficulty level MILRs.

	Conv-A n = 37	Conv-B n = 13	p Value
Operative time, minutes	210 (170–280)	250 (190–300)	0.227
Blood loss, mL	400 (270–520)	700 (400–900)	0.029
Red blood cell transfusion, n (%)	2 (5.4%)	1 (7.7%)	0.034
Fresh frozen plasma transfusion, n (%)	9 (24.3%)	5 (38.5%)	0.007
R0, n (%)	36 (97.3%)	12 (92.3%)	0.905
Use of Pringle maneuver, n (%)	34 (91.9%)	11 (84.6%)	0.076
Duration of Pringle maneuver, minutes	45 ± 25	40 ± 10	0.765
Total morbidity, n (%)	9 (24.3%)	5 (38.5%)	0.038
Grade 1	1 (2.7%)	2 (15.4%)	0.020
Grade 2	5 (13.5%)	3 (23.1%)	0.031
Grade 3	3 (8.1%)	0	NC
Grade 4	0	0	NC
Grade 5	0	0	NC
90-days mortality, n (%)	0	0	NC
Bleeding	0	1 (7.7%)	NC
Bile leak	3 (8.1%)	0	NC
Ascites	8 (21.6%)	4 (30.8%)	0.025
Postoperative liver failure	5 (13.5%)	2 (15.4%)	0.535
Collection	1 (2.7%)	1 (7.7%)	0.034
Chest infection	1 (2.7%)	0	NC
Pleural effusion	4 (10.8%)	2 (15.4%)	0.037
Length of stay, days	6 (5–10)	9 (4–10)	0.022
Readmissions, n (%)	3 (8.1%)	1 (7.7%)	0.809

4. Discussion

MILRs in cirrhosis are universally recognized as challenging. It must be considered that several risk factors for the conversion and difficulty of MILRs have been investigated and various studies have reported the independent role of cirrhosis in both contexts [26,27]. Therefore, MILRs in cirrhosis are regarded as among the most complex minimally invasive liver operations and simultaneously exposed to a relevant possibility of conversion. The need to analyze MILRs is based on the fact that current trends are to increasingly implement MILRs worldwide. This is due to its favorable effects of reduced blood loss, morbidity, hospitalization and favoured pain control, together with less postoperative inflammatory response. There is no evidence that MILRs can prevent HCC development and an oncological long-term advantage cannot be accounted among the demonstrated benefits. However, MILR for HCC is specifically associated with important short-term benefits which are the reduced incidence of postoperative ascites and hepatic insufficiency. These advantages have led HCC to constitute the prevalent indication for MILR [10–13]. Indeed, despite the disadvantages of MILR, which are technical hurdles for the surgeon linked to the loss of direct manual action as challenging bleeding control and intraoperative staging, many studies have shown adequate and favorable results provided the learning curve is completed. The status of current widely used techniques other than MILR include open liver resection, liver transplantation and ablation as options for HCC according to tumor- and liver-related factors. Minimally invasive approaches have entered this scenario not only as an alternative technique to perform curative treatments but also as a potential means of extending the indications to HCC resection. With these premises, this study specifically investigated the outcomes associated with MILR conversion in patients with HCC and liver cirrhosis, with the purpose of specifically investigating outcomes in the setting of advanced cirrhosis given that conversion is not avoidable in a certain proportion of MILRs and considering its potentially harmful effect. The novelty is that this knowledge would help in the mindful process of the refinement of outcomes and indications according to technical and technological development.

Compared to successfully completed MILRs, conversion is known to be associated with worse perioperative outcomes and also inferior overall survival in case of malignant diagnosis [17–20,23,24]. To our knowledge, three previous studies published between 2019 and 2021 investigated the impact of conversion in the specific oncological context of HCC. Stiles and colleagues [23] identified nearly 1000 patients undergoing attempted MILR within a national American cancer database, whereas Lee and Shin and their colleagues [24,25] analyzed nearly 300 MILRs performed at two separate Korean institutions. In all three studies, successfully completed MILRs were compared with patients converted. Despite comparable mortality rates, these were associated with poorer perioperative outcomes including longer postoperative hospitalization, higher blood loss and transfusion rates, longer operative times and higher readmission and morbidity rates including ascites. Although it is clear from these data that converted MILRs for HCC may lose some of the benefits of the minimally invasive approach such as in other disease contexts, the issue of the impact of conversion in relationship with the severity of cirrhosis remained unexplored. Thus, the question persisted unanswered whether MILR conversion in advanced cirrhosis may be held to even inferior outcomes than in the setting of compensated liver disease.

By separately comparing successfully completed with converted MILRs for compensated and advanced cirrhosis, this study confirmed that conversion has inferior results for both compensated and advanced cirrhotic patients. In both cases, converted patients exhibited greater blood loss, higher transfusion rates, longer hospitalization and higher morbidity and readmission rates. Notably, the incidence of pleural effusion, ascites and postoperative liver failure was higher, which are major concerns for patients affected by chronic liver disease given the potential negative impact of short-term survival. Always, when allocating a patient to liver resection in consideration of the possible beneficial course linked to a minimally invasive approach, the possibility of conversion, which is expected to provide a postoperative course similar to that of open resection, has to be considered. This is of utmost importance when the feasibility of a minimally invasive approach weighs significantly in favor of liver resection as the therapeutic choice. Progressive literature has demonstrated the significant advantages of the minimally invasive approach for HCC surgery, precisely in terms of the reduction of ascites and postoperative liver failure, i.e., the elements that traditionally most limit the choice of resection as the treatment option. Moreover, during the years, this advantage has also resulted in patients with advanced cirrhosis, leading them to have a postoperative course similar to that of compensated patients [8,12,45]. This evidence has led to hypothesize and also consider a formal expansion of resective indications for more fragile patients [13]. However, a tendency of this type cannot disregard the consideration that the possibility of conversion exists and cannot be canceled, nor can its possible effects. Therefore, the choice of allocating a patient to resection by virtue of the feasibility of a minimally invasive operation must be a criterion proposed with an awareness of the limits and applied to selected patients if this is based on an extension of the indications.

This study took the available evidence a step further: it showed that conversion in patients with advanced cirrhosis can have similar—and not inferior—results to patients with compensated cirrhosis, provided adequate patient selection is applied. In fact, the comparative analysis between the two groups of converted patients (entire cohort) resulted in non-significant statistical differences regarding perioperative outcomes (the only exception was the incidence of grade 1 complications, which was higher in patients with advanced cirrhosis). Although well accepted, this finding was not entirely expected on the assumption that a laparotomy in the patient with decompensated cirrhosis or with portal hypertension is generally associated with less brilliant results than in the patient with compensated cirrhosis, in particular with a higher rate of postoperative complications and a prolonged stay. Therefore, in interpreting the result of this analysis, the difficulty profile of the resections performed has a logical explanatory role. It is immediate to note that only an extremely limited portion of the cohort of patients with advanced cirrhosis underwent complex resections (understood as advanced or expert level) with a clear prevalence of resections of low and intermediate difficulty; at the same time, the complexity of the resections was much more homogeneous in the cohort of patients with compensated cirrhosis, of which more than 30% received a complex resection. A more contained difficulty profile of resections appears able to counteract the clinical effect that conversion can have in patients with advanced cirrhosis, keeping the average impact similar to that of compensated patients undergoing a wider and less restrictive range of procedures. This is further supported by the results of the analysis comparing conversion in patients with compensated and advanced cirrhosis when resections are stratified for difficulty. Indeed, the comparative analysis between the two groups of converted low difficulty MILRs resulted in non-significant statistical differences regarding perioperative outcomes (the only exception was again the incidence of grade 1 complications, which was higher in patients with advanced cirrhosis). Instead, the comparison of converted more difficult MILRs (intermediate/advanced/expert) resulted in several worse perioperative outcomes for patients with advanced cirrhosis such as higher blood loss, transfusion rates, global morbidity and grade 2 complications rates including ascites, collection and pleural effusion, as well as a longer length of stay. As such, it is clear that advanced cirrhotics undergoing intermediate/advanced/expert MILR is a category of patients that pays a significant price of conversion and that the difficulty of MILR is a factor that should be taken into significant account in the process of patient selection. It follows that the difficulty scoring system can be a very useful tool in the decision-making of proposing minimally invasive surgery to patients with advanced cirrhosis: it may help identify those patients for whom broadening the indications allows maintaining satisfactory outcomes, including the potential conversion effect (patients elected to low difficulty MILR), and may be at the basis of reasoned and aware modern resective indications. The significance of these novel results support the idea that the process of proposing expanded resective indications for HCC in view of the feasibility of minimally invasive operations must include criteria proposed with an awareness of the limitations and applied to selected patients, and a difficulty scoring system for MILR can play a useful role for patient selection.

Regarding the incidence of MILR conversions in HCC, the rates reported in the literature vary greatly as for MILR in general. Stiles, Shin and Lee reported rates of 18.0%, 6% and 4%, respectively, and our study's rate falls somewhere between these values at 11%. We found the conversion rate was not different between the two groups as well as the incidence of bleeding as a cause, despite—as in the other studies—being the most frequent reason for conversion. This is obviously related to the aptitude of cirrhotic parenchyma to bleed more than healthy liver and to the known frequent coagulation disorders observed in cirrhotic patients. [24,25]. It has been also reported that patients who experience emergent conversion due to an intraoperative complication suffered even worse perioperative outcomes than those undergoing elective conversion [21]. The limited number of conversions, due to the single-center design of this study, precluded this specific analysis which can be the subject of a multi-center analysis together with the reasons of conversion. We cannot exclude that larger sample sizes could find higher rates of conversions in the advanced cirrhotic group, especially due to difficult hemostasis or bleeding, highlighting the role of cirrhosis status rather than the presence of cirrhosis itself in this setting. The other limitation to be acknowledged for this study is the retrospective design, which carries in itself the burden of selection bias and a possible influence on some results. However, it is clear that selection bias is itself a premise for satisfactory outcomes in these particular categories of patients.

This study sets the stage for a systematization of patient selection, and we believe that future studies should continue in this direction in order to achieve a thoughtful and accurate expansion of the indications, ideally validated within guidelines.

5. Conclusions

In conclusion, conversion during MILR for HCC represents a loss of advantage with respect to successfully completed MILRs, and the risk and impact of conversion should be accurately estimated when proposing to expand the indications to liver resection for HCC in view of a minimally invasive approach. Conversion in the setting of advanced cirrhosis can be associated with non-inferior outcomes compared to compensated cirrhosis, provided careful patient selection is applied (patients elected to low difficulty MILR). Difficulty scoring systems may help identify the most appropriate candidates to maintain satisfactory outcomes, even in case of conversion, and become useful in multidisciplinary treatment decisions.

Author Contributions: Conceptualization, L.A. and F.C.; methodology, L.A. and F.C.; formal analysis, F.C.; data curation, F.R., G.F., R.M., A.T. and M.C.; writing—original draft preparation, F.C.; writing—review and editing, F.R., G.F., R.M., A.T. and M.C.; visualization, F.R., G.F., R.M., A.T. and M.C.; supervision, L.A. All authors have read and agreed to the published version of the manuscript.

Funding: This research received no external funding.

Institutional Review Board Statement: This study was conducted in accordance with the Declaration of Helsinki and approved by the Institutional Review Board of San Raffaele Hospital Ethical Committee (ethics code: IGOMILS Protocol; approval date: 6 March 2014).

Informed Consent Statement: Consents from subjects were waived.

Data Availability Statement: The data presented in this study are available on request from the corresponding author. The data are not publicly available due to privacy restrictions.

Conflicts of Interest: The authors declare no conflict of interest.

References

1. Ratti, F.; Cipriani, F.; Ariotti, R.; Giannone, F.; Paganelli, M.; Aldrighetti, L. Laparoscopic major hepatectomies: Current trends and indications. A comparison with the open technique. *Updates Surg.* **2015**, *67*, 157–167. [CrossRef] [PubMed]
2. Ciria, R.; Ocaña, S.; Gomez-Luque, I.; Cipriani, F.; Halls, M.; Fretland, A.; Okuda, Y.; Aroori, S.; Briceño, J.; Aldrighetti, L.; et al. A systematic review and meta-analysis comparing the short- and long-term outcomes for laparoscopic and open liver resections for liver metastases from colorectal cancer. *Surg. Endosc.* **2020**, *34*, 349–360. [CrossRef] [PubMed]
3. Berardi, G.; Van Cleven, S.; Fretland, A.; Barkhatov, L.; Halls, M.; Cipriani, F.; Aldrighetti, L.; Abu Hilal, M.; Edwin, B.; Troisi, R.I. Evolution of Laparoscopic Liver Surgery from Innovation to Implementation to Mastery: Perioperative and Oncologic Outcomes of 2,238 Patients from 4 European Specialized Centers. *J. Am. Coll. Surg.* **2017**, *225*, 639–649. [CrossRef] [PubMed]
4. van der Poel, M.J.; Barkhatov, L.; Fuks, D.; Berardi, G.; Cipriani, F.; Aljaiuossi, A.; Lainas, P.; Dagher, I.; D'Hondt, M.; Rotellar, F.; et al. Multicentre propensity score-matched study of laparoscopic versus open repeat liver resection for colorectal liver metastases. *Br. J. Surg.* **2019**, *106*, 783–789. [CrossRef]
5. Morise, Z.; Aldrighetti, L.; Belli, G.; Ratti, F.; Belli, A.; Cherqui, D.; Tanabe, M.; Wakabayashi, G.; Cheung, T.T.; Lo, C.M.; et al. Laparoscopic repeat liver resection for hepatocellular carcinoma: A multicentre propensity score-based study. *Br. J. Surg.* **2020**, *107*, 889–895. [CrossRef]
6. Aldrighetti, L.; Guzzetti, E.; Pulitanò, C.; Cipriani, F.; Catena, M.; Paganelli, M.; Ferla, G. Case-matched analysis of totally laparoscopic versus open liver resection for HCC: Short and middle term results. *J. Surg. Oncol.* **2010**, *102*, 82–86. [CrossRef]
7. Tranchart, H.; Di Giuro, G.; Lainas, P.; Roudie, J.; Agostini, H.; Franco, D.; Dagher, I. Laparoscopic resection for hepatocellular carcinoma: A matched-pair comparative study. *Surg. Endosc.* **2010**, *24*, 1170–1176. [CrossRef]
8. Troisi, R.; Berardi, G.; Morise, Z.; Cipriani, F.; Ariizumi, S.; Sposito, C.; Panetta, V.; Simonelli, I.; Kim, S.; Goh, B.K.P.; et al. Laparoscopic and open liver resection for hepatocellular carcinoma with Child-Pugh B cirrhosis: Multicentre propensity score-matched study. *Br. J. Surg.* **2021**, *108*, 196–204. [CrossRef]

9. Morise, Z.; Ciria, R.; Cherqui, D.; Chen, K.-H.; Belli, G.; Wakabayashi, G. Can we expand the indications for laparoscopic liver resection? A systematic review and meta-analysis of laparoscopic liver resection for patients with hepatocellular carcinoma and chronic liver disease. *J. Hepatobiliary Pancreat. Sci.* 2015, *22*, 342–352. [CrossRef]
10. Aldrighetti, L.; Italian Group of Minimally Invasive Liver Surgery (I GO MILS); Belli, G.; Boni, L.; Cillo, U.; Ettorre, G.M.; De Carlis, L.; Pinna, A.; Casciola, L.; Calise, F. Italian Group of Minimally Invasive Liver Surgery (I GO MILS). Italian experience in minimally invasive liver surgery: A national survey. *Updates Surg.* 2015, *67*, 129–140. [CrossRef]
11. Ciria, R.; Cherqui, D.; Geller, D.A.; Briceno, J.; Wakabayashi, G. Comparative Short-term Benefits of Laparoscopic Liver Resection: 9000 Cases and Climbing. *Ann. Surg.* 2016, *263*, 761–777. [CrossRef] [PubMed]
12. Cipriani, F.; Fantini, C.; Ratti, F.; Lauro, R.; Tranchart, H.; Halls, M.; Scuderi, V.; Barkhatov, L.; Edwin, B.; Troisi, R.I.; et al. Laparoscopic liver resections for hepatocellular carcinoma. Can we extend the surgical indication in cirrhotic patients? *Surg. Endosc.* 2018, *32*, 617–626. [CrossRef] [PubMed]
13. Reig, M.; Forner, A.; Rimola, J.; Ferrer-Fàbrega, J.; Burrel, M.; Garcia-Criado, Á.; Kelley, R.K.; Galle, P.R.; Mazzaferro, V.; Salem, R.; et al. BCLC strategy for prognosis prediction and treatment recommendation: The 2022 update. *J. Hepatol.* 2022, *76*, 681–693. [CrossRef] [PubMed]
14. Cipriani, F.; Ratti, F.; Fiorentini, G.; Catena, M.; Paganelli, M.; Aldrighetti, L. Effect of Previous Abdominal Surgery on Laparoscopic Liver Resection: Analysis of Feasibility and Risk Factors for Conversion. *J. Laparosc. Adv. Surg. Tech. A* 2018, *28*, 785–791. [CrossRef]
15. Goh, B.K.P.; Chan, C.-Y.; Wong, J.-S.; Lee, S.-Y.; Lee, V.T.W.; Cheow, P.-C.; Chow, P.K.H.; Ooi, L.L.P.J.; Chung, A.Y.F. Factors associated with and outcomes of open conversion after laparoscopic minor hepatectomy: Initial experience at a single institution. *Surg. Endosc.* 2015, *29*, 2636–2642. [CrossRef]
16. Cipriani, F.; Ratti, F.; Fiorentini, G.; Catena, M.; Paganelli, M.; Aldrighetti, L. Pure laparoscopic right hepatectomy: A risk score for conversion for the paradigm of difficult laparoscopic liver resections. A single centre case series. *Int. J. Surg.* 2020, *82*, 108–115. [CrossRef]
17. Costi, R.; Scatton, O.; Haddad, L.; Randone, B.; Andraus, W.; Massault, P.-P.; Soubrane, O. Lessons learned from the first 100 laparoscopic liver resections: Not delaying conversion may allow reduced blood loss and operative time. *J. Laparosc. Adv. Surg. Tech. A* 2012, *22*, 425–431. [CrossRef]
18. Wang, H.P.; Yong, C.C.; Wu, A.G.; Cherqui, D.; Troisi, R.I.; Cipriani, F.; Aghayan, D.; Marino, M.V.; Belli, A.; Chiow, A.K.; et al. Factors associated with and impact of open conversion on the outcomes of minimally invasive left lateral sectionectomies: An international multicenter study. *Surgery* 2022, *172*, 617–624. [CrossRef]
19. Cauchy, F.; Fuks, D.; Nomi, T.; Schwarz, L.; Barbier, L.; Dokmak, S.; Scatton, O.; Belghiti, J.; Soubrane, O.; Gayet, B. Risk factors and consequences of conversion in laparoscopic major liver resection. *Br. J. Surg.* 2015, *102*, 785–795. [CrossRef]
20. Stiles, Z.E.; Behrman, S.W.; Glazer, E.S.; Deneve, J.L.; Dong, L.; Wan, J.Y.; Dickson, P.V. Predictors and implications of unplanned conversion during minimally invasive hepatectomy: An analysis of the ACS-NSQIP database. *HPB* 2017, *19*, 957–965. [CrossRef] [PubMed]
21. Halls, M.C.; Cipriani, F.; Berardi, G.; Barkhatov, L.; Lainas, P.; Alzoubi, M.; D'Hondt, M.; Rotellar, F.; Dagher, I.; Aldrighetti, L.; et al. Conversion for Unfavorable Intraoperative Events Results in Significantly Worst Outcomes During Laparoscopic Liver Resection: Lessons Learned from a Multicenter Review of 2861 Cases. *Ann. Surg.* 2018, *268*, 1051–1057. [CrossRef] [PubMed]
22. Cipriani, F.; Ratti, F.; Cardella, A.; Catena, M.; Paganelli, M.; Aldrighetti, L. Laparoscopic Versus Open Major Hepatectomy: Analysis of Clinical Outcomes and Cost Effectiveness in a High-Volume Center. *J. Gastrointest. Surg.* 2019, *23*, 2163–2173. [CrossRef] [PubMed]
23. Stiles, Z.E.; Glazer, E.S.; DeNeve, J.L.; Shibata, D.; Behrman, S.W.; Dickson, P.V. Long-term implications of unplanned conversion during laparoscopic liver resection for hepatocellular carcinoma. *Ann. Surg. Oncol.* 2019, *26*, 282–289. [CrossRef] [PubMed]
24. Shin, H.; Cho, J.Y.; Han, H.-S.; Yoon, Y.-S.; Lee, H.W.; Lee, J.S.; Lee, B.; Kim, M.; Jo, Y. Risk factors and long-term implications of unplanned conversion during laparoscopic liver resection for hepatocellular carcinoma located in anterolateral liver segments. *J. Minim. Invasive Surg.* 2021, *24*, 191–199. [CrossRef] [PubMed]
25. Lee, J.Y.; Rho, S.Y.; Han, D.H.; Choi, J.S.; Choi, G.H. Unplanned conversion during minimally invasive liver resection for hepatocellular carcinoma: Risk factors and surgical outcomes. *Ann. Surg. Treat Res.* 2020, *98*, 23–30. [CrossRef] [PubMed]
26. Wakabayashi, G. What has changed after the Morioka consensus conference 2014 on laparoscopic liver resection? *Hepatobiliary Surg. Nutr.* 2016, *5*, 281–289. [CrossRef]
27. Li, L.; Xu, L.; Wang, P.; Zhang, M.; Li, B. The risk factors of intraoperative conversion during laparoscopic hepatectomy: A systematic review and meta-analysis. *Langenbecks Arch. Surg.* 2022, *407*, 469–478. [CrossRef]
28. Lin, H.; Bai, Y.; Yin, M.; Chen, Z.; Yu, S. External validation of different difficulty scoring systems of laparoscopic liver resection for hepatocellular carcinoma. *Surg. Endosc.* 2022, *36*, 3732–3749. [CrossRef]
29. Pugh, R.N.H.; Murray-Lyon, I.M.; Dawson, J.L.; Pietroni, M.C.; Williams, R. Transection of the oesophagus for bleeding oesophageal varices. *Br. J. Surg.* 1973, *60*, 646–649. [CrossRef]
30. Llovet, J.M.; Brú, C.; Bruix, J. Prognosis of hepatocellular carcinoma: The BCLC staging classification. *Semin. Liver. Dis.* 1999, *19*, 329–338. [CrossRef]
31. Ratti, F.; Cipriani, F.; Catena, M.; Paganelli, M.; Aldrighetti, L. Approach to hepatocaval confluence during laparoscopic right hepatectomy: Three variations on a theme. *Surg. Endosc.* 2017, *31*, 949. [CrossRef] [PubMed]

32. Cipriani, F.; Ratti, F.; Paganelli, M.; Reineke, R.; Catena, M.; Aldrighetti, L. Laparoscopic or open approaches for posterosuperior and anterolateral liver resections? A propensity score based analysis of the degree of advantage. *HPB* **2019**, *21*, 1676–1686. [CrossRef] [PubMed]
33. Aldrighetti, L.; Pulitanò, C.; Arru, M.; Catena, M.; Guzzetti, E.; Casati, M.; Ferla, G. Ultrasonic-mediated laparoscopic liver transection. *Am. J. Surg.* **2008**, *195*, 270–272. [CrossRef]
34. Aldrighetti, L.; Catena, M.; Ratti, F. Maximizing Performance in Complex Minimally Invasive Surgery of the Liver: The RoboLap Approach. *J. Gastrointest. Surg.* **2022**, *26*, 1811–1813. [CrossRef] [PubMed]
35. Abu Hilal, M.; Aldrighetti, L.; Dagher, I.; Edwin, B.; Troisi, R.I.; Alikhanov, R.; Aroori, S.; Belli, G.; Besselink, M.; Briceno, J.; et al. The Southampton Consensus Guidelines for Laparoscopic Liver Surgery: From Indication to Implementation. *Ann. Surg.* **2018**, *268*, 11–18. [CrossRef]
36. Ratti, F.; Cipriani, F.; Reineke, R.; Catena, M.; Comotti, L.; Beretta, L.; Aldrighetti, L. Impact of ERAS approach and minimally-invasive techniques on outcome of patients undergoing liver surgery for hepatocellular carcinoma. *Dig. Liver. Dis.* **2016**, *48*, 1243–1248. [CrossRef] [PubMed]
37. Ratti, F.; Cipriani, F.; Reineke, R.; Comotti, L.; Paganelli, M.; Catena, M.; Beretta, L.; Aldrighetti, L. The clinical and biological impacts of the implementation of fast track perioperative programs in complex liver resections: A propensity score-based analysis between the open and laparoscopic approaches. *Surgery* **2018**, *164*, 395–403. [CrossRef]
38. Pulitanò, C.; Arru, M.; Bellio, L.; Rossini, S.; Ferla, G.; Aldrighetti, L. A risk score for predicting perioperative blood transfusion in liver Surgery. *Br. J. Surg.* **2007**, *94*, 860–865. [CrossRef]
39. Strasberg, S.M. Nomenclature of hepatic anatomy and resections: A review of the Brisbane 2000 system. *J. Hepatobiliary Pancreat. Surg.* **2005**, *12*, 351–355. [CrossRef]
40. Dindo, D.; Demartines, N.; Clavien, P.-A. Classification of surgical complications: A new proposal with evaluation in a cohort of 6336 patients and results of a survey. *Ann. Surg.* **2004**, *240*, 205–213. [CrossRef]
41. Rahbari, N.N.; Garden, O.J.; Padbury, R.; Brooke-Smith, M.; Crawford, M.; Adam, R.; Koch, M.; Makuuchi, M.; Dematteo, R.P.; Christophi, C.; et al. Posthepatectomy liver failure: A definition and grading by the International Study Group of Liver Surgery (ISGLS). *Surgery* **2011**, *149*, 713–724. [CrossRef] [PubMed]
42. Ishizawa, T.; Hasegawa, K.; Kokudo, N.; Sano, K.; Imamura, H.; Beck, Y.; Sugawara, Y.; Makuuchi, M. Risk factors and management of ascites after liver resection to treat hepatocellular carcinoma. *Arch. Surg.* **2009**, *144*, 46–51. [CrossRef] [PubMed]
43. Koch, M.; Garden, O.J.; Padbury, R.; Rahbari, N.N.; Adam, R.; Capussotti, L.; Fan, S.T.; Yokoyama, Y.; Crawford, M.; Makuuchi, M.; et al. Bile leakage after hepatobiliary and pancreatic surgery: A definition and grading of severity by the International Study Group of Liver Surgery. *Surgery* **2011**, *149*, 680–688. [CrossRef] [PubMed]
44. Cucchetti, A.; Ercolani, G.; Vivarelli, M.; Cescon, M.; Ravaioli, M.; La Barba, G.; Zanello, M.; Grazi, G.L.; Pinna, A.D. Impact of model for end-stage liver disease (MELD) score on prognosis after hepatectomy for hepatocellular carcinoma on cirrhosis. *Liver Transpl.* **2006**, *12*, 966–971. [CrossRef]
45. Watanabe, Y.; Aikawa, M.; Kato, T.; Takase, K.; Okada, K.; Okamoto, K.; Koyama, I. Influence of Child-Pugh B7 and B8/9 cirrhosis on laparoscopic liver resection for hepatocellular carcinoma: A retrospective cohort study. *Surg. Endosc.* **2022**, *37*, 1316–1333. [CrossRef]

Disclaimer/Publisher's Note: The statements, opinions and data contained in all publications are solely those of the individual author(s) and contributor(s) and not of MDPI and/or the editor(s). MDPI and/or the editor(s) disclaim responsibility for any injury to people or property resulting from any ideas, methods, instructions or products referred to in the content.

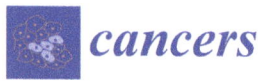

Systematic Review

Challenging Scenarios and Debated Indications for Laparoscopic Liver Resections for Hepatocellular Carcinoma

Giammauro Berardi [1,*], Edoardo Maria Muttillo [2], Marco Colasanti [1], Germano Mariano [1], Roberto Luca Meniconi [1], Stefano Ferretti [1], Nicola Guglielmo [1], Marco Angrisani [1], Alessio Lucarini [1], Eleonora Garofalo [1], Davide Chiappori [1], Ludovica Di Cesare [1], Damiano Vallati [1], Paolo Mercantini [2] and Giuseppe Maria Ettorre [1]

[1] Department of General, Hepatobiliary and Pancreatic Surgery, Liver Transplantation Service, San Camillo Forlanini Hospital of Rome, 00152 Rome, Italy
[2] Surgical and Medical Department of Translational Medicine, Sant'Andrea Hospital, Sapienza University of Rome, 00189 Rome, Italy
* Correspondence: gberardi2@scamilloforlanini.rm.it; Tel.: +39-065-870-5816

Simple Summary: Minimally invasive liver resections are nowadays performed worldwide for both benign and malignant lesions. Good short-term and safe long-term outcomes have been reported. Despite this growing implementation of the technique, challenging scenarios and debated indications still exist. There is currently a lack of high-quality evidence regarding minimally invasive liver resections in portal hypertension, advanced cirrhosis, lesions in the posterosuperior segments and large and recurrent tumors.

Abstract: Laparoscopic liver resections (LLRs) have been increasingly adopted for the treatment of hepatocellular carcinoma (HCC), with safe short- and long-term outcomes reported worldwide. Despite this, lesions in the posterosuperior segments, large and recurrent tumors, portal hypertension, and advanced cirrhosis currently represent challenging scenarios in which the safety and efficacy of the laparoscopic approach are still controversial. In this systematic review, we pooled the available evidence on the short-term outcomes of LLRs for HCC in challenging clinical scenarios. All randomized and non-randomized studies reporting LLRs for HCC in the above-mentioned settings were included. The literature search was run in the Scopus, WoS, and Pubmed databases. Case reports, reviews, meta-analyses, studies including fewer than 10 patients, non-English language studies, and studies analyzing histology other than HCC were excluded. From 566 articles, 36 studies dated between 2006 and 2022 fulfilled the selection criteria and were included in the analysis. A total of 1859 patients were included, of whom 156 had advanced cirrhosis, 194 had portal hypertension, 436 had large HCCs, 477 had lesions located in the posterosuperior segments, and 596 had recurrent HCCs. Overall, the conversion rate ranged between 4.6% and 15.5%. Mortality and morbidity ranged between 0.0% and 5.1%, and 18.6% and 34.6%, respectively. Full results according to subgroups are described in the study. Advanced cirrhosis and portal hypertension, large and recurrent tumors, and lesions located in the posterosuperior segments are challenging clinical scenarios that should be carefully approached by laparoscopy. Safe short-term outcomes can be achieved provided experienced surgeons and high-volume centers.

Keywords: laparoscopic liver resection; hepatocellular carcinoma; advanced cirrhosis; portal hypertension; large HCC; posterosuperior segments; recurrent HCC

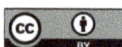

1. Introduction

Hepatocellular carcinoma (HCC) is the most common primary liver tumor and the third leading cause of cancer-related deaths worldwide [1,2]. Whenever feasible, liver resection (LR) is one of the treatments of choice in very early and early-stage disease, offering long-term survivals exceeding 50% at 5 years [3]. Since 1992, when the first laparoscopic liver resection (LLR) was described, minimally invasive approaches have been increasingly employed for both benign and malignant liver diseases [4]. Indeed, despite the initial skepticism from the oncological point of view, nowadays, LLRs are considered safe for the treatment of malignant tumors and are widely adopted in experienced centers for colorectal liver metastases, intrahepatic cholangiocarcinomas, and HCCs [5]. Recent meta-analyses disclosed improved short- and comparable long-term outcomes of LLRs compared to open in the setting of HCC [6,7]. However, a variety of different patients and tumor presentations were included, eventually analyzing a heterogeneous population with different risk factors from both the perioperative and long-term standpoint.

Conditions such as advanced cirrhosis (AC), portal hypertension (PH), lesions located in the posterosuperior (PS) segments, large tumors, and recurrent HCCs represent unique clinical scenarios that require careful and specific considerations in the setting of minimally invasive approaches. Indeed, these conditions are associated with increased perioperative morbidity and mortality and were initially considered as contraindications to LLRs as recommended in the Southampton Consensus Guidelines for Laparoscopic liver surgery [8]. Despite this, experienced centers have been pushing the indications in these challenging scenarios, reporting safe outcomes both in the perioperative setting and long-term survivals [9–11]. Nevertheless, the evidence is still limited to small studies, which have been mostly singe center and retrospective in nature. This systematic review aimed to pool all the available literature regarding LLRs in these challenging scenarios and to summarize the evidence.

2. Material and Methods

2.1. Literature Search

Preferred Reporting Items for Systematic Reviews and Meta-Analyses (PRISMA) statement guidelines were followed for conducting and reporting this systematic review. A systematic literature search was performed independently by two of the authors (E.M.M. and G.B.) using PubMed, WoS, and Scopus databases. The search was limited to studies in humans and published in English. Case reports, reviews, and meta-analyses were excluded. No restrictions were set for the date of publication. The search strategy was based on different combinations of words for each database. For the PubMed database, the following combination was used: (repeat hepatectomy OR recurrent HCC) AND (large HCC OR large hepatocellular carcinoma) AND (laparoscopic liver resections OR minimally invasive) AND (portal hypertension) AND (advanced liver cirrhosis) AND (posterosuperior segments). The same keywords were inserted in the search manager fields of Scopus. Extensive crosschecking of the reference lists of all retrieved articles that fulfilled the inclusion criteria further broadened the search. This systematic review was registered in the PROSPERO database with the number CRD42023396942.

2.2. Study Selection

The same two authors independently screened the titles and abstracts of the studies that were identified with the electronic search. Duplicate studies were excluded. The following criteria were set: (1) studies reporting laparoscopic liver resections for the above-mentioned indications; (2) studies reporting at least one perioperative outcome. The following exclusion criteria were set: (1) studies reporting non-laparoscopic liver resections, (2) studies not reporting separate outcomes for laparoscopic liver resections and (3) studies in which it was impossible to retrieve or calculate the data of interest. In the case of more than one report from the same center, only the most recent or the highest-quality study was included in the review. Advanced cirrhosis was defined as a Child–Pugh score of B or more [12]. Portal hypertension was defined as the presence of indirect signs of clinically significant portosystemic shunts (radiological or biochemical) or by a portosystemic gradient of more than 10 mmHg [13]. Segments VII, VIII, and IVa were considered posterosuperior [14]. A size of >5 cm was considered a large HCC [15].

2.3. Data Extraction

The same two authors extracted the main data as follows: (1) first author, study type, and subgroup; (2) number and characteristics of patients including Child–Pugh and/or MELD score; (3) intraoperative characteristics including the number of major/minor hepatectomies, anatomic or non-anatomic resections, operative time, blood loss, Pringle maneuver, conversion rates, and (4) postoperative outcomes including complications, Clavien–Dindo et al. [16] grade, liver-specific complications (bile leak, ascites, and liver failure) and mortality. Liver failure was defined according to the classification of International Study Group of Liver Surgery (ISGLS) [17] Major complications were defined as Clavien–Dindo > II. Relevant texts, tables, and figures were reviewed for data extraction, and whenever further information was required, the corresponding authors of the papers were contacted by e-mail. Discrepancies between the two reviewers were resolved by consensus discussion. Quality assessment was performed according to the Newcastle–Ottawa Scale (Table 1) [18].

Table 1. Newcastle–Ottawa scale for quality assessment of the included studies.

Study Authors	Selection	Comparability	Outcome	Total
Cipriani et al. [19]	***	**	***	8
Troisi et al. [20]	****	**	***	9
Cai et al. [21]	***	**	***	8
Beard et al. [22]	****	**	***	9
Lim et al. [23]	****	**	***	9
Guo et al. [24]	****	**	**	8
Molina et al. [25]	***	**	***	8
Zheng et al. [26]	***	**	***	8
Casellas et al. [27]	****	**	***	9
Ruzzenente et al. [28]	****	**	***	9
Kwon et al. [29]	***	**	**	7
Chiang et al. [30]	***	**	***	8
Fu et al. [31]	**	**	***	7
Xu et al. [32]	***	**	***	8
Xiang et al. [33]	****	**	***	9
Levi Sandri et al. [34]	****	**	***	9
Ai et al. [35]	****	**	***	9
Casaccia et al. [36]	****	**	**	8
Xiang et al. [37]	****	**	***	9
Lee et al. [38]	***	**	**	7
Tagaytay et al. [39]	***	**	***	8
Kwon et al. [40]	***	**	***	8
Yoon et al. [41]	****	**	**	8
Xiao et al. [42]	****	**	***	9
Cherqui et al. [43]	***	**	**	7
Levi Sandri et al. [44]	****	**	***	9
Liu et al. [45]	***	**	***	8
Belli et al. [46]	**	**	***	7

Table 1. *Cont.*

Study Authors	Selection	Comparability	Outcome	Total
Goh et al. [47]	***	**	**	7
Levi Sandri et al. [48]	****	**	***	9
Gon et al. [49]	***	**	***	8
Zhang et al. [50]	***	**	**	7
Morise et al. [51]	***	**	**	7
Kanazawa et al. [52]	***	**	*	6
Onoe et al. [53]	***	**	***	8
Miyama et al. [54]	***	**	***	8

Each * counts as 1 point.

3. Results

The literature search yielded 566 articles; after duplicate removal, 401 titles and abstracts were reviewed (Figure 1). Of these, 226 papers were excluded based on abstract and title; 175 articles were assessed for eligibility and full text screened. Of these, 139 articles were excluded. Finally, a total of 36 articles dated between 2006 and 2022 fulfilled the selection criteria and were included in this systematic review [19–54]. There was no disagreement between the authors regarding eligibility. The articles consisted of 33 retrospective and three prospective reports, gathering a total of 1859 patients. Characteristics of the included studies are summarized in Table 2.

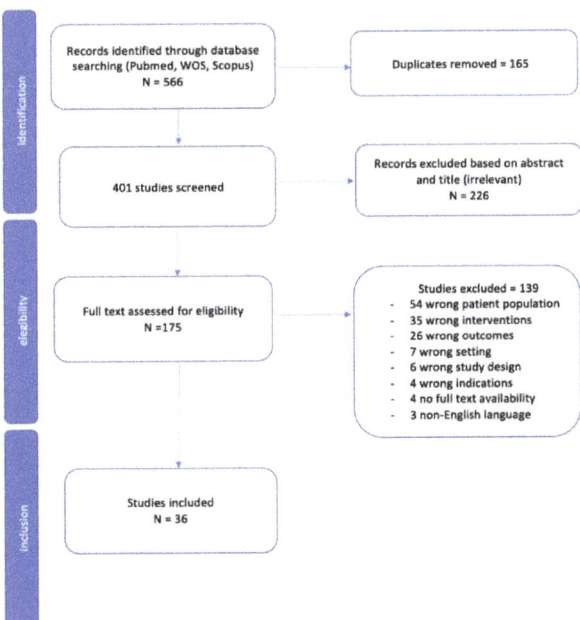

Figure 1. Prisma flow diagram.

Table 2. Baseline characteristics of the included studies.

First Author	Subgroup	Country	Type of Study	No. of Patients	Age	Gender M/F	Child–Pugh A/B/C	MELD Score
Cipriani et al. [19]	Advanced cirrhosis	Italy	Retro	25	66 (23–88)	14/11	0/25/0	NR
Troisi et al. [20]	Advanced cirrhosis	Italy	Retro	100	68 (27–84)	75/25	0/100/0	9 (4–22)
Cai et al. [21]	Advanced cirrhosis	China	Retro	5	60 (27–79)	5/0	0/5/0	NR
Beard et al. [22]	Advanced cirrhosis	USA	Retro	26	60.5 (49–77)	22/4	0/20/6	NR
Lim et al. [23]	Portal hypertension	France	Prosp	18	64 (52–83)	11/7	18/0/0	8 (6–11)
Guo et al. [24]	Portal hypertension	China	Retro	16	50 (29–70)	9/7	12/4/0	NR
Molina et al. [25]	Portal hypertension	Spain	Retro	16	64 (50–75)	11/5	16/0/0	NR
Zheng et al. [26]	Portal hypertension	China	Retro	24	58.5 (54–68)	21/3	18/6/0	NR
Casellas et al. [27]	Portal hypertension	Spain	Retro	31	64 ± 8 *	20/11	31/0/0	NR
Ruzzenente et al. [28]	Portal hypertension	Italy	Retro	89	NR	67/22	67/19/3	NR
Kwon et al. [29]	Large HCC	Republic of Korea	Retro	20	56.1 ± 12.6 *	16/4	NR	NR
Chiang et al. [30]	Large HCC	Taiwan	Retro	37	58 ± 11.7 *	30/7	36/1/0	NR
Fu et al. [31]	Large HCC	China	Retro	14	61.5 (28–77)	10/4	NR	6 (6–7)
Xu et al. [32]	Large HCC	China	Retro	102	52.5 (25–80)	80/22	NR	NR
Xiang et al. [33]	Large HCC	China	Prosp	128	51 ± 11.9 *	109/19	108/20/0	NR
Levi Sandri et al. [34]	Large HCC	Italy	Retro	38	71 (61–77)	25/13	38/0/0	7 (6–8)
Ai et al. [35]	Large HCC	China	Retro	97	52 (14–77)	75/22	59/38/0	NR
Casaccia et al. [36]	Posterosuperior segments	Italy	Retro	22	66 (47–76)	13/9	19/3/0	NR
Xiang et al. [37]	Posterosuperior segments	China	Retro	56	51.6 ± 10.2	47/9	NR	NR
Lee et al. [38]	Posterosuperior segments	Republic of Korea	Retro	58	56 (33–74)	37/21	56/2/0	NR
Tagaytay et al. [39]	Posterosuperior segments	Republic of Korea	Retro	37	60 ± 10.58 *	28/9	NR	NR
Kwon et al. [40]	Posterosuperior segments	Republic of Korea	Retro	149	57 ± 10.4 *	115/34	146/1/2	NR
Yoon et al. [41]	Posterosuperior segments	Republic of Korea	Retro	25	53 ± 10 *	14/11	23/2/0	NR
Xiao et al. [42]	Posterosuperior segments	China	Retro	41	52 ± 11.62 *	34/7	39/2/0	NR
Cherqui et al. [43]	Posterosuperior segments	France	Retro	27	63 (40–76)	22/5	27/0/0	NR
Levi Sandri et al. [44]	Posterosuperior segments	Italy	Retro	62	71 (59.5–75)	50/12	62/0/0	7 (6–8)
Liu et al. [45]	Recurrent HCC	China	Retro	30	56.5 (27–79)	23/7	30/0/0	NR
Belli et al. [46]	Recurrent HCC	Italy	Retro	15	68 (58–75)	NR	15/0/0	NR
Goh et al. [47]	Recurrent HCC	Singapore	Retro	20	68.5 (67–71)	18/2	NR	NR
Levi Sandri et al. [48]	Recurrent HCC	Italy	Retro	74	72 (65–76)	55/19	66/8/0	7 (7–9)
Gon et al. [49]	Recurrent HCC	Japan	Retro	23	72 (67–79)	18/5	23/0/0	NR
Zhang et al. [50]	Recurrent HCC	China	Prosp	31	54 (37–66)	26/5	NR	NR

Table 2. *Cont.*

First Author	Subgroup	Country	Type of Study	No. of Patients	Age	Gender M/F	Child–Pugh A/B/C	MELD Score
Morise et al. [51]	Recurrent HCC	Japan	Retro	238	67 ± 11.8 *	181/57	NR	NR
Kanazawa et al. [52]	Recurrent HCC	Japan	Retro	20	70 (46–83)	15/5	19/1/0	NR
Onoe et al. [53]	Recurrent HCC	Japan	Retro	30	71(50–85)	23/7	30/0/0	5 (4–13)
Miyama et al. [54]	Recurrent HCC	Japan	Retro	115	68 ± 10.8 *	91/24	NR	NR

Data are expressed as median (min; max). NR, not reported. HCC, hepatocellular carcinoma. Retro, retrospective. Prosp, prospective. * Data expressed as mean ± standard deviation.

3.1. Advanced Cirrhosis

Four studies were included in the subgroup of LLRs in patients with advanced cirrhosis gathering a total of 156 patients, of whom 116 (74.4%) were male and 40 (25.6%) were female (Table 2). Median age ranged between 60 (27–79) and 68 (27–84). One-hundred and fifty patients (96.1%) were scored as Child–Pugh B and 6 (3.9%) as Child–Pugh C with a MELD score of 9 (4–22) that was reported only in one study [20]. Three studies reported the number of minor/major hepatectomies and anatomic/non-anatomic resections (Table 3). Minor hepatectomies were more frequently performed (117/131, 89.3%) as compared to major hepatectomies (14/131, 10.7%). Non-anatomic resections were performed in 74/131 (56.5%) cases, while anatomic hepatectomies were carried out in 57/131 (43.5%). Only one study described tumor localization (62% anterolateral and 38% posterosuperior segments) [20]. Operative time ranged between 99 (43–354) and 235 (84–605) minutes, while blood loss was between 50 (10–4750) and 800 (240–1000) mL (Table 3). Concerning hilar clamping, no Pringle maneuver was used in two studies, while 63/156 (40.4%) of the hepatectomies were performed under clamping among the remaining studies. Overall, 8/151 (5.3%) patients required intraoperative blood transfusions. Thirteen cases (8.3%) were converted to open. Concerning postoperative outcomes, 54 (34.6%) patients developed postoperative complications, of which 44 (81.5%) were minor and 10 (18.5%) were major (Table 4). Liver-specific morbidity was observed in 34 (21.8%) cases, with 3 (1.9%) patients experiencing liver failure, 29 (18.6%) patients experiencing ascites, and 2 (1.3%) patients experiencing bile leaks. Median hospital stay ranged between 2 (1–19) and 10 (7–15) days. Eight (5.1%) patients died within 90 days of surgery (Table 4).

Table 3. Intraoperative characteristics of the included studies.

First Author	Subgroup	Type of Hepatectomy Major/Minor	Type of Resection Non-Anatomic/Anatomic	Operative Time (min)	Pringle n (%)	Conversion n (%)	Blood Loss (mL)	Intraoperative Transfusions n (%)
Cipriani et al. [19]	Advanced cirrhosis	NR	NR	210 (120–280)	7 (28%)	4 (16%)	350 (200–1000)	3 (12%)
Troisi et al. [20]	Advanced cirrhosis	14/86	51/49	235 (84–605)	56 (56%)	6 (6%)	110 (0–3270)	1 (1–4)
Cai et al. [21]	Advanced cirrhosis	0/5	5/0	135 (80–170)	0	2 (40%)	800 (240–1000)	NR
Beard et al. [22]	Advanced cirrhosis	0/26	18/8	99 (43–354)	0	1 (4%)	50 (10–4750)	4 (15%)
Lim et al. [23]	Portal hypertension	2/16	12/6	240 (100–360)	NR	2 (11%)	300 (20–1700)	0 (0%)
Guo et al. [24]	Portal hypertension	0/16	16/0	336 ± 18 *	NR	NR	337 ± 351 *	NR
Molina et al. [25]	Portal hypertension	0/15	4/12	150 (90–215)	6 (40)	3 (20%)	90 (80–1000)	1 (7%)

Table 3. Cont.

First Author	Subgroup	Type of Hepatectomy Major/Minor	Type of Resection Non-Anatomic/Anatomic	Operative Time (min)	Pringle n (%)	Conversion n (%)	Blood Loss (mL)	Intraoperative Transfusions n (%)
Zheng et al. [26]	Portal hypertension	12/12	15/9	180 (150–250)	12 (50%)	2 (8.3%)	200 (100–400)	5 (21%)
Casellas et al. [27]	Portal hypertension	1/30	17/14	280 (202–338)	25 (81%)	1 (3%)	415 (200–731)	1 (3%)
Ruzzenente et al. [28]	Portal hypertension	14/75	NR	NR	NR	NR	NR	NR
Kwon et al. [29]	Large HCC	11/9	1/19	358.8 ± 136 *	0 (0%)	2 (10%)	600 (NR)	5 (25%)
Chiang et al. [30]	Large HCC	19/18	4/33	232 ± 91.2 *	NR	1 (2.7%)	623 ± 841.75 *	NR
Fu et al. [31]	Large HCC	0/14	0/14	195 (90–390)	NR	1 (7%)	50 (10–1200)	13 (93%)
Xu et al. [32]	Large HCC	28/74	51/51	217.5 (55–470)	50 (0–115) **	3 (3%)	175 (10–1000)	3 (3%)
Xiang et al. [33]	Large HCC	28/100	70/58	234 (105–501)	NR	12 (9.4%)	456 (50–2000)	23 (18%)
Levi Sandri et al. [34]	Large HCC	12/26	9/29	225 (159–270)	10 (26%)	7 (18.4%)	300 (75–800)	NR
Ai et al. [35]	Large HCC	5/92	24/73	245 ± 105 *	NR	9 (9%)	460 ± 426 *	5 (4.5%)
Casaccia et al. [36]	Posterosuperior segments	0/22	15/7	300 (120–560)	1 (4.5%)	1 (4.5%)	55 (20–1400)	10 (45.4%)
Xiang et al. [37]	Posterosuperior segments	14/42	31/25	217.5 ± 63.7 *	NR	10 (17.9%)	295 ± 187 *	9 (16.1%)
Lee et al. [38]	Posterosuperior segments	8/50	16/42	355 (165–930)	NR	8 (13.8%)	600 (130–14,300)	NR
Tagaytay et al. [39]	Posterosuperior segments	0/37	25/12	215 ± 70 *	NR	1 (2.7%)	201 ± 254 *	1 (1.8%)
Kwon et al. [40]	Posterosuperior segments	28/121	73/76	362 ± 180.7 *	60 (40%)	28 (19%)	1376 ± 2509 *	22 (15%)
Yoon et al. [41]	Posterosuperior segments	6/19	7/18	347 ± 117.9 *	NR	4 (16%)	986 ± 920.8 *	10 (40%)
Xiao et al. [42]	Posterosuperior segments	6/35	7/34	242 ± 73.6 *	NR	3 (7.3%)	272 ± 170 *	3 (7.3%)
Cherqui et al. [43]	Posterosuperior segments	1/26	10/17	240 (150–360)	NR	7 (26%)	338 ± 182 *	3 (15%)
Levi Sandri et al. [44]	Posterosuperior segments	12/50	32/30	240 (172–300)	32 (18–45) **	12 (18%)	200 (50–300)	5 (8%)
Liu et al. [45]	Recurrent HCC	1/29	19/11	200.5 (68–525)	0	4 (13.3%)	100 (10–600)	0 (0%)
Belli et al. [46]	Recurrent HCC	0/15	7/8	84 (40–130)	9	1 (6.6%)	NR	NR
Goh et al. [47]	Recurrent HCC	2/18	0/20	315 (181–395)	4 (20%)	3 (15%)	200 (100–450)	2 (10%)
Levi Sandri et al. [48]	Recurrent HCC	5/69	47/27	210 (150–300)	NR	9 (12.1%)	100 (50–225)	5 (6.7%)
Gon et al. [49]	Recurrent HCC	0/23	21/2	286 (251–417)	NR	1 (4%)	10 (10–50)	0 (0%)
Zhang et al. [50]	Recurrent HCC	0/31	19/12	116 ± 37.5 *	NR	0 (0%)	117.5 ± 35.5 *	NR
Morise et al. [51]	Recurrent HCC	9/229	NR	272 ± 187 *	NR	0 (0%)	268 ± 730 *	22 (9%)
Kanazawa et al. [52]	Recurrent HCC	0/20	NR	239 (69–658)	NR	2 (10%)	78 (1–1500)	0 (0%)
Onoe et al. [53]	Recurrent HCC	0/30	27/3	276 (125–589)	NR	2 (6.75%)	100 (0–1050)	NR
Miyama et al. [54]	Recurrent HCC	1/114	108/7	260 ± 158 *	NR	NR	283 ± 823 *	12 (10%)

Data are expressed as median (min–max). NR, not reported. HCC, hepatocellular carcinoma. * Data expressed as mean ± standard deviation. ** Mean time of clamping.

Table 4. Post operative outcomes of the included studies.

First Author	Subgroup	Morbidity n (%)	CD 0-II n (%)	CD III-IV n (%)	Liver Failure n (%)	Ascites n (%)	Bile Leak n (%)	Mortality n (%)
Cipriani et al. [19]	Advanced cirrhosis	9 (36%)	7 (78%)	2 (22%)	1 (4%)	3 (12%)	1 (4%)	4 (16%)
Troisi et al. [20]	Advanced cirrhosis	38 (38%)	31 (81.5%)	7 (18.5%)	2 (5%)	26 (68.4%)	1 (3%)	2 (2%)
Cai et al. [21]	Advanced cirrhosis	1 (20%)	1 (100%)	0 (0%)	0 (0%)	0 (0%)	0 (0%)	0 (0%)
Beard et al. [22]	Advanced cirrhosis	6 (23%)	5 (19%)	1 (4%)	0 (0%)	0 (0%)	0 (0%)	2 (8%)
Lim et al. [23]	Portal hypertension	7 (39%)	7 (100%)	0 (0%)	2 (28.5%)	2 (28.5%)	0 (0%)	0 (0%)
Guo et al. [24]	Portal hypertension	6 (37.5%)	NR	NR	NR	NR	NR	0 (0%)
Molina et al. [25]	Portal hypertension	6 (40%)	4 (67%)	2 (33%)	0 (0%)	1 (17%)	0 (0%)	0 (0%)
Zheng et al. [26]	Portal hypertension	8 (33%)	5 (62.5%)	3 (37.5%)	1 (12.5%)	2 (25%)	0 (0%)	0 (0%)
Casellas et al. [27]	Portal hypertension	16 (52%)	14 (93%)	2 (7%)	3 (19%)	5 (31%)	0 (0%)	0 (0%)
Ruzzenente et al. [28]	Portal hypertension	26 (29%)	15 (57%)	11 (42%)	NR	NR	NR	0 (0%)
Kwon et al. [29]	Large HCC	3 (15%)	3 (100%)	0 (0%)	0 (0%)	0 (0%)	0 (0%)	0 (0%)
Chiang et al. [30]	Large HCC	7 (18.9%)	6 (85%)	1 (15%)	1 (14%)	3 (43%)	1 (14%)	0 (0%)
Fu et al. [31]	Large HCC	1 (7%)	1 (100%)	0 (0%)	0 (0%)	0 (0%)	0 (0%)	0 (0%)
Xu et al. [32]	Large HCC	20 (19%)	15 (75%)	5 (25%)	4 (20%)	5 (25%)	4 (20%)	0 (0%)
Xiang et al. [33]	Large HCC	26 (20.3%)	13 (50%)	13 (50%)	2 (7.7%)	0 (0%)	0 (0%)	1 (0.78%)
Levi Sandri et al. [34]	Large HCC	20 (52%)	17 (85%)	3 (15%)	0 (0%)	NR	NR	0 (0%)
Ai et al. [35]	Large HCC	10 (10%)	10 (100%)	0 (0%)	0 (0%)	0 (0%)	0 (0%)	0 (0%)
Casaccia et al. [36]	Posterosuperior segments	4 (18%)	4 (100%)	0 (0%)	NR	NR	NR	0 (0%)
Xiang et al. [37]	Posterosuperior segments	9 (16.1%)	9 (100%)	0 (0%)	0 (0%)	1 (11%)	1 (11%)	0 (0%)
Lee et al. [38]	Posterosuperior segments	10 (17.2%)	4 (40%)	6 (60%)	NR	NR	NR	0 (0%)
Tagaytay et al. [39]	Posterosuperior segments	3 (8.1%)	2 (67%)	1 (33%)	0 (0%)	0 (0%)	0 (0%)	0 (0%)
Kwon et al. [40]	Posterosuperior segments	28 (19%)	14 (50%)	14 (50%)	NR	NR	NR	0 (0%)

Table 4. Cont.

First Author	Subgroup	Morbidity n (%)	CD 0-II n (%)	CD III-IV n (%)	Liver Failure n (%)	Ascites n (%)	Bile Leak n (%)	Mortality n (%)
Yoon et al. [41]	Posterosuperior segments	7 (28%)	7 (100%)	0 (0%)	NR	NR	NR	0 (0%)
Xiao et al. [42]	Posterosuperior segments	7 (17%)	5 (71%)	2 (29%)	0 (0%)	1 (14%)	1 (14%)	0 (0%)
Cherqui et al. [43]	Posterosuperior segments	9 (33%)	NR	NR	1 (4%)	2 (7%)	0 (0%)	0 (0%)
Levi Sandri et al. [44]	Posterosuperior segments	NR	NR	NR	NR	NR	NR	0 (0%)
Liu et al. [45]	Recurrent HCC	2 (6.7%)	1 (50%)	1 (50%)	0 (0%)	0 (0%)	1 (50%)	0 (0%)
Belli et al. [46]	Recurrent HCC	4 (26.6%)	4 (100%)	0 (0%)	0 (0%)	1 (25%)	0 (0%)	0 (0%)
Goh et al. [47]	Recurrent HCC	2 (10%)	2 (100%)	0 (0%)	NR	NR	NR	0 (0%)
Levi Sandri et al. [48]	Recurrent HCC	17 (22.9%)	5 (29%)	12 (71%)	NR	3 (3.7%)	1 (1.7%)	0 (0%)
Gon et al. [49]	Recurrent HCC	2 (9%)	1 (50%)	1 (50%)	0 (0%)	0 (0%)	0 (0%)	0 (0%)
Zhang et al. [50]	Recurrent HCC	NR	NR	0 (0%)	NR	NR	NR	1 (3%)
Morise et al. [51]	Recurrent HCC	36 (15%)	7 (19%)	29 (81%)	2 (5.5%)	5 (14%)	15 (42%)	1 (0.4%)
Kanazawa et al. [52]	Recurrent HCC	1 (5%)	0 (0%)	1 (100%)	0 (0%)	1 (100%)	0 (0%)	0 (0%)
Onoe et al. [53]	Recurrent HCC	30 (100%)	28 (93.3%)	2 (6.7%)	0 (0%)	0 (0%)	0 (0%)	0 (0%)
Miyama et al. [54]	Recurrent HCC	15 (13%)	10 (67%)	5 (22%)	NR	NR	NR	0 (0%)

Data are expressed as median (range). NR, not reported. HCC, hepatocellular carcinoma. CD, Clavien–Dindo.

Comparative Results between Open vs. Minimally Invasive Surgery in Advanced Cirrhosis

Only Troisi et al. compared open vs. laparoscopic surgery in advanced cirrhosis. All patients were scored as Child–Pugh B. Laparoscopy was associated with lower blood loss (median 110 mL versus 400 mL in the open group; $p = 0.004$), lower morbidity (38% vs. 51%; $p = 0.041$) and fewer major complications (7% vs. 21%; $p = 0.010$) [20].

3.2. Portal Hypertension

Six studies were included in the subgroup of LLRs in patients with portal hypertension with a total of 194 patients, 139 (71.6%) male and 55 (28.4%) female with a median age between 50 (29–70) and 64 (52–83). One-hundred and sixty-two (83.5%) patients were scored as Child–Pugh A, 29 (14.9%) were scored as Child–Pugh B, and 3 (1.5%) were scored as Child–Pugh C, with a MELD score of 8 (6–11) that was reported only in one study [23] (Table 2). Tumor size ranged between 2.0 (1.1–5.7) and 3.3 (2.0–4.8) cm. The majority of patients underwent a minor hepatectomy (165, 85.1%), while major hepatectomies were performed in 29 (14.9%) cases. Non-anatomic resections were conducted in 64/105 (61.0%) patients, while 41/105 (39.0%) underwent an anatomical hepatectomy (Table 3). Only one study reported tumor's location (77% anterolateral and 23% posterosuperior segments) [27].

Operative time ranged between 150 (90–215) and 336 ± 18 min. Blood loss ranged between 90 (80–1000) and 415 (200–731) mL. Pringle maneuver was performed in 43/71 cases (60.6%). Intraoperative blood transfusions were needed in 7/89 patients (7.9%). Conversion to open happened in 8/89 (9.0%) cases (Table 3). Regarding postoperative outcomes, 69 (35.5%) patients developed postoperative complications of which 45 (71.4%) were minor and 18 (28.6%) were major. Liver-specific morbidity was reported in 16/89 (17.9%) cases with 89 (6.7%) patients developing liver failure and 10/89 (11.2%) experiencing ascites. Hospital stays ranged between 3 (2–20) and 13.5 (9–24) days. In this subgroup, neither bile leak nor 90-day mortality was observed (Table 4).

Comparative Results between Open vs. Minimally Invasive Surgery in Portal Hypertension

Only Ruzzenente et al. reported comparative results between laparoscopic and open surgery in portal hypertension. They found that patients undergoing laparoscopic approach had shorter hospital stay (>7 days: open 55% vs. laparoscopic 29%, $p < 0.001$) as well as lower morbidity (open: 42% vs. laparoscopic: 29%, $p = 0.001$) [28].

3.3. Large HCC

Seven studies were included in the subgroup of patients with large HCC, with a total of 436 individuals, 345 (79.1%) males, and 91 (20.9%) females. Age ranged between 51 ± 11.9 and 71 (61–77). Two hundred and forty-one patients (80.3%) were scored as Child–Pugh A, and 59/300 (19.7%) were scored as Child–Pugh B (Table 2). No Child–Pugh C patients were reported in this subgroup. Tumor size ranged between 6 (5.5–10) and 7.8 ± 2.15 cm. Only one study described tumor locations (73 (71.56%) anterolateral and 29 (28.44%) posterosuperior segments) [32]. Three hundred and thirty-three patients (76.4%) underwent a minor hepatectomy, while 103 (23.6%) were submitted to a major resection. Anatomic hepatectomies were performed in 277 patients (63.5%) (Table 3). Operative time ranged between 195 (90–390) and 358 ± 136 min. Pringle maneuver was applied in 10/58 (17.2%) cases. Blood loss ranged between 50 (10–1200) and 623 ± 841.7 mL. Forty-nine (13.6%) patients required intraoperative blood transfusions. Thirty five (8.0%) cases were converted to laparotomy (Table 3). Only one study described the reason for conversion (four cases for uncontrollable bleeding, two cases for oncological safety and three cases for tumor encroaching on the diaphragmatic muscle) [35]. Regarding postoperative outcomes, 87 (19.9%) patients developed complications, of which 65 (74.7%) were minor and 22 (25.3%) were major (Table 4). Liver-specific morbidity was observed in 20/398 (5.0%) cases, with 7/436 patients (1.6%) developing liver failure, 8/398 (2.0%) developing ascites, and 5/398 (1.3%) developing bile leak. Median hospital stay ranged between 6 (4–8) and 11.4 ± 3.1 days. One patient (0.2%) died within 90 days of surgery.

Comparative Results between Open vs. Minimally Invasive Surgery in Large HCC

Four studies compared the postoperative results of open vs. laparoscopic surgery [30,31,33,35] in the setting of large lesions. All of them showed shorter hospital stay in the laparoscopic group. Xiang et al. and Ai et al. showed lower rates of postoperative complications in the laparoscopic group [33,35]. Chiang et al. and Fu et al. found a lower blood loss [30,31]. No differences were found in terms of postoperative mortality.

3.4. Posterosuperior Segments

Nine studies were included in the subgroup of LLRs in patients with HCC located in the posterosuperior segments with a total of 477 patients, 360 (75.5%) male and 117 (24.5%) female with an age ranging between 51.6 ± 10.2 and 71 (59.5–75) (Table 2). Three hundred and seventy-two patients (96.9%) were scored as Child–Pugh A, 10/384 (2.6%) were scored as Child–Pugh B and 2/384 (0.5%) were scored as Child–Pugh C. Tumor size ranged between 2.31 ± 0.78 and 4.22 ± 2.05 cm. Major hepatectomies were performed in 75 (15.7%) cases, while 402 (84.3%) underwent a minor resection. In 216 (45.2%) cases, a non-anatomic resection was performed as compared to 261 (54.8%) in which the resection was anatomic (Table 3). Operative time ranged between 215 ± 70 and 362 ± 180.7 min. Pringle maneuver was applied in 61/171 (35.7%) cases. Blood loss ranged between 55 (20–1400) and 1376 ± 2509 mL. Sixty-three (15.0%) patients required an intraoperative blood transfusion, and conversion to open was necessary in 15.5% of cases (Table 3). Regarding postoperative outcomes, 77/415 (18.6%) patients had complications of which 45 (66.2%) were minor and 23 (33.8%) were major. Liver-specific morbidity was observed in 7/161 (4.3%) cases, with 1/161 (0.6%) patient developing liver failure, 4/161 (2.4%) experiencing ascites, and 2 (1.2%) experiencing bile leaks (Table 4). Hospital stay ranged between 5 (3–7) and 10.5 ± 2.7 days. Mortality at 90 days was 0%.

Comparative Results between Open vs. Minimally Invasive Surgery for Lesions Located in Posterosuperior Segments

Three studies compare the results of laparoscopic and open surgery for HCC located in posterosuperior segments [39,40,42]. All of the studies showed a lower morbidity rate and shorter hospital stay in the laparoscopic group. Only Tagaytay et al. found lower blood loss (218.11 vs. 358.92 mL, $p = 0.046$) and shorter operative time (7.03 vs. 11.78 days, $p = 0.001$) in the laparoscopic group. No differences were found in terms of 90-day mortality.

3.5. Recurrent HCC

Ten studies were included in the subgroup of repeat LLRs in patients with recurrent HCC with a total of 596 patients, 450 (77.4%) male and 131 (22.6%) female with a median age between 54 (37–66) and 72 (67–79). One hundred and eighty-three patients (95.3%) were Child–Pugh A, and 9/192 (4.7%) were Child–Pugh B. No Child–Pugh C patients were reported in this subgroup (Table 2). Tumor size ranged between 1.25 (0.8–3.5) and 3.8 (3.3–4.5) cm. Only two studies reported on the location of tumors (254 (71.95%) anterior segments and 99 (28.05%) posterior segments) [51,54]. Minor hepatectomies were performed in the vast majority of cases (578, 97.0%) and 248/338 (73.4%) patients underwent a non-anatomic resection. The median time interval from the first operation ranged between 3.9 (0.2–16) and 32 (3–136) months. In 318 (77%) cases, the first operation was performed by open and in 95 (23%), it was performed by laparoscopy. The site of recurrence was described only in two studies and was shown to be ipsilateral in 40 (65.5%) cases and controlateral in 21 (34.5%) cases [49,50]. Operative time ranged between 84 (40–130) and 315 (181–395) min (Table 3). Pringle maneuver was applied in 13/65 (0.2%) cases, which was probably due to difficult surgical anatomy because of re-operation. Blood loss ranged between 10 (10–50) and 283 ± 823 mL, and 41/520 (7.9%) patients required intraoperative blood transfusions. Conversion to laparotomy happened in 22/481 (4.6%). Regarding postoperative outcomes, 109/565 (19.3%) patients developed complications of which 58 (53.3%) were minor and 51 (46.7%) were major (Table 4). Two patients (0.5%) experienced liver failure, 10 (2.3%) developed ascites, and 17 (3.9%) developed a bile leak. The hospital stay ranged between 4 (3–5) and 11.7 ± 11.5 days. Two patients died within 90 days from surgery with a mortality rate of 0.34%.

Comparative Results between Open vs. Minimally Invasive Surgery for Recurrent HCC

Eight studies compared the results of laparoscopic vs. open surgery for recurrent HCCs [45,47,49–54]. All of them showed a shorter hospital stay in the laparoscopic group. The majority found lower blood loss [45,49–51,53] and only three studies reported lower postoperative morbidity rate in the laparoscopic group [45,52,54]. Concerning operative time, Morise et al. and Goh et al. reported longer operative time, while Zhang et al. reported shorter operative time in the laparoscopic group [47,50,51]. Gon et al. showed shorter operative time in the laparoscopic group only if the recurrent HCC was located in the controlateral parenchyma from the previous resection [49]. No statistically significant differences in 90-day mortality was observed.

4. Discussion

Despite the recent advances in surgical techniques and the widespread adoption of minimally invasive approaches for liver resections, patients with advanced cirrhosis, portal hypertension, large and recurrent lesions, and tumors located in the posterosuperior segments still represent a challenge even in the most experienced hands. Indeed, perioperative complications in the above-mentioned settings are potentially high, and long-term outcomes are still under investigation [15]. Careful preoperative evaluation and assessment of potential risk factors is key to guide a thorough discussion of potential risks and benefits, thereby selecting patients and minimizing unexpected events.

Patients with advanced cirrhosis and portal hypertension represent one of the most difficult clinical scenarios in the management of HCC [3]. Indeed, these patients may present with impaired performance status, sarcopenia, encephalopathy, ascites, and severe portosystemic shunts. Therapeutic alternatives such as liver transplantation and locoregional options might come into play, but many patients still undergo resection. The decision of whether to operate on patients with such advanced conditions represents a dilemma. Perioperative risks are high, with increased rates of postoperative morbidity, especially liver failure and ascites [17,55,56]. In this setting, minimally invasive approaches could be beneficial to improve postoperative outcomes [7,9,21]. Indeed, the abdominal cavity is respected as compared to a large open incision, avoiding the interruption of portosystemic shunts, manipulation of the liver is reduced, and the abdominal cavity is not exposed to the air, thus avoiding electrolyte imbalances [57]. However, the LLRs in such patients are technically more challenging. Adhesions are well vascularized, there is an increased bleeding during the transection, and the parenchyma is stiff, thus limiting exposure. According to our review, only four papers have been reported describing LLRs on AC, thus limiting the evidence in this setting. Furthermore, most patients with advanced cirrhosis were scored as Child–Pugh B, while only six patients were scored as C. The literature on liver resection in Child–Pugh C patients is limited both in open and laparoscopic surgery because of the questionable postoperative outcomes [15]. In our opinion, therapeutic alternatives should be well discussed in such patients, as no sufficient data are available so far to support resection, especially in laparoscopy. Although minor and non-anatomical resections were more frequent in these subgroups, intraoperative blood loss was high, the Pringle maneuver was frequently applied (40.4% in AC and 60.6% in PH), and conversion rates were high (8.3% in AC and 9.0% in PH), confirming the technical complexity of these procedures. Despite the potential advantages of the minimally invasive approach, according to our review, AC and PH had the highest rates of morbidity, especially postoperative liver failure (up to 6.7% in PH), ascites production (up to 18.6% in AC) and the highest chance of dying after surgery (5.1% mortality in AC). This confirms that the presence of clinically significant portal hypertension and advanced cirrhosis are important prognostic factors for worse postoperative outcomes, especially in terms of liver decompensation surrogates. For this reason, these very high-risk patients, when considered for surgery, should be managed by experienced surgeons in high volume centers and should be well selected to improve the outcomes.

Large HCCs represent another common surgical dilemma to approach by laparoscopy. These lesions frequently require major hepatectomies and/or anatomic resections. The dissection of the hilar structures, the large parenchymal transection, the major vasculobiliary structures encountered and the extensive mobilizations require specific learning curve, as each of these steps have specific technical challenges [8,58,59]. This is enhanced when dealing with large lesions, since exposure and mobilization are further limited [60]. Notwithstanding, perioperative outcomes were good with no major blood loss or high rates of conversions to open, and only 20% of patients were developing postoperative morbidity, mostly minor in severity. A cutoff of 5 cm was applied by most of the included studies to define large lesions [29–35]. Together with the dimensions of the tumor that should be further categorized, we also believe that localization of the lesion should be considered in future studies, as perioperative outcomes could be very different between a lesion located close to the hilum or at the periphery. Dimensions and localization would therefore allow for a more precise selection of patients, thereby improving outcomes.

Posterosuperior segments were initially considered as a contraindication to the laparoscopic approach, being defined as the non-laparoscopic segments [61]. Thanks to the widespread adoption of minimally invasive approaches and to the learning curves, nowadays, lesions in the PS segments are frequently approached by laparoscopy, with good short and long-term outcomes for both benign and malignant lesions [62,63]. However, few reports on HCCs in the PS segments exist, as this still represents a challenging indication, especially in cirrhotic patients. According to our review, intraoperative and postoperative outcomes were good, with a morbidity rate as high as 18.6%, thereby disclosing the safety and efficacy of such approach. However, conversion to open was high (15.5%) as was the need for Pringle maneuver (36%), again stressing the technical complexity and thereby confirming the need for advanced technical skills.

Despite the good long-term outcomes of liver resections for HCC, as much as 70% of patients will experience recurrence of their tumor [3,64]. Salvage liver transplantation, for those eligible, represents a valid treatment. However, repeat liver resection could also be used in selected patients, as outcomes are good both in the short and long-term. According to our review, most resections were minor, reflecting the fact that a parenchymal sparing policy is very important in these patients that have already undergone a previous resection. Unnecessary sacrifice of healthy parenchyma should be minimized. We found that repeat resections for recurrent HCCs require long operative time. This is reasonable considering adhesions from previous surgery that can often be vascularized in cirrhotic patients, thereby prolonging the dissection and exposure as well as preparation of the Pringle maneuver. Indeed, the Pringle maneuver was rarely applied (only 0.2% of cases), reflecting the fact that during repeat resections, the pedicle is difficult to sling given previous maneuvers in the area. This makes the liver transection phase potentially riskier, as bleeding cannot be controlled by hilar clamping.

This systematic review has some limitations; first, it is mainly based on retrospective studies, including mostly small and single-center studies. While the evidence is limited for advanced cirrhosis and portal hypertension, more patients have been reported in the setting of large and recurrent lesions and in posterosuperior segments. The wide inclusion period of the studies might also limit the conclusions, since technical evolutions have happened and are still happening in the field of LLRs. Therefore, we need more data to compare minimally invasive surgery and open surgery in the mentioned situations. In this setting, robotics has been increasingly used in the most recent years: from initial skepticism due to the lack of substantial literature to a worldwide adoption of this technique with similar outcomes as compared to laparoscopy [65]. This review was limited to patients operated on by laparoscopy, and conclusions should therefore not be generalized to robotics. Future studies investigating the role of robotic liver resections in challenging scenarios such as the ones depicted in this review are warranted. Long-term outcomes also have been rarely disclosed in these settings [66–68]. Further studies should clarify the oncological safety. To our knowledge, this is the first review that includes all the challenging indications for LLRs for HCC. Only Yin et al. explored the role of LLRs in posterosuperior segments, but no pooled evidence exists concerning AC, PH, large lesions, tumors in the PS segments and repeat LLRs [69].

5. Conclusions

Laparoscopic liver resections for HCC have good short- and long-term outcomes. Advanced cirrhosis and portal hypertension, large and recurrent tumors and lesions located in the posterosuperior segments are challenging clinical scenarios that should be carefully approached by laparoscopy. Safe short-term outcomes can be achieved provided experienced surgeons and high-volume centers. Advanced cirrhosis and portal hypertension are the riskiest scenarios. The selection of patients is key in these settings.

Author Contributions: Conceptualization, G.B. and E.M.M.; methodology, M.C.; software, G.M.; validation, R.L.M., S.F. and N.G.; formal analysis, M.A.; investigation, A.L.; resources, E.G.; data curation, D.C.; writing—original draft preparation, L.D.C.; writing—review and editing, E.M.M. and G.B.; visualization, D.V.; supervision, G.B.; project administration, G.M.E.; funding acquisition, P.M. All authors have read and agreed to the published version of the manuscript.

Funding: This research received no external funding.

Data Availability Statement: Not applicable.

Acknowledgments: The authors would like to thank Matilde Berardi for her substantial support during manuscript drafting.

Conflicts of Interest: The authors declare no conflict of interest.

References

1. Ferlay, J.; Soerjomataram, I.; Dikshit, R.; Eser, S.; Mathers, C.; Rebelo, M.; Parkin, D.M.; Forman, D.; Bray, F. Cancer incidence and mortality worldwide: Sources, methods and major patterns in GLOBOCAN 2012. *Int. J. Cancer* **2015**, *136*, E359–E386. [CrossRef] [PubMed]
2. Siegel, R.L.; Miller, K.D.; Jemal, A. Cancer statistics, 2020. *CA Cancer J. Clin.* **2020**, *70*, 7–30. [CrossRef] [PubMed]
3. Reig, M.; Forner, A.; Rimola, J.; Ferrer-Fàbrega, J.; Burrel, M.; Garcia-Criado, Á.; Kelley, R.K.; Galle, P.R.; Mazzaferro, V.; Salem, R.; et al. BCLC strategy for prognosis prediction and treatment recommendation: The 2022 update. *J. Hepatol.* **2022**, *76*, 681–693. [CrossRef] [PubMed]
4. Gagner, M.; Rheault, M.; Dubuc, J. Laparoscopic partial hepatectomy for liver tumor. *Surg. Endosc.* **1992**, *6*, 97–98.
5. Ciria, R.; Cherqui, D.; Geller, D.A.; Briceno, J.; Wakabayashi, G. Comparative Short-term Benefits of Laparoscopic Liver Resection: 9000 Cases and Climbing. *Ann. Surg.* **2016**, *263*, 761–777. [CrossRef]
6. Ciria, R.; Gomez-Luque, I.; Ocaña, S.; Cipriani, F.; Halls, M.; Briceño, J.; Okuda, Y.; Troisi, R.; Rotellar, F.; Soubrane, O.; et al. A Systematic Review and Meta-Analysis Comparing the Short- and Long-Term Outcomes for Laparoscopic and Open Liver Resections for Hepatocellular Carcinoma: Updated Results from the European Guidelines Meeting on Laparoscopic Liver Surgery, Southampton, UK, 2017. *Ann. Surg. Oncol.* **2019**, *26*, 252–263. [CrossRef]
7. Morise, Z.; Ciria, R.; Cherqui, D.; Chen, K.-H.; Belli, G.; Wakabayashi, G. Can we expand the indications for laparoscopic liver resection? A systematic review and meta-analysis of laparoscopic liver resection for patients with hepatocellular carcinoma and chronic liver disease. *J. Hepato-Biliary-Pancreatic Sci.* **2015**, *22*, 342–352. [CrossRef]
8. Abu Hilal, M.; Aldrighetti, L.; Dagher, I.; Edwin, B.; Troisi, R.I.; Alikhanov, R.; Aroori, S.; Belli, G.; Besselink, M.; Briceno, J.; et al. The Southampton Consensus Guidelines for Laparoscopic Liver Surgery: From Indication to Implementation. *Ann. Surg.* **2018**, *268*, 11–18. [CrossRef]
9. Berardi, G.; Morise, Z.; Sposito, C.; Igarashi, K.; Panetta, V.; Simonelli, I.; Kim, S.; Goh, B.K.; Kubo, S.; Tanaka, S.; et al. Development of a nomogram to predict outcome after liver resection for hepatocellular carcinoma in Child-Pugh B cirrhosis. *J. Hepatol.* **2020**, *72*, 75–84. [CrossRef]
10. D'Hondt, M.; Ovaere, S.; Knol, J.; Vandeputte, M.; Parmentier, I.; De Meyere, C.; Vansteenkiste, F.; Besselink, M.; Pottel, H.; Verslype, C. Laparoscopic right posterior sectionectomy: Single-center experience and technical aspects. *Langenbeck's Arch. Surg.* **2019**, *404*, 21–29. [CrossRef]
11. Azoulay, D.; Ramos, E.; Casellas-Robert, M.; Salloum, C.; Lladó, L.; Nadler, R.; Busquets, J.; Caula-Freixa, C.; Mils, K.; Lopez-Ben, S.; et al. Liver resection for hepatocellular carcinoma in patients with clinically significant portal hypertension. *JHEP Rep.* **2020**, *3*, 100190. [CrossRef]
12. Child, C.G.; Turcotte, J.G. Surgery and portal hypertension. *Major Probl. Clin. Surg.* **1964**, *1*, 1–85.
13. Berzigotti, A.; Reig, M.; Abraldes, J.G.; Bosch, J.; Bruix, J. Portal hypertension and the outcome of surgery for hepatocellular carcinoma in compensated cirrhosis: A systematic review and meta-analysis. *Hepatology* **2015**, *61*, 526–536. [CrossRef]
14. Berardi, G.; Aghayan, D.; Fretland, Å.A.; Elberm, H.; Cipriani, F.; Spagnoli, A.; Montalti, R.; Ceelen, W.P.; Aldrighetti, L.; Abu Hilal, M.; et al. Multicentre analysis of the learning curve for laparoscopic liver resection of the posterosuperior segments. *Br. J. Surg.* **2019**, *106*, 1512–1522. [CrossRef]
15. European Association for the Study of the Liver. EASL Clinical Practice Guidelines: Management of hepatocellular carcinoma. *J. Hepatol.* **2018**, *69*, 182–236. [CrossRef]
16. Dindo, D.; Demartines, N.; Clavien, P.A. Classification of surgical complications: A new proposal with evaluation in a cohort of 6336 patients and results of a survey. *Ann. Surg.* **2004**, *240*, 205–213. [CrossRef]
17. Rahbari, N.N.; Garden, O.J.; Padbury, R.; Brooke-Smith, M.; Crawford, M.; Adam, R.; Koch, M.; Makuuchi, M.; Dematteo, R.P.; Christophi, C.; et al. Posthepatectomy liver failure: A definition and grading by the International Study Group of Liver Surgery (ISGLS). *Surgery* **2011**, *149*, 713–724. [CrossRef]
18. Stang, A. Critical evaluation of the Newcastle-Ottawa scale for the assessment of the quality of nonrandomized studies in meta-analyses. *Eur. J. Epidemiol.* **2010**, *25*, 603–605. [CrossRef]

19. Cipriani, F.; Fantini, C.; Ratti, F.; Lauro, R.; Tranchart, H.; Halls, M.; Scuderi, V.; Barkhatov, L.; Edwin, B.; Troisi, R.I.; et al. Laparoscopic liver resections for hepatocellular carcinoma. Can we extend the surgical indication in cirrhotic patients? *Surg. Endosc.* **2018**, *32*, 617–626. [CrossRef]
20. Troisi, R.I.; Berardi, G.; Morise, Z.; Cipriani, F.; Ariizumi, S.; Sposito, C.; Panetta, V.; Simonelli, I.; Kim, S.; Goh, B.K.P.; et al. Laparoscopic and open liver resection for hepatocellular carcinoma with Child–Pugh B cirrhosis: Multicentre propensity score-matched study. *Br. J. Surg.* **2021**, *108*, 196–204. [CrossRef]
21. Cai, X.; Liang, X.; Yu, T.; Liang, Y.; Jing, R.; Jiang, W.; Li, J.; Ying, H. Liver cirrhosis grading Child-Pugh class B: A Goliath to challenge in laparoscopic liver resection?—Prior experience and matched comparisons. *HepatoBiliary Surg. Nutr.* **2015**, *4*, 391–397. [CrossRef] [PubMed]
22. Beard, R.E.; Wang, Y.; Khan, S.; Marsh, J.W.; Tsung, A.; Geller, D.A. Laparoscopic liver resection for hepatocellular carcinoma in early and advanced cirrhosis. *HPB* **2018**, *20*, 521–529. [CrossRef]
23. Lim, C.; Osseis, M.; Lahat, E.; Doussot, A.; Sotirov, D.; Hemery, F.; Lantéri-Minet, M.; Feray, C.; Salloum, C.; Azoulay, D. Safety of laparoscopic hepatectomy in patients with hepatocellular carcinoma and portal hypertension: Interim analysis of an open prospective study. *Surg. Endosc.* **2019**, *33*, 811–820. [CrossRef] [PubMed]
24. Guo, P.; Liao, S.; Li, J.; Zheng, S. Clinical application of combined laparoscopic surgery in the treatment of primary hepatocellular carcinoma with portal hypertension: A report of 16 cases. *Transl. Cancer Res.* **2019**, *8*, 330–337. [CrossRef] [PubMed]
25. Molina, V.; Sampson-Dávila, J.; Ferrer, J.; Fondevila, C.; del Gobbo, R.D.; Calatayud, D.; Bruix, J.; García-Valdecasas, J.C.; Fuster, J. Benefits of laparoscopic liver resection in patients with hepatocellular carcinoma and portal hypertension: A case-matched study. *Surg. Endosc.* **2018**, *32*, 2345–2354. [CrossRef]
26. Zheng, J.; Feng, X.; Liang, Y.; Cai, J.; Shi, Z.; Kirih, M.A.; Tao, L.; Liang, X. Safety and feasibility of laparoscopic liver resection for hepatocellular carcinoma with clinically significant portal hypertension: A propensity score-matched study. *Surg. Endosc.* **2021**, *35*, 3267–3278. [CrossRef]
27. Casellas-Robert, M.; Lim, C.; Lopez-Ben, S.; Lladó, L.; Salloum, C.; Codina-Font, J.; Comas-Cufí, M.; Ramos, E.; Figueras, J.; Azoulay, D. Laparoscopic Liver Resection for Hepatocellular Carcinoma in Child–Pugh A Patients with and Without Portal Hypertension: A Multicentre Study. *World J. Surg.* **2020**, *44*, 3915–3922. [CrossRef]
28. Ruzzenente, A.; Bagante, F.; Ratti, F.; Alaimo, L.; Marques, H.P.; da Silva, S.G.; Soubrane, O.; Endo, I.; Sahara, K.; Beal, E.; et al. Minimally Invasive Versus Open Liver Resection for Hepatocellular Carcinoma in the Setting of Portal Vein Hypertension: Results of an International Multi-institutional Analysis. *Ann. Surg. Oncol.* **2020**, *27*, 3360–3371. [CrossRef]
29. Kwon, Y.; Han, H.-S.; Yoon, Y.-S.; Cho, J.Y. Are Large Hepatocellular Carcinomas Still a Contraindication for Laparoscopic Liver Resection? *J. Laparoendosc. Adv. Surg. Tech. A* **2015**, *25*, 98–102. [CrossRef]
30. Chiang, M.-H.; Tsai, K.-Y.; Chen, H.-A.; Wang, W.-Y.; Huang, M.-T. Comparison of surgical outcomes for laparoscopic liver resection of large hepatocellular carcinomas: A retrospective observation from single-center experience. *Asian J. Surg.* **2021**, *44*, 1376–1382. [CrossRef]
31. Fu, X.-T.; Tang, Z.; Shi, Y.-H.; Zhou, J.; Liu, W.-R.; Gao, Q.; Ding, G.-Y.; Chen, J.-F.; Song, K.; Wang, X.-Y.; et al. Laparoscopic Versus Open Left Lateral Segmentectomy for Large Hepatocellular Carcinoma: A Propensity Score–Matched Analysis. *Surg. Laparosc. Endosc. Percutaneous Tech.* **2019**, *29*, 513–519. [CrossRef]
32. Xu, H.; Liu, F.; Hao, X.; Wei, Y.; Li, B.; Wen, T.; Wang, W.; Yang, J. Laparoscopically anatomical versus non-anatomical liver resection for large hepatocellular carcinoma. *HPB* **2020**, *22*, 136–143. [CrossRef]
33. Xiang, L.; Li, J.; Chen, J.; Wang, X.; Guo, P.; Fan, Y.; Zheng, S. Prospective cohort study of laparoscopic and open hepatectomy for hepatocellular carcinoma. *Br. J. Surg.* **2016**, *103*, 1895–1901. [CrossRef]
34. Sandri, G.B.L.; Spoletini, G.; Vennarecci, G.; Francone, E.; Abu Hilal, M.; Ettorre, G.M. Laparoscopic liver resection for large HCC: Short- and long-term outcomes in relation to tumor size. *Surg. Endosc.* **2018**, *32*, 4772–4779. [CrossRef]
35. Ai, J.-H.; Li, J.-W.; Chen, J.; Bie, P.; Wang, S.-G.; Zheng, S.-G. Feasibility and Safety of Laparoscopic Liver Resection for Hepatocellular Carcinoma with a Tumor Size of 5–10 cm. *PLoS ONE* **2013**, *8*, e72328. [CrossRef]
36. Casaccia, M.; Andorno, E.; Di Domenico, S.; Nardi, I.; Bottino, G.; Gelli, M.; Valente, U. Laparoscopic liver resection for hepatocellular carcinoma in cirrhotic patients. Feasibility of nonanatomic resection in difficult tumor locations. *J. Minimal Access Surg.* **2011**, *7*, 222–226. [CrossRef]
37. Xiang, L.; Xiao, L.; Li, J.; Chen, J.; Fan, Y.; Zheng, S. Safety and Feasibility of Laparoscopic Hepatectomy for Hepatocellular Carcinoma in the Posterosuperior Liver Segments. *World J. Surg.* **2015**, *39*, 1202–1209. [CrossRef]
38. Lee, W.; Han, H.-S.; Yoon, Y.-S.; Cho, J.Y.; Choi, Y.; Shin, H.K.; Jang, J.Y.; Choi, H.; Kwon, S.U. Comparison of laparoscopic liver resection for hepatocellular carcinoma located in the posterosuperior segments or anterolateral segments: A case-matched analysis. *Surgery* **2016**, *160*, 1219–1226. [CrossRef]
39. Tagaytay, T.G.; Han, D.H.; Chong, J.U.; Hwang, H.S.; Choi, G.H.; Kim, K.S. Laparoscopic Minor Liver Resections for Hepatocellular Carcinoma in the Posterosuperior Segments Using the Rubber Band Technique. *World J. Surg.* **2022**, *46*, 1151–1160. [CrossRef]
40. Kwon, Y.; Cho, J.Y.; Han, H.-S.; Yoon, Y.-S.; Lee, H.W.; Lee, J.S.; Lee, B.; Kim, M. Improved Outcomes of Laparoscopic Liver Resection for Hepatocellular Carcinoma Located in Posterosuperior Segments of the Liver. *World J. Surg.* **2021**, *45*, 1178–1185. [CrossRef]
41. Yoon, Y.-S.; Han, H.-S.; Cho, J.Y.; Ahn, K.S. Total laparoscopic liver resection for hepatocellular carcinoma located in all segments of the liver. *Surg. Endosc.* **2010**, *24*, 1630–1637. [CrossRef] [PubMed]

42. Xiao, L.; Xiang, L.-J.; Li, J.-W.; Chen, J.; Fan, Y.-D.; Zheng, S.-G. Laparoscopic versus open liver resection for hepatocellular carcinoma in posterosuperior segments. *Surg. Endosc.* **2015**, *29*, 2994–3001. [CrossRef] [PubMed]
43. Cherqui, D.; Laurent, A.; Tayar, C.; Chang, S.; Van Nhieu, J.T.; Loriau, J.; Karoui, M.; Duvoux, C.; Dhumeaux, D.; Fagniez, P.-L. Laparoscopic Liver Resection for Peripheral Hepatocellular Carcinoma in Patients with Chronic Liver Disease: Midterm results and per-spectives. *Ann. Surg.* **2006**, *243*, 499–506. [CrossRef] [PubMed]
44. Sandri, G.B.L.; Ettorre, G.M.; Aldrighetti, L.; Cillo, U.; Valle, R.D.; Guglielmi, A.; Mazzaferro, V.; Ferrero, A.; Di Benedetto, F.; I Go MILS Group on HCC. Laparoscopic liver resection of hepatocellular carcinoma located in unfavorable segments: A propensity score-matched analysis from the I Go MILS (Italian Group of Minimally Invasive Liver Surgery) Registry. *Surg. Endosc.* **2019**, *33*, 1451–1458. [CrossRef]
45. Liu, K.; Chen, Y.; Wu, X.; Huang, Z.; Lin, Z.; Jiang, J.; Tan, W.; Zhang, L. Laparoscopic liver re-resection is feasible for patients with posthepatectomy hepatocellular carcinoma recurrence: A propensity score matching study. *Surg. Endosc.* **2017**, *31*, 4790–4798. [CrossRef]
46. Belli, G.; Cioffi, L.; Fantini, C.; D'Agostino, A.; Russo, G.; Limongelli, P.; Belli, A. Laparoscopic redo surgery for recurrent hepatocellular carcinoma in cirrhotic patients: Feasibility, safety, and results. *Surg. Endosc.* **2009**, *23*, 1807–1811. [CrossRef]
47. Goh, B.K.P.; Syn, N.; Teo, J.-Y.; Guo, Y.-X.; Lee, S.-Y.; Cheow, P.-C.; Chow, P.K.H.; Ooi, L.L.P.J.; Chung, A.Y.F.; Chan, C.-Y. Perioperative Outcomes of Laparoscopic Repeat Liver Resection for Recurrent HCC: Comparison with Open Repeat Liver Resection for Recurrent HCC and Laparoscopic Resection for Primary HCC. *World J. Surg.* **2019**, *43*, 878–885. [CrossRef]
48. Sandri, G.B.L.; Colasanti, M.; Aldrighetti, L.; Guglielmi, A.; Cillo, U.; Mazzaferro, V.; Valle, R.D.; De Carlis, L.; Gruttadauria, S.; Di Benedetto, F.; et al. Is minimally invasive liver surgery a reasonable option in recurrent HCC? A snapshot from the I Go MILS registry. *Updat. Surg.* **2022**, *74*, 87–96. [CrossRef]
49. Gon, H.; Kido, M.; Tanaka, M.; Kuramitsu, K.; Komatsu, S.; Awazu, M.; So, S.; Toyama, H.; Fukumoto, T. Laparoscopic repeat hepatectomy is a more favorable treatment than open repeat hepatectomy for contralateral recurrent hepatocellular carcinoma cases. *Surg. Endosc.* **2021**, *35*, 2896–2906. [CrossRef]
50. Zhang, J.; Zhou, Z.-G.; Huang, Z.-X.; Yang, K.-L.; Chen, J.-C.; Chen, J.-B.; Xu, L.; Chen, M.-S.; Zhang, Y.-J. Prospective, single-center cohort study analyzing the efficacy of complete laparoscopic resection on recurrent hepatocellular carcinoma. *Chin. J. Cancer* **2016**, *35*, 25. [CrossRef]
51. Morise, Z.; Aldrighetti, L.; Belli, G.; Ratti, F.; Belli, A.; Cherqui, D.; Tanabe, M.; Wakabayashi, G.; Cheung, T.T.; Lo, C.M.; et al. Laparoscopic repeat liver resection for hepatocellular carcinoma: A multicentre propensity score-based study. *Br. J. Surg.* **2020**, *107*, 889–895. [CrossRef]
52. Kanazawa, A.; Tsukamoto, T.; Shimizu, S.; Kodai, S.; Yamamoto, S.; Yamazoe, S.; Ohira, G.; Nakajima, T. Laparoscopic liver resection for treating recurrent hepatocellular carcinoma. *J. Hepato-Biliary-Pancreatic Sci.* **2013**, *20*, 512–517. [CrossRef]
53. Onoe, T.; Yamaguchi, M.; Irei, T.; Ishiyama, K.; Sudo, T.; Hadano, N.; Kojima, M.; Kubota, H.; Ide, R.; Tazawa, H.; et al. Feasibility and efficacy of repeat laparoscopic liver resection for recurrent hepatocellular carcinoma. *Surg. Endosc.* **2020**, *34*, 4574–4581. [CrossRef]
54. Miyama, A.; Morise, Z.; Aldrighetti, L.; Belli, G.; Ratti, F.; Cheung, T.-T.; Lo, C.-M.; Tanaka, S.; Kubo, S.; Okamura, Y.; et al. Multicenter Propensity Score-Based Study of Laparoscopic Repeat Liver Resection for Hepatocellular Carcinoma: A Subgroup Analysis of Cases with Tumors Far from Major Vessels. *Cancers* **2021**, *13*, 3187. [CrossRef]
55. Bruix, J.; Castells, A.; Bosch, J.; Feu, F.; Fuster, J.; Garcia-Pagan, J.C.; Visa, J.; Bru, C.; Rodes, J. Surgical resection of hepatocellular carcinoma in cirrhotic patients: Prognostic value of preoperative portal pressure. *Gastroenterology* **1996**, *111*, 1018–1022. [CrossRef]
56. Northup, P.G.; Wanamaker, R.C.; Lee, V.D.; Adams, R.B.; Berg, C.L. Model for End-Stage Liver Disease (MELD) Predicts Nontransplant Surgical Mortality in Patients with Cirrhosis. *Ann. Surg.* **2005**, *242*, 244–251. [CrossRef]
57. Morise, Z.; Sugioka, A.; Kawabe, N.; Umemoto, S.; Nagata, H.; Ohshima, H.; Kawase, J.; Arakawa, S.; Yoshida, R. Pure laparoscopic hepatectomy for hepatocellular carcinoma patients with severe liver cirrhosis. *Asian J. Endosc. Surg.* **2011**, *4*, 143–146. [CrossRef]
58. Wakabayashi, G.; Cherqui, D.; A Geller, D.; Buell, J.F.; Kaneko, H.; Han, H.S.; Asbun, H.; O'rourke, N.; Tanabe, M.; Koffron, A.J.; et al. Recommendations for laparoscopic liver resection: A report from the second international consensus conference held in Morioka. *Ann. Surg.* **2015**, *261*, 619–629. [CrossRef]
59. Pietrasz, D.; Fuks, D.; Subar, D.; Donatelli, G.; Ferretti, C.; Lamer, C.; Portigliotti, L.; Ward, M.; Cowan, J.; Nomi, T.; et al. Laparoscopic extended liver resection: Are postoperative outcomes different? *Surg. Endosc.* **2018**, *32*, 4833–4840. [CrossRef]
60. Martin, A.N.; Narayanan, S.; Turrentine, F.E.; Bauer, T.W.; Adams, R.B.; Stukenborg, G.J.; Zaydfudim, V.M. Clinical Factors and Postoperative Impact of Bile Leak After Liver Resection. *J. Gastrointest. Surg.* **2018**, *22*, 661–667. [CrossRef]
61. Buell, J.F.; Cherqui, D.; Geller, D.A.; O'Rourke, N.; Iannitti, D.; Dagher, I.; Koffron, A.J.; Thomas, M.; Gayet, B.; Han, H.S.; et al. The International Position on Laparoscopic Liver Surgery: The Louisville Statement, 2008. *Ann. Surg.* **2009**, *250*, 825–830. [CrossRef] [PubMed]
62. Berardi, G.; Wakabayashi, G.; Igarashi, K.; Ozaki, T.; Toyota, N.; Tsuchiya, A.; Nishikawa, K. Full Laparoscopic Anatomical Segment 8 Resection for Hepatocellular Carcinoma Using the Glissonian Approach with Indocyanine Green Dye Fluorescence. *Ann. Surg. Oncol.* **2019**, *26*, 2577–2578. [CrossRef] [PubMed]
63. Van der Poel, M.J.; Huisman, F.; Busch, O.R.; Abu Hilal, M.; van Gulik, T.M.; Tanis, P.J.; Besselink, M.G. Stepwise introduction of laparoscopic liver surgery: Validation of guideline recommendations. *HPB* **2017**, *19*, 894–900. [CrossRef] [PubMed]

64. Tabrizian, P.; Jibara, G.; Shrager, B.; Schwartz, M.; Roayaie, S. Recurrence of Hepatocellular Cancer After Resection: Patterns, treat-ments, and prognosis. *Ann. Surg.* **2015**, *261*, 947–955. [CrossRef]
65. Ciria, R.; Berardi, G.; Alconchel, F.; Briceño, J.; Choi, G.H.; Wu, Y.; Sugioka, A.; Troisi, R.I.; Salloum, C.; Soubrane, O.; et al. The impact of robotics in liver surgery: A worldwide systematic review and short-term outcomes meta-analysis on 2,728 cases. *J. Hepato-Biliary-Pancreatic Sci.* **2022**, *29*, 181–197. [CrossRef]
66. Nomi, T.; Kaibori, M.; Tanaka, S.; Hirokawa, F.; Hokuto, D.; Noda, T.; Ueno, M.; Nakai, T.; Ikoma, H.; Iida, H.; et al. Short- and long-term outcomes of laparoscopic versus open repeat liver resection for hepatocellular carcinoma: A multicenter study. *J. Hepato-Biliary-Pancreat. Sci.* [CrossRef]
67. Zhang, K.-J.; Liang, L.; Diao, Y.-K.; Xie, Y.-M.; Wang, D.-D.; Xu, F.-Q.; Ye, T.-W.; Lu, W.-F.; Cheng, J.; Shen, G.-L.; et al. Short- and long-term outcomes of laparoscopic versus open liver resection for large hepatocellular carcinoma: A propensity score study. *Surg. Today* **2022**, *53*, 322–331. [CrossRef]
68. Belli, G.; Fantini, C.; Belli, A.; Limongelli, P. Laparoscopic Liver Resection for Hepatocellular Carcinoma in Cirrhosis: Long-Term Outcomes. *Dig. Surg.* **2011**, *28*, 134–140. [CrossRef]
69. Yin, Z.; Jin, H.; Ma, T.; Wang, H.; Huang, B.; Jian, Z. Laparoscopic hepatectomy versus open hepatectomy in the management of posterosuperior segments of the Liver: A systematic review and meta-analysis. *Int. J. Surg.* **2018**, *60*, 101–110. [CrossRef]

Disclaimer/Publisher's Note: The statements, opinions and data contained in all publications are solely those of the individual author(s) and contributor(s) and not of MDPI and/or the editor(s). MDPI and/or the editor(s) disclaim responsibility for any injury to people or property resulting from any ideas, methods, instructions or products referred to in the content.

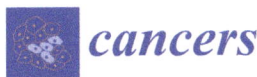

Perspective

Positioning of Minimally Invasive Liver Surgery for Hepatocellular Carcinoma: From Laparoscopic to Robot-Assisted Liver Resection

Shogo Tanaka *, Shoji Kubo and Takeaki Ishizawa

Department of Hepato-Biliary-Pancreatic Surgery, Osaka Metropolitan University Graduate School of Medicine, Osaka 545-8585, Japan
* Correspondence: shogotanaka@omu.ac.jp; Tel.: +81-6-6645-3841; Fax: +81-6-6646-6057

Simple Summary: Laparoscopic liver resection is widely accepted in the surgical treatment of hepatocellular carcinoma. Laparoscopic liver resection has been reported to result in earlier postoperative recovery and fewer postoperative complications than open liver resection for hepatocellular carcinoma. Laparoscopic liver resection is technically feasible for selected patients with hepatocellular carcinoma even under several situations such as the prevalence of liver cirrhosis, obesity, elderly, hepatocellular carcinoma recurrence (repeat liver resection), and major resection that led to better intra- and post-operative outcomes than open liver resection. In recent years, robot-assisted liver resection has gradually become popular, and its short- and long-term results for hepatocellular carcinoma are reported to be not different from those of laparoscopic liver resection. Robot-assisted liver resection is expected to become the mainstay of minimally invasive surgery in the future.

Abstract: Laparoscopic liver resection (LLR) is widely accepted in the surgical treatment of hepatocellular carcinoma (HCC) through international consensus conferences and the development of difficulty classifications. LLR has been reported to result in earlier postoperative recovery and fewer postoperative complications than open liver resection (OLR) for HCC. However, the prevalence of liver cirrhosis, obesity, the elderly, HCC recurrence (repeat liver resection), and major resection must be considered for LLR for HCC. Some systematic reviews, meta-analysis studies, and large cohort studies indicated that LLR is technically feasible for selected patients with HCC with these factors that led to less intraoperative blood loss, fewer transfusions and postoperative complication incidences, and shorter hospital stays than OLR. Furthermore, some reported LLR prevents postoperative loss of independence. No difference was reported in long-term outcomes among patients with HCC who underwent LLR and OLR; however, some recent reports indicated better long-term outcomes with LLR. In recent years, robot-assisted liver resection (RALR) has gradually become popular, and its short- and long-term results for HCC are not different from those of LLR. Additionally, RALR is expected to become the mainstay of minimally invasive surgery in the future.

Keywords: hepatocellular carcinoma; laparoscopic liver resection; long-term outcomes; robot-assisted

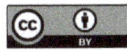

1. Introduction

Hepatocellular carcinoma (HCC) is the most common primary liver tumor and the third leading cause of cancer-related death worldwide [1,2]. Liver resection is a valuable treatment modality in patients with HCC with preserved liver function [3,4]. The first laparoscopic liver resection (LLR) was reported in 1992, whereas the first LLR for HCC was in 1995 [5]. The LLR application was considered controversial for many years. Progress in laparoscopic techniques and expertise in combination with technological advances have led to more widespread adoption of minimally invasive approaches for HCC resection over the last 15 years [6]. Subsequently, the number of LLR cases increased due to the roadmap advocacy for the widespread use of safe LLR at numerous international consensus conferences [7–10] and the development of a difficulty scale classification [11–14]. Additionally, in Japan, the number and the proportion of LLR for the total number of liver resections increased from 1848 cases (9.9%) in 2011 to 5648 (24.8%) in 2017 [15]. At present, solitary lesions (≤5 cm) located in segments 2 through 6, which was the most acceptable LLR indication, as well as laparoscopic major liver resection, have been performed [7,8,14,16–20]. With these LLR developments, perioperative outcomes are better in patients with HCC who underwent LLR than those who underwent OLR, with no difference in long-term outcomes [16,17,21–23], whereas a recent systematic review and meta-analysis study indicated better long-term outcomes after minimal invasive liver resection (MILR), including LLR (48 articles) and robot-assisted liver resection (RALR, 2 articles) for HCC than OLR among the recently published data [24]. The pooled analysis revealed an 18% decrease in disease-specific 3-year mortality after MILR (almost, LLR) compared with OLR (Figure 1), and the sensitivity analysis of contemporary studies from 2010 to 2019 revealed a significantly lower 5-year all-cause mortality and 3-year disease-specific mortality in MILR compared to OLR. Thus, the overall picture is important in the surgical HCC treatment; however, factors such as cirrhosis due to background liver disease, repeat liver resection for HCC recurrence, advanced age, and obesity must be considered.

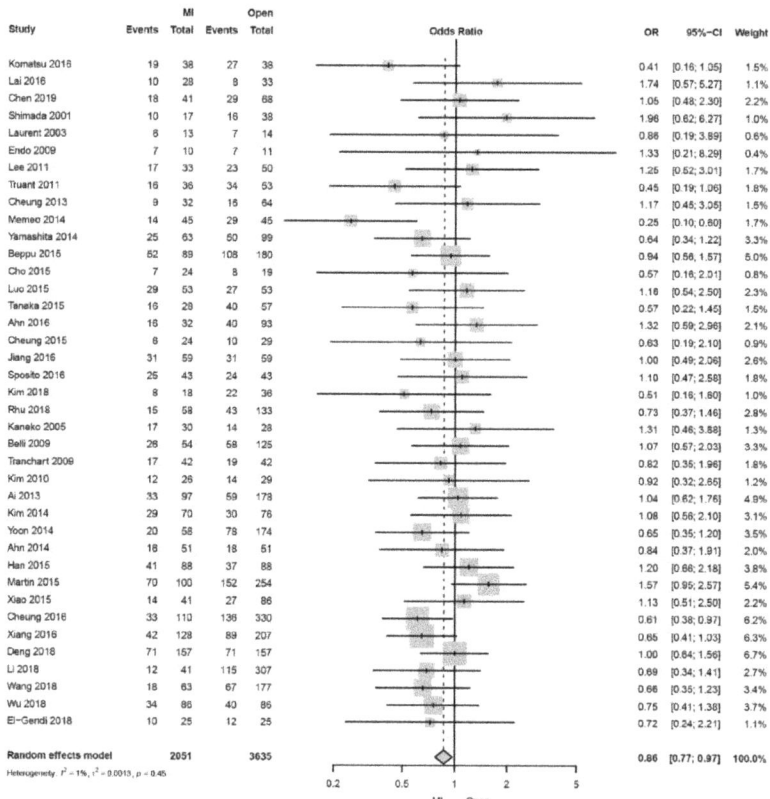

Figure 1. Forest plot of disease-specific 3-year mortality comparing minimally invasive and open liver resection for hepatocellular carcinoma. The studies shown in this figure can be found as references [6,21,23,25–58]. Reprinted/adapted with permission from Ref. [24]. 2021, SAGE Publications.

We reviewed the short- and long-term results of LLR usefulness (vs. OLR) with a special focus on these factors. Additionally, the usefulness of RALR, which has become increasingly popular in recent years, is discussed.

2. Liver Cirrhosis

Most patients with HCC commonly have chronic hepatitis and cirrhosis. Liver resection for patients with cirrhosis is challenging due to elevated portal pressure and impaired coagulation function. One systematic review and meta-analysis [59], one systematic review [60], and two meta-analyses [61,62] compared LLR with OLR for patients with cirrhosis with HCC. These reports revealed no difference in operation time among patients who underwent LLR and OLR; however, LLR reports decreased blood loss, transfusion rate, postoperative complications (including postoperative ascites and liver failure), and length of hospital stay. Moreover, LLR gains better 1-year overall survival (OS) [61,62] and 5-year OS [60–62]. Only one report revealed better 1-year disease-free survival (DFS) in LLR than in OLR [61]. However, among patients with cirrhosis, patients with Child-Pugh class B were reported to have more complications and deaths in the hospital and poorer long-term outcomes than patients with Child-Pugh class A [63–67], but the effect of LLR remains controversial because of the small number of patients [68,69]. Recently, Berardi et al. [70] reported an international multicenter study of 253 patients with Child-Pugh class B regarding short- and long-term outcomes. The comorbidity prevalence, increased Child-Pugh score (7 to 9), decreased preoperative hemoglobin and platelet count, and preoperative ascites and portal hypertension prevalence, increased the risk for postoperative complication within 90 days postoperatively (Figure 2). Moreover, minimally invasive surgery, including LLR and minor liver resection, decreased the risk for postoperative complications. Additionally, LLR did not affect DFS or OS rates. Liver cirrhosis is a well-known risk factor for postoperative liver failure-related mortality [71]. However, the development of devices, hemostasis techniques, and pneumoperitoneum and minimization of delamination in the LLR has controlled the bleeding and prevented postoperative ascites [25,72], which might lead to postoperative early recovery even for patients with Child-Pugh class B cirrhosis. Some better LLR prognoses might be caused by less compression during laparoscopic manipulation, which prevented tumor cell metastasis [62]. However, several reports revealed that LLR has no effect on long-term prognosis (no difference from OLR) [25,73], and only tumor factors were found to determine DFS in a study of Child-Pugh class B, while tumor factors and systemic status, including cirrhosis, determine OS [70]. LLR may be a useful treatment for patients who may not have previously been candidates for open surgery and may even prolong survival. However, further study is needed on the efficacy of LLR on long-term outcomes after cirrhotic liver resection.

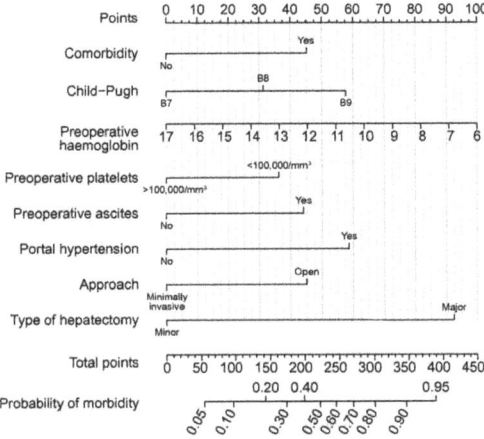

Figure 2. Nomogram for predicting 90-day morbidity after liver resection for hepatocellular carcinoma in patients with Child-Pugh class B. Nomogram was drawn using the multivariable logistic model for 90-day morbidity. Reprinted/adapted with permission from Ref. [70]. 2019, Elsevier.

3. Laparoscopic Repeat Liver Resection (LRLR) for Recurrent HCC

High recurrence even after curative liver resection for the initial HCC is a significant oncologic feature of HCC [74–77]. Additionally, hepatic resection is recommended for HCC recurrences (HCCR), as well as primary cases, if HCC has ≤3 nodules [4]. However, adhesions after initial hepatectomy are not only seen on the liver dissection surface, but also on the dissection surface and hepatoduodenal mesentery at a certain frequency, which makes repeat liver resection difficult, leading to unexpected blood loss and vascular or biliary structure intraoperative injury [78–80]. Conversely, some reported the remits of LRLR, such as minimalization of dissection of the adhesion under high magnification directly from the caudal direction [13,81] and small targeted area without damages to the surrounding area in the LRLR [79]. Some highly experienced centers reported feasible and safe LRLR for HCCR in the single-arm study [81–84]. A meta-analysis revealed that LRLR (n = 145) had a lower rate of in-hospital complication, much less blood loss, and a shorter hospital stay than open repeat liver resection (ORLR, n = 190) [85]. However, these studies were very small in number. Recently, an international collaborative study by Morise et al. [86] examined the usefulness of LRLR (n = 648) for HCCR and compared ORLR (n = 934) using propensity score matching (PSM, each, n = 238). The operation time was longer in the PSM cohort (mean, 273 min vs. 232 min, p = 0.007), but blood loss was lower (mean, 268 mL vs. 497 mL, p = 0.001) in patients who underwent LRLR than in those who did ORLR. No differences were found in the incidence of postoperative 90-day complications, 90-day mortality, length of hospital stay, or long-term survival. Therefore, case selection that would benefit from LRLR would be important. Kinoshita, et al. [87] reported the difficulty of LRLR in 60 patients with HCCR. Additionally, (1) an open approach during previous liver resection, (2) two or more previous liver resections, (3) a history of previous liver resection with not less than a sectionectomy, (4) a tumor near the resected site of the previous liver resection, and (5) intermediate or high difficulty in the difficulty scoring system [11] were independent risk factors for prolonged operative time and/or severe adhesion of LRLR. Thereafter, they validated less blood loss and lower postoperative complication incidence in LRLR than in ORLR among patients with ≤3 applicable risk factors; however, the operation time was longer in LRLR than in ORLR, and no difference was observed in other intra- and postoperative outcomes among LRLR and ORLR in patients with ≥4 of these 5 variables, suggesting that LRLR has no advantage in these patients [88]. On the basis of these findings, LRLR may have better short-term results than ORLR, but preoperative evaluation, such as details of prior surgeries, will be needed to determine whether it can be safely applied.

4. Elderly

The geriatric population has dramatically increased, and the number of elderly patients who undergo liver resection has even more rapidly increased [89]. Some reports revealed that the incidences of postoperative complication and mortality were comparable between elderly and non-elderly patients in OLR [90,91], but others have revealed an increased mortality incidence in elderly patients [92]. The reported incidence of overall postoperative complications in the elderly (aged 65–75 years) ranged from 29% to 59%, that of major complications (Clavien–Dindo grade ≥ IIIa) ranged from 16% to 41%, and that of mortality ranged from 0% to 9% [90–93]. Large-scale data from the Diagnosis Procedure Combination database, a national administrative database in Japan (2007–2012, n = 27,094), indicated the incidence of postoperative complication and mortality after liver resection increased up until the 70 s; however, no differences were found among patients aged in their 70 s, 80–84 years, and ≥85 years [94]. These results may be attributed to the fact that the adaptation is strictly handled for the elderly. Nomi et al. [95] reported a lower incidence of overall postoperative and major complications in elderly patients (aged ≥75 years) with HCC who underwent LLR than in those who underwent OLR, but others reported no difference among LLR and OLR [96,97]. However, LLR shortened the length of hospital stay [95–97]. One systematic review and meta-analysis using 12 studies (LLR: $n = 831$ and OLR; $n = 931$) indicated that LLR decreased the intraoperative blood loss, incidence of overall postoperative complications, including liver failure, ascites, and surgical site infection, major complication, and length of hospital stay although it includes all diseases, not just HCC [98]. Therefore, age would not be a determining factor for surgery. However, the high incidence of "elderly-related events", including respiratory complications (pneumonia and respiratory failure requiring reintubation) [91], cardiac events [90], delirium [90,99], and discharge to rehabilitation facilities [99] are a major problem for liver resection in the elderly. LLR was reported to decrease the incidence of elderly-related events such as cardiopulmonary complications [95,96,100]. Moreover, maintenance of independence after liver resection is very important for elderly patients who underwent liver resection. Our previous study indicated that LLR decreased the incidence of postoperative loss of independence during the early postoperative period, including transfer to rehabilitation facilities, readmission within 30 days, discharge with any health care supports, and/or death within 90 days except cancer-related death, and at 1 year after liver resection, including the need of any healthcare supports and/or death due to deterioration of physical function [101,102]. A few studies reported regarding long-term survival; however, no differences were found in DFS or OS rate among elderly patients with HCC who underwent LLR or OLR [97]. LLR for the elderly has better intraoperative outcomes and fewer postoperative complications than OLR. In addition, LLR may have advantages to reduce elderly-related events and maintain independent living.

5. Obesity

The prevalence of obesity and its associated diseases has remained increasing worldwide. The prevalence of obesity (body mass index [BMI] of ≥ 30 kg/m^2) is 40% in the United States [103] and approximately 20% in Europe [104]. In Japan, obesity is defined by a BMI of ≥ 25 kg/m^2 [105]. As of 2018, 32.2% of males and 21.9% of females aged ≥ 20 years were classified as obese [106]. Furthermore, several reports revealed that patients with obesity are at high risk of developing HCC [107,108]. Thus, a higher prevalence of obesity and expansion of liver resection indications could increase the number of liver resections among patients with obesity with HCC in the future. Obesity is correlated with comorbidities and technical difficulties in open surgery and is considered a risk factor for postoperative complications in several surgical fields [109,110]. Countermeasures for the depth of the surgical field and large volume of intraperitoneal fat are important in abdominal surgery, including liver resection, in patients who are overweight and obese [111,112]. These situations are associated with increased operation time, blood loss, and postoperative complications in the OLR [113–115]. Liver parenchyma dissection and hepatic hilum treatment are sometimes challenging despite a large skin incision and gastrointestinal tract and greater momentum compression in OLR [116–118]. In contrast, pneumoperitoneum, head-up position, and high magnification—even at deep portions in the caudal view—can provide sufficient free space to control the forceps in LLR, even in patients who are overweight and obese (Caudal approach, Figure 3) [119–121]. There is some disagreement as to whether obesity increases the risk of conversion [12,111,113,122,123], but the LLR is reported to decrease intraoperative blood loss and postoperative complications compared with OLR even in obesity [113,118,121,124]. Moreover, obesity did not affect conversion rate, operation time, or blood loss in the LLR compared with non-obesity [113,122,123]. There is some disagreement regarding conversion to open surgery, but LLR has better short-term outcomes than OLR. Therefore, LLR for obesity would be feasible and safe.

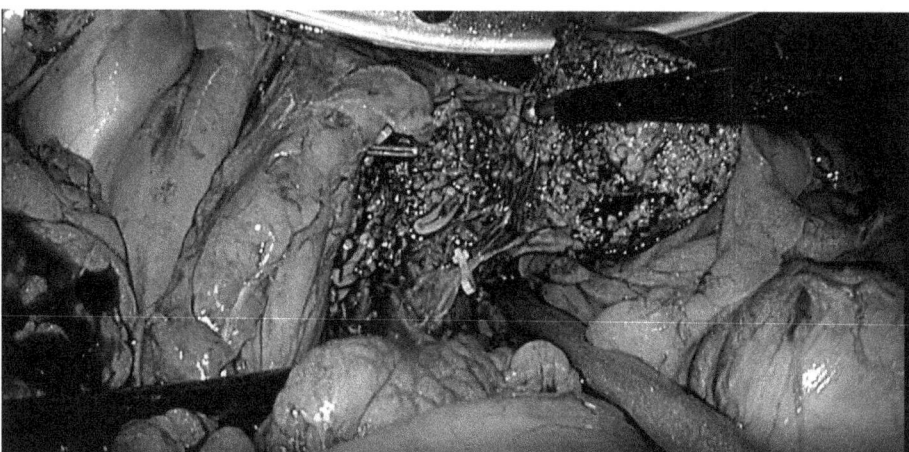

Figure 3. Laparoscopic liver resection for tumor located at segment I in a patient with obesity. Taking advantage of the Caudal approach of laparoscopic surgery, liver resection was performed with a good field of view despite the surgical depth.

6. Robot-Assisted Liver Resection (RALR)

RALRs are slowly spreading, although at a slower speed than LLRs [125,126]. In 2018, an international expert panel published a consensus guideline on the use of robotics in liver surgery, concluding that "RALR is as safe and feasible as LLR and OLR" for both major and minor liver resection [127]. Advantages of RALR include stability and magnification of a three-dimensional view, the best possible ergonomics, enhanced suturing capacity, the ability to complete more extensive or complex minimally invasive operations, integrated fluorescence guidance, and a shortened learning curve. However, the robotic platform remains limited by a paucity of parenchymal transection devices, a complete lack of hepatic feedback, and an additional operation time associated with docking and instrument exchange [128,129].

Some reported learning curves for LLR in 35 to 75 cases regarding operation time and incidence of liver injury (liver ischemia, congestion, or portal vein thrombosis) [130–133]. Conversely, early proponents of the robotic platform felt that robotic operations would be easier to learn than their laparoscopic counterparts due to the intentionally intuitive nature of robotic instrument us even for novice surgeons [134–136]. Some studies indicated shortened learning curves of 15 to 52 cases in RALR [137–139]. Additionally, the best possible ergonomics would increase the number of major hepatectomies and/or highly difficult cases [140–142]. However, RALR may become mainstream in the future. Some meta-analyses indicated less blood loss and a lower proportion of transfusion and incidence of postoperative complications in patients who underwent RALR than OLR [143–145]. Moreover, Kamarajah et al. [146] reported a systematic review and meta-analysis that included 26 articles and 2630 patients (RARL: 950 patients and LLR: 1680 patients) and revealed that blood loss was less (median, 286 mL vs. 301 mL, $p < 0.001$) and operation time was longer (median, 281 min vs. 221 min, $p < 0.001$) in patients who underwent RALR than in those who underwent LLR. Additionally, no difference was found in the incidence of postoperative complications, mortality, or length of hospital stay among patients who underwent RALR and LLR although readmission was lower in patients who underwent RALR than in those who underwent LLR. Moreover, a meta-analysis for major hepatectomy revealed an association between RALR and lower blood loss and conversion rate but with a slightly longer hospital stay compared to LLR [147]. Zhu et al. [148] revealed intra- and postoperative outcomes among patients who underwent RALR ($n = 71$), LLR ($n = 141$), and OLR ($n = 157$) for HCC; operation time was shortest and the length of hospital stay was longest in patients who underwent OLR, and similar results were demonstrated between those who did RALR and LLR. Conversely, some studies reported a higher incidence of postoperative bile leakage after RALR [149–151]. RALR is easy to manipulate in the hepatic hilum, but the lack of tactile sensation may cause inadvertent bile duct injury. In contrast, careful infraphrenic dissection was reported to reduce the incidence of postoperative pleural effusions [150]. Therefore, RALR does not significantly differ from LLR and is considered less invasive than OLR in terms of short-term results. Few studies reported on long-term outcomes after RALR; however, Zhu et al. [148] revealed no difference in DFS or OS among patients who underwent RALR, LLR, and OLR. Hence, RALR is as good as LLR as MIS. RALR may provide better perioperative results than LLR with further equipment development.

7. Conclusions

In conclusion, liver resection for HCC requires consideration of various situations, such as liver cirrhosis, repeat liver resection, obesity, and the elderly, but LLR overcomes these situations and has equal or better outcomes compared to OLR. In the future, RALR is expected to develop as an MIS alongside LLR.

Author Contributions: Conceptualization S.T. and T.I.; methodology S.T. and S.K.; validation S.T. and T.I.; investigation S.T.; writing—original draft preparation S.T. and S.K.; writing—review and editing, S.T., S.K. and T.I.; supervision S.T. and T.I.; funding acquisition S.T; final revision S.T., S.K. and T.I. All authors have read and agreed to the published version of the manuscript.

Funding: This study was funded by MEXT/JSPS KAKENHI (Grant Number 19K09152).

Data Availability Statement: Data sharing is not applicable to this article as no datasets were generated or analyzed during the current study.

Conflicts of Interest: The authors declare no conflict of interest. The funders had no role in the design of the study; in the collection, analyses, or interpretation of data; in the writing of the manuscript, or in the decision to publish the results.

References

1. Ferlay, J.; Soerjomataram, I.; Dikshit, R.; Eser, S.; Mathers, C.; Rebelo, M.; Parkin, D.M.; Forman, D.; Bray, F. Cancer incidence and mortality worldwide: Sources, methods and major patterns in GLOBOCAN 2012. *Int. J. Cancer* **2015**, *136*, E359–E386. [CrossRef] [PubMed]
2. Siegel, R.L.; Miller, K.D.; Jemal, A. Cancer statistics, 2018. *CA Cancer J. Clin.* **2018**, *68*, 7–30. [CrossRef] [PubMed]
3. Kokudo, N.; Takemura, N.; Hasegawa, K.; Takayama, T.; Kubo, S.; Shimada, M.; Nagano, H.; Hatano, E.; Izumi, N.; Kaneko, S.; et al. Clinical practice guidelines for hepatocellular carcinoma: The Japan Society of Hepatology 2017 (4th JSH-HCC guidelines) 2019 update. *Hepatol. Res.* **2019**, *49*, 1109–1113. [CrossRef] [PubMed]
4. European Association for the Study of the Liver. EASL Clinical Practice Guidelines: Management of hepatocellular carcinoma. *J. Hepatol.* **2018**, *69*, 182–236. [CrossRef] [PubMed]
5. Hashizume, M.; Takenaka, K.; Yanaga, K.; Ohta, M.; Kajiyama, K.; Shirabe, K.; Itasaka, H.; Nishizaki, T.; Sugimachi, K. Laparoscopic hepatic resection for hepatocellular carcinoma. *Surg. Endosc.* **1995**, *9*, 1289–1291. [CrossRef]
6. Laurent, A. Laparoscopic Liver Resection for Subcapsular Hepatocellular Carcinoma Complicating Chronic Liver Disease. *Arch. Surg.* **2003**, *138*, 763. [CrossRef]
7. Buell, J.F.; Cherqui, D.; Geller, D.A.; O'Rourke, N.; Iannitti, D.; Dagher, I.; Koffron, A.J.; Thomas, M.; Gayet, B.; Han, H.S.; et al. The international position on laparoscopic liver surgery: The Louisville Statement, 2008. *Ann. Surg.* **2009**, *250*, 825–830. [CrossRef]
8. Wakabayashi, G.; Cherqui, D.; Geller, D.A.; Buell, J.F.; Kaneko, H.; Han, H.S.; Asbun, H.; O'rourke, N.; Tanabe, M.; Koffron, A.J.; et al. Recommendations for laparoscopic liver resection: A report from the second international consensus conference held in Morioka. *Ann. Surg.* **2015**, *261*, 619–629. [CrossRef]
9. Cheung, T.T.; Han, H.-S.; She, W.H.; Chen, K.-H.; Chow, P.; Yoong, B.K.; Lee, K.F.; Kubo, S.; Tang, C.N.; Wakabayashi, G. The Asia Pacific Consensus Statement on Laparoscopic Liver Resection for Hepatocellular Carcinoma: A Report from the 7th Asia-Pacific Primary Liver Cancer Expert Meeting Held in Hong Kong. *Liver Cancer* **2017**, *7*, 28–39. [CrossRef]
10. Abu Hilal, M.; Aldrighetti, L.; Dagher, I.; Edwin, B.; Troisi, R.I.; Alikhanov, R.; Aroori, S.; Belli, G.; Besselink, M.; Briceno, J.; et al. The Southampton Consensus Guidelines for Laparoscopic Liver Surgery. *Ann. Surg.* **2018**, *268*, 11–18. [CrossRef]
11. Ban, D.; Tanabe, M.; Ito, H.; Otsuka, Y.; Nitta, H.; Abe, Y.; Hasegawa, Y.; Katagiri, T.; Takagi, C.; Itano, O.; et al. A novel difficulty scoring system for laparoscopic liver resection. *J. Hepato-Biliary-Pancreat. Sci.* **2014**, *21*, 745–753. [CrossRef] [PubMed]

12. Hasegawa, Y.; Wakabayashi, G.; Nitta, H.; Takahara, T.; Katagiri, H.; Umemura, A.; Makabe, K.; Sasaki, A. A novel model for prediction of pure laparoscopic liver resection surgical difficulty. *Surg. Endosc.* **2017**, *31*, 5356–5363. [CrossRef] [PubMed]
13. Wakabayashi, G.; Cherqui, D.; Geller, D.A.; Han, H.-S.; Kaneko, H.; Buell, J.F. Laparoscopic hepatectomy is theoretically better than open hepatectomy: Preparing for the 2nd International Consensus Conference on Laparoscopic Liver Resection. *J. Hepato-Biliary-Pancreat. Sci.* **2014**, *21*, 723–731. [CrossRef]
14. Kawaguchi, Y.; Fuks, D.; Kokudo, N.; Gayet, B. Difficulty of Laparoscopic Liver Resection. *Ann. Surg.* **2018**, *267*, 13–17. [CrossRef] [PubMed]
15. Ban, D.; Tanabe, M.; Kumamaru, H.; Nitta, H.; Otsuka, Y.; Miyata, H.; Kakeji, Y.; Kitagawa, Y.; Kaneko, H.; Wakabayashi, G.; et al. Safe Dissemination of Laparoscopic Liver Resection in 27,146 Cases Between 2011 and 2017 From the National Clinical Database of Japan. *Ann. Surg.* **2020**, *274*, 1043–1050. [CrossRef]
16. Han, H.-S.; Shehta, A.; Ahn, S.; Yoon, Y.-S.; Cho, J.Y.; Choi, Y. Laparoscopic versus open liver resection for hepatocellular carcinoma: Case-matched study with propensity score matching. *J. Hepatol.* **2015**, *63*, 643–650. [CrossRef]
17. Takahara, T.; Wakabayashi, G.; Beppu, T.; Aihara, A.; Hasegawa, K.; Gotohda, N.; Hatano, E.; Tanahashi, Y.; Mizuguchi, T.; Kamiyama, T.; et al. Long-term and perioperative outcomes of laparoscopic versus open liver resection for hepatocellular carcinoma with propensity score matching: A multi-institutional Japanese study. *J. Hepato-Biliary-Pancreat. Sci.* **2015**, *22*, 721–727. [CrossRef]
18. Takahara, T.; Wakabayashi, G.; Konno, H.; Gotoh, M.; Yamaue, H.; Yanaga, K.; Fujimoto, J.; Kaneko, H.; Unno, M.; Endo, I.; et al. Comparison of laparoscopic major hepatectomy with propensity score matched open cases from the National Clinical Database in Japan. *J. Hepato-Biliary-Pancreat. Sci.* **2016**, *23*, 721–734. [CrossRef]
19. Tanaka, S.; Kawaguchi, Y.; Kubo, S.; Kanazawa, A.; Takeda, Y.; Hirokawa, F.; Nitta, H.; Nakajima, T.; Kaizu, T.; Kaibori, M.; et al. Validation of index-based IWATE criteria as an improved difficulty scoring system for laparoscopic liver resection. *Surgery* **2019**, *165*, 731–740. [CrossRef]
20. Tanaka, S.; Kubo, S.; Kanazawa, A.; Takeda, Y.; Hirokawa, F.; Nitta, H.; Nakajima, T.; Kaizu, T.; Kaneko, H.; Wakabayashi, G. Validation of a Difficulty Scoring System for Laparoscopic Liver Resection: A Multicenter Analysis by the Endoscopic Liver Surgery Study Group in Japan. *J. Am. Coll. Surg.* **2017**, *225*, 249–258e1. [CrossRef]
21. Li, W.; Han, J.; Xie, G.; Xiao, Y.; Sun, K.; Yuan, K.; Wu, H. Laparoscopic versus open mesohepatectomy for patients with centrally located hepatocellular carcinoma: A propensity score matched analysis. *Surg. Endosc.* **2018**, *33*, 2916–2926. [CrossRef]
22. Meguro, M.; Mizuguchi, T.; Kawamoto, M.; Ota, S.; Ishii, M.; Nishidate, T.; Okita, K.; Kimura, Y.; Hirata, K. Clinical comparison of laparoscopic and open liver resection after propensity matching selection. *Surgery* **2015**, *158*, 573–587. [CrossRef]
23. Xiang, L.; Li, J.; Chen, J.; Wang, X.; Guo, P.; Fan, Y.; Zheng, S. Prospective cohort study of laparoscopic and open hepatectomy for hepatocellular carcinoma. *Br. J. Surg.* **2016**, *103*, 1895–1901. [CrossRef]
24. Kamarajah, S.K.; Gujjuri, R.R.; Hilal, M.A.; Manas, D.M.; White, S.A. Does minimally invasive liver resection improve long-term survival compared to open resection for hepatocellular carcinoma? A systematic review and meta-analysis. *Scand. J. Surg.* **2021**, *111*, 14574969211042455. [CrossRef]
25. Tanaka, S.; Takemura, S.; Shinkawa, H.; Nishioka, T.; Hamano, G.; Kinoshita, M.; Ito, T.; Kubo, S. Outcomes of Pure Laparoscopic versus Open Hepatic Resection for Hepatocellular Carcinoma in Cirrhotic Patients: A Case-Control Study with Propensity Score Matching. *Eur. Surg. Res.* **2015**, *55*, 291–301. [CrossRef]
26. Komatsu, S.; Brustia, R.; Goumard, C.; Perdigao, F.; Soubrane, O.; Scatton, O. Laparoscopic versus open major hepatectomy for hepatocellular carcinoma: A matched pair analysis. *Surg. Endosc.* **2015**, *30*, 1965–1974. [CrossRef]
27. Lai, C.; Jin, R.-A.; Liang, X.; Cai, X.-J. Comparison of laparoscopic hepatectomy, percutaneous radiofrequency ablation and open hepatectomy in the treatment of small hepatocellular carcinoma. *J. Zhejiang Univ. B* **2016**, *17*, 236–246. [CrossRef]
28. Chen, K.; Pan, Y.; Wang, Y.-F.; Zheng, X.-Y.; Liang, X.; Yu, H.; Cai, X.-J. Laparoscopic Right Hepatectomy for Hepatocellular Carcinoma: A Propensity Score Matching Analysis of Outcomes Compared with Conventional Open Surgery. *J. Laparoendosc. Adv. Surg. Tech.* **2019**, *29*, 503–512. [CrossRef]
29. Shimada, M.; Hashizume, M.; Maehara, S.; Tsujita, E.; Rikimaru, T.; Yamashita, Y.; Tanaka, S.; Adachi, E.; Sugimachi, K. Laparoscopic hepatectomy for hepatocellular carcinoma. *Surg. Endosc.* **2001**, *15*, 541–544. [CrossRef]
30. Endo, Y.; Ohta, M.; Sasaki, A.; Kai, S.; Eguchi, H.; Iwaki, K.; Shibata, K.; Kitano, S. A Comparative Study of the Long-term Outcomes After Laparoscopy-assisted and Open Left Lateral Hepatectomy for Hepatocellular Carcinoma. *Surg. Laparosc. Endosc. Percutaneous Tech.* **2009**, *19*, e171–e174. [CrossRef]
31. Lee, K.F.; Chong, C.N.; Wong, J.; Cheung, Y.S.; Wong, J.; Lai, P. Long-Term Results of Laparoscopic Hepatectomy Versus Open Hepatectomy for Hepatocellular Carcinoma: A Case-Matched Analysis. *World J. Surg.* **2011**, *35*, 2268–2274. [CrossRef] [PubMed]
32. Truant, S.; Bouras, A.F.; Hebbar, M.; Boleslawski, E.; Fromont, G.; Dharancy, S.; Leteurtre, E.; Zerbib, P.; Pruvot, F.R. Laparoscopic resection vs. open liver resection for peripheral hepatocellular carcinoma in patients with chronic liver disease: A case-matched study. *Surg. Endosc.* **2011**, *25*, 3668–3677. [CrossRef] [PubMed]
33. Cheung, T.T.; Poon, R.T.P.; Yuen, W.K.; Chok, K.S.H.; Jenkins, C.R.; Chan, S.C.; Fan, S.T.; Lo, C.M. Long-Term Survival Analysis of Pure Laparoscopic Versus Open Hepatectomy for Hepatocellular Carcinoma in Patients with Cirrhosis. *Ann. Surg.* **2013**, *257*, 506–511. [CrossRef]
34. Memeo, R.; De'Angelis, N.; Compagnon, P.; Salloum, C.; Cherqui, D.; Laurent, A.; Azoulay, D. Laparoscopic vs. Open Liver Resection for Hepatocellular Carcinoma of Cirrhotic Liver: A Case–Control Study. *World J. Surg.* **2014**, *38*, 2919–2926. [CrossRef]

35. Yamashita, Y.-I.; Ikeda, T.; Kurihara, T.; Yoshida, Y.; Takeishi, K.; Itoh, S.; Harimoto, N.; Kawanaka, H.; Shirabe, K.; Maehara, Y. Long-Term Favorable Surgical Results of Laparoscopic Hepatic Resection for Hepatocellular Carcinoma in Patients with Cirrhosis: A Single-Center Experience over a 10-Year Period. *J. Am. Coll. Surg.* **2014**, *219*, 1117–1123. [CrossRef] [PubMed]
36. Beppu, T.; Wakabayashi, G.; Hasegawa, K.; Gotohda, N.; Mizuguchi, T.; Takahashi, Y.; Hirokawa, F.; Taniai, N.; Watanabe, M.; Katou, M.; et al. Long-term and perioperative outcomes of laparoscopic versus open liver resection for colorectal liver metastases with propensity score matching: A multi-institutional Japanese study. *J. Hepato-Biliary-Pancreat. Sci.* **2015**, *22*, 711–720. [CrossRef]
37. Cho, J.Y.; Han, H.-S.; Yoon, Y.-S.; Choi, Y.; Lee, W. Outcomes of laparoscopic right posterior sectionectomy in patients with hepatocellular carcinoma in the era of laparoscopic surgery. *Surgery* **2015**, *158*, 135–141. [CrossRef]
38. Luo, L.; Zou, H.; Yao, Y.; Huang, X. Laparoscopic versus open hepatectomy for hepatocellular carcinoma: Short- and long-term outcomes comparison. *Int. J. Clin. Exp. Med.* **2015**, *8*, 18772–18778.
39. Ahn, S.; Cho, A.; Kim, E.K.; Paik, K.Y. Favorable Long-Term Oncologic Outcomes of Hepatocellular Carcinoma Following Laparoscopic Liver Resection. *J. Laparoendosc. Adv. Surg. Tech.* **2016**, *26*, 447–452. [CrossRef]
40. Cheung, T.T.; Poon, R.T.P.; Dai, W.C.; Chok, K.S.H.; Chan, S.C.; Lo, C.M. Pure Laparoscopic Versus Open Left Lateral Sectionectomy for Hepatocellular Carcinoma: A Single-Center Experience. *World J. Surg.* **2015**, *40*, 198–205. [CrossRef]
41. Jiang, X.; Liu, L.; Zhang, Q.; Jiang, Y.; Huang, J.; Zhou, H.; Zeng, L. Laparoscopic versus open hepatectomy for hepatocellular carcinoma: Long-term outcomes. *J. BUON* **2016**, *21*, 135–141. [PubMed]
42. Sposito, C.; Battiston, C.; Facciorusso, A.; Mazzola, M.; Muscarà, C.; Scotti, M.; Romito, R.; Mariani, L.; Mazzaferro, V. Propensity score analysis of outcomes following laparoscopic or open liver resection for hepatocellular carcinoma. *Br. J. Surg.* **2016**, *103*, 871–880. [CrossRef] [PubMed]
43. Kim, W.-J.; Kim, K.-H.; Kim, S.-H.; Kang, W.-H.; Lee, S.-G. Laparoscopic Versus Open Liver Resection for Centrally Located Hepatocellular Carcinoma in Patients with Cirrhosis: A Propensity Score-matching Analysis. *Surg. Laparosc. Endosc. Percutaneous Tech.* **2018**, *28*, 394–400. [CrossRef] [PubMed]
44. Rhu, J.; Kim, S.J.; Choi, G.S.; Kim, J.M.; Joh, J.-W.; Kwon, C.H.D. Laparoscopic Versus Open Right Posterior Sectionectomy for Hepatocellular Carcinoma in a High-Volume Center: A Propensity Score Matched Analysis. *World J. Surg.* **2018**, *42*, 2930–2937. [CrossRef]
45. Kaneko, H.; Takagi, S.; Otsuka, Y.; Tsuchiya, M.; Tamura, A.; Katagiri, T.; Maeda, T.; Shiba, T. Laparoscopic liver resection of hepatocellular carcinoma. *Am. J. Surg.* **2005**, *189*, 190–194. [CrossRef]
46. Belli, G.; Limongelli, P.; Fantini, C.; D'Agostino, A.; Cioffi, L.; Belli, A.; Russo, G. Laparoscopic and open treatment of hepatocellular carcinoma in patients with cirrhosis. *Br. J. Surg.* **2009**, *96*, 1041–1048. [CrossRef]
47. Tranchart, H.; Di Giuro, G.; Lainas, P.; Roudie, J.; Agostini, H.; Franco, D.; Dagher, I. Laparoscopic resection for hepatocellular carcinoma: A matched-pair comparative study. *Surg. Endosc.* **2009**, *24*, 1170–1176. [CrossRef]
48. Kim, H.-H.; Park, E.K.; Seoung, J.S.; Hur, Y.H.; Koh, Y.S.; Kim, J.C.; Cho, C.K.; Kim, H.J. Liver resection for hepatocellular carcinoma: Case-matched analysis of laparoscopic versus open resection. *J. Korean Surg. Soc.* **2011**, *80*, 412–419. [CrossRef]
49. Ai, J.-H.; Li, J.-W.; Chen, J.; Bie, P.; Wang, S.-G.; Zheng, S.-G. Feasibility and Safety of Laparoscopic Liver Resection for Hepatocellular Carcinoma with a Tumor Size of 5–10 cm. *PLoS ONE* **2013**, *8*, e72328. [CrossRef]
50. Kim, S.-J.; Jung, H.-K.; Lee, D.-S.; Yun, S.-S.; Kim, H.-J. The comparison of oncologic and clinical outcomes of laparoscopic liver resection for hepatocellular carcinoma. *Ann. Surg. Treat. Res.* **2014**, *86*, 61–67. [CrossRef]
51. Yoon, S.-Y.; Kim, K.-H.; Jung, D.-H.; Yu, A.; Lee, S.-G. Oncological and surgical results of laparoscopic versus open liver resection for HCC less than 5 cm: Case-matched analysis. *Surg. Endosc.* **2014**, *29*, 2628–2634. [CrossRef] [PubMed]
52. Ahn, K.S.; Kang, K.J.; Kim, Y.H.; Kim, T.-S.; Lim, T.J. A Propensity Score-Matched Case-Control Comparative Study of Laparoscopic and Open Liver Resection for Hepatocellular Carcinoma. *J. Laparoendosc. Adv. Surg. Tech.* **2014**, *24*, 872–877. [CrossRef] [PubMed]
53. Martin, R.C.G.; Mbah, N.A.; Hill, R.S.; Kooby, D.; Weber, S.; Scoggins, C.R.; Maithel, S.K. Laparoscopic Versus Open Hepatic Resection for Hepatocellular Carcinoma: Improvement in Outcomes and Similar Cost. *World J. Surg.* **2015**, *39*, 1519–1526. [CrossRef] [PubMed]
54. Xiao, L.; Xiang, L.-J.; Li, J.-W.; Chen, J.; Fan, Y.-D.; Zheng, S.-G. Laparoscopic versus open liver resection for hepatocellular carcinoma in posterosuperior segments. *Surg. Endosc.* **2015**, *29*, 2994–3001. [CrossRef] [PubMed]
55. Deng, Z.-C.; Jiang, W.-Z.; Tang, X.-D.; Liu, S.-H.; Qin, L.; Qian, H.-X. Laparoscopic hepatectomy versus open hepatectomy for hepatocellular carcinoma in 157 patients: A case controlled study with propensity score matching at two Chinese centres. *Int. J. Surg.* **2018**, *56*, 203–207. [CrossRef]
56. Wang, W.-H.; Kuo, K.-K.; Wang, S.-N.; Lee, K.-T. Oncological and surgical result of hepatoma after robot surgery. *Surg. Endosc.* **2018**, *32*, 3918–3924. [CrossRef]
57. Wu, X.; Huang, Z.; Lau, W.Y.; Li, W.; Lin, P.; Zhang, L.; Chen, Y. Perioperative and long-term outcomes of laparoscopic versus open liver resection for hepatocellular carcinoma with well-preserved liver function and cirrhotic background: A propensity score matching study. *Surg. Endosc.* **2018**, *33*, 206–215. [CrossRef]
58. El-Gendi, A.; El-Shafei, M.; El-Gendi, S.; Shawky, A. Laparoscopic Versus Open Hepatic Resection for Solitary Hepatocellular Carcinoma Less Than 5 cm in Cirrhotic Patients: A Randomized Controlled Study. *J. Laparoendosc. Adv. Surg. Tech.* **2018**, *28*, 302–310. [CrossRef]

59. Twaij, A. Laparoscopic vs open approach to resection of hepatocellular carcinoma in patients with known cirrhosis: Systematic review and meta-analysis. *World J. Gastroenterol.* **2014**, *20*, 8274–8281. [CrossRef]
60. Chen, J.; Bai, T.; Zhang, Y.; Xie, Z.-B.; Wang, X.-B.; Wu, F.-X.; Li, L.-Q. The safety and efficacy of laparoscopic and open hepatectomy in hepatocellular carcinoma patients with liver cirrhosis: A systematic review. *Int. J. Clin. Exp. Med.* **2015**, *8*, 20679–20689.
61. Goh, E.L.; Chidambaram, S.; Ma, S. Laparoscopic vs open hepatectomy for hepatocellular carcinoma in patients with cirrhosis: A meta-analysis of the long-term survival outcomes. *Int. J. Surg.* **2018**, *50*, 35–42. [CrossRef]
62. Pan, Y.; Xia, S.; Cai, J.; Chen, K.; Cai, X. Efficacy of Laparoscopic Hepatectomy versus Open Surgery for Hepatocellular Carcinoma With Cirrhosis: A Meta-analysis of Case-Matched Studies. *Front. Oncol.* **2021**, *11*. [CrossRef]
63. Kusano, T.; Sasaki, A.; Kai, S.; Endo, Y.; Iwaki, K.; Shibata, K.; Ohta, M.; Kitano, S. Predictors and prognostic significance of operative complications in patients with hepatocellular carcinoma who underwent hepatic resection. *Eur. J. Surg. Oncol. (EJSO)* **2009**, *35*, 1179–1185. [CrossRef]
64. Giuliante, F.; Ardito, F.; Pinna, A.D.; Sarno, G.; Giulini, S.M.; Ercolani, G.; Portolani, N.; Torzilli, G.; Donadon, M.; Aldrighetti, L.; et al. Liver Resection for Hepatocellular Carcinoma ≤3 cm: Results of an Italian Multicenter Study on 588 Patients. *J. Am. Coll. Surg.* **2012**, *215*, 244–254. [CrossRef]
65. Kabir, T.; Syn, N.L.; Tan, Z.Z.; Tan, H.-J.; Yen, C.; Koh, Y.-X.; Kam, J.H.; Teo, J.-Y.; Lee, S.-Y.; Cheow, P.-C.; et al. Predictors of post-operative complications after surgical resection of hepatocellular carcinoma and their prognostic effects on outcome and survival: A propensity-score matched and structural equation modelling study. *Eur. J. Surg. Oncol. (EJSO)* **2020**, *46*, 1756–1765. [CrossRef]
66. Koh, Y.X.; Tan, H.J.; Liew, Y.X.; Syn, N.; Teo, J.Y.; Lee, S.Y.; Goh, B.K.; Goh, G.B.; Chan, C.Y. Liver Resection for Nonalcoholic Fatty Liver Disease-Associated Hepatocellular Carcinoma. *J. Am. Coll. Surg.* **2019**, *229*, 467–478e1. [CrossRef]
67. Chen, Y.-S.; Hsieh, P.-M.; Lin, H.-Y.; Hung, C.-M.; Lo, G.-H.; Hsu, Y.-C.; Lu, I.-C.; Lee, C.-Y.; Wu, T.-C.; Yeh, J.-H.; et al. Surgical resection significantly promotes the overall survival of patients with hepatocellular carcinoma: A propensity score matching analysis. *BMC Gastroenterol.* **2021**, *21*, 220. [CrossRef]
68. Brytska, N.; Han, H.-S.; Shehta, A.; Yoon, Y.-S.; Cho, J.Y.; Choi, Y. Laparoscopic liver resection for hepatitis B and C virus-related hepatocellular carcinoma in patients with Child B or C cirrhosis. *HepatoBiliary Surg. Nutr.* **2015**, *4*, 373–378. [CrossRef]
69. Cai, X.; Liang, X.; Yu, T.; Liang, Y.; Jing, R.; Jiang, W.; Li, J.; Ying, H. Liver cirrhosis grading Child-Pugh class B: A Goliath to challenge in laparoscopic liver resection?—Prior experience and matched comparisons. *HepatoBiliary Surg. Nutr.* **2015**, *4*, 391–397. [CrossRef]
70. Berardi, G.; Morise, Z.; Sposito, C.; Igarashi, K.; Panetta, V.; Simonelli, I.; Kim, S.; Goh, B.K.; Kubo, S.; Tanaka, S.; et al. Development of a nomogram to predict outcome after liver resection for hepatocellular carcinoma in Child-Pugh B cirrhosis. *J. Hepatol.* **2019**, *72*, 75–84. [CrossRef]
71. Kubo, S.; Tsukamoto, T.; Hirohashi, K.; Tanaka, H.; Shuto, T.; Takemura, S.; Yamamoto, T.; Uenishi, T.; Ogawa, M.; Kinoshita, H. Correlation Between Preoperative Serum Concentration of Type IV Collagen 7s Domain and Hepatic Failure Following Resection of Hepatocellular Carcinoma. *Ann. Surg.* **2004**, *239*, 186–193. [CrossRef]
72. Kanazawa, A.; Tsukamoto, T.; Shimizu, S.; Kodai, S.; Yamazoe, S.; Yamamoto, S.; Kubo, S. Impact of laparoscopic liver resection for hepatocellular carcinoma with F4-liver cirrhosis. *Surg. Endosc.* **2013**, *27*, 2592–2597. [CrossRef]
73. Cheung, T.T.; Dai, W.C.; Tsang, S.H.Y.; Chan, A.C.Y.; Chok, K.S.H.; Chan, S.C.; Lo, C.M. Pure Laparoscopic Hepatectomy Versus Open Hepatectomy for Hepatocellular Carcinoma in 110 Patients with Liver Cirrhosis. *Ann. Surg.* **2016**, *264*, 612–620. [CrossRef]
74. Koda, M.; Tanaka, S.; Takemura, S.; Shinkawa, H.; Kinoshita, M.; Hamano, G.; Ito, T.; Kawada, N.; Shibata, T.; Kubo, S. Long-Term Prognostic Factors after Hepatic Resection for Hepatitis C Virus-Related Hepatocellular Carcinoma, with a Special Reference to Viral Status. *Liver Cancer* **2018**, *7*, 261–276. [CrossRef]
75. Tanaka, S.; Iimuro, Y.; Hirano, T.; Hai, S.; Suzumura, K.; Fujimoto, J. Outcomes of Hepatic Resection for Large Hepatocellular Carcinoma: Special Reference to Postoperative Recurrence. *Am. Surg.* **2015**, *81*, 64–73. [CrossRef]
76. Tanaka, S.; Shinkawa, H.; Tamori, A.; Takemura, S.; Takahashi, S.; Amano, R.; Kimura, K.; Ohira, G.; Kawada, N.; Kubo, S. Surgical outcomes for hepatocellular carcinoma detected after hepatitis C virus eradication by direct-acting antivirals. *J. Surg. Oncol.* **2020**, *122*, 1543–1552. [CrossRef]
77. Tanaka, S.; Shinkawa, H.; Tamori, A.; Takemura, S.; Uchida-Kobayashi, S.; Amano, R.; Kimura, K.; Ohira, G.; Nishio, K.; Tauchi, J.; et al. Postoperative direct-acting antiviral treatment after liver resection in patients with hepatitis C virus-related hepatocellular carcinoma. *Hepatol. Res.* **2021**, *51*, 1102–1114. [CrossRef]
78. Kinoshita, M.; Tanaka, S.; Kodai, S.; Takemura, S.; Shinkawa, H.; Ohira, G.; Nishio, K.; Tauchi, J.; Kanazawa, A.; Kubo, S. Increasing incidence and severity of post-hepatectomy adhesion around the liver may be influenced by the hepatectomy-related operative procedures. *Asian J. Surg.* **2023**, *46*, 228–235. [CrossRef]
79. Morise, Z. Status and perspective of laparoscopic repeat liver resection. *World J. Hepatol.* **2018**, *10*, 479–484. [CrossRef]
80. Szomstein, S.; Menzo, E.L.; Simpfendorfer, C.; Zundel, N.; Rosenthal, R.J. Laparoscopic Lysis of Adhesions. *World J. Surg.* **2006**, *30*, 535–540. [CrossRef]
81. Hu, M.; Zhao, G.; Xu, D.; Liu, R. Laparoscopic Repeat Resection of Recurrent Hepatocellular Carcinoma. *World J. Surg.* **2010**, *35*, 648–655. [CrossRef]
82. Belli, G.; Cioffi, L.; Fantini, C.; D'Agostino, A.; Russo, G.; Limongelli, P.; Belli, A. Laparoscopic redo surgery for recurrent hepatocellular carcinoma in cirrhotic patients: Feasibility, safety, and results. *Surg. Endosc.* **2009**, *23*, 1807–1811. [CrossRef]

83. Goh, B.K.P.; Teo, J.; Chan, C.; Lee, S.; Cheow, P.; Chung, A.Y.F. Laparoscopic repeat liver resection for recurrent hepatocellular carcinoma. *ANZ J. Surg.* **2016**, *87*, E143–E146. [CrossRef]
84. Tsuchiya, M.; Otsuka, Y.; Maeda, T.; Ishii, J.; Tamura, A.; Kaneko, H. Efficacy of Laparoscopic Surgery for Recurrent Hepatocellular Carcinoma. *Hepatogastroenterology* **2012**, *59*, 1333–1337. [CrossRef]
85. Cai, W.; Liu, Z.; Xiao, Y.; Zhang, W.; Tang, D.; Cheng, B.; Li, Q. Comparison of clinical outcomes of laparoscopic versus open surgery for recurrent hepatocellular carcinoma: A meta-analysis. *Surg. Endosc.* **2019**, *33*, 3550–3557. [CrossRef]
86. Morise, Z.; Aldrighetti, L.; Belli, G.; Ratti, F.; Belli, A.; Cherqui, D.; Tanabe, M.; Wakabayashi, G.; Cheung, T.T.; Lo, C.M.; et al. Laparoscopic repeat liver resection for hepatocellular carcinoma: A multicentre propensity score-based study. *Br. J. Surg.* **2020**, *107*, 889–895. [CrossRef]
87. Kinoshita, M.; Kanazawa, A.; Kodai, S.; Shimizu, S.; Murata, A.; Nishio, K.; Hamano, G.; Shinkawa, H.; Tanaka, S.; Takemura, S.; et al. Difficulty classifications of laparoscopic repeated liver resection in patients with recurrent hepatocellular carcinoma. *Asian J. Endosc. Surg.* **2019**, *13*, 366–374. [CrossRef]
88. Kinoshita, M.; Kanazawa, A.; Tanaka, S.; Takemura, S.; Amano, R.; Kimura, K.; Shinkawa, H.; Ohira, G.; Nishio, K.; Kubo, S. Indications of Laparoscopic Repeat Liver Resection for Recurrent Hepatocellular Carcinoma. *Ann. Gastroenterol. Surg.* **2021**, *6*, 119–126. [CrossRef]
89. Nanashima, A.; Abo, T.; Nonaka, T.; Fukuoka, H.; Hidaka, S.; Takeshita, H.; Ichikawa, T.; Sawai, T.; Yasutake, T.; Nakao, K.; et al. Prognosis of patients with hepatocellular carcinoma after hepatic resection: Are elderly patients suitable for surgery? *J. Surg. Oncol.* **2011**, *104*, 284–291. [CrossRef]
90. Nozawa, A.; Kubo, S.; Takemura, S.; Sakata, C.; Urata, Y.; Nishioka, T.; Kinoshita, M.; Hamano, G.; Uenishi, T.; Suehiro, S. Hepatic resection for hepatocellular carcinoma in super-elderly patients aged 80 years and older in the first decade of the 21st century. *Surg. Today* **2014**, *45*, 851–857. [CrossRef]
91. Wang, W.-L.; Zhu, Y.; Cheng, J.-W.; Li, M.-X.; Xia, J.-M.; Hao, J.; Yu, L.; Lv, Y.; Wu, Z.; Wang, B. Major hepatectomy is safe for hepatocellular carcinoma in elderly patients with cirrhosis. *Eur. J. Gastroenterol. Hepatol.* **2014**, *26*, 444–451. [CrossRef] [PubMed]
92. Cook, E.J.; Welsh, F.K.S.; Chandrakumaran, K.; John, T.G.; Rees, M. Resection of colorectal liver metastases in the elderly: Does age matter? *Color. Dis.* **2012**, *14*, 1210–1216. [CrossRef] [PubMed]
93. Kishida, N.; Hibi, T.; Itano, O.; Okabayashi, K.; Shinoda, M.; Kitago, M.; Abe, Y.; Yagi, H.; Kitagawa, Y. Validation of Hepatectomy for Elderly Patients with Hepatocellular Carcinoma. *Ann. Surg. Oncol.* **2015**, *22*, 3094–3101. [CrossRef] [PubMed]
94. Okinaga, H.; Yasunaga, H.; Hasegawa, K.; Fushimi, K.; Kokudo, N. Short-Term Outcomes following Hepatectomy in Elderly Patients with Hepatocellular Carcinoma: An Analysis of 10,805 Septuagenarians and 2,381 Octo- and Nonagenarians in Japan. *Liver Cancer* **2017**, *7*, 55–64. [CrossRef]
95. Nomi, T.; Hirokawa, F.; Kaibori, M.; Ueno, M.; Tanaka, S.; Hokuto, D.; Noda, T.; Nakai, T.; Ikoma, H.; Iida, H.; et al. Laparoscopic versus open liver resection for hepatocellular carcinoma in elderly patients: A multi-centre propensity score-based analysis. *Surg. Endosc.* **2019**, *34*, 658–666. [CrossRef]
96. Goh, B.K.P.; Chua, D.; Syn, N.; Teo, J.-Y.; Chan, C.-Y.; Lee, S.-Y.; Jeyaraj, P.R.; Cheow, P.-C.; Chow, P.K.H.; Ooi, L.L.P.J.; et al. Perioperative Outcomes of Laparoscopic Minor Hepatectomy for Hepatocellular Carcinoma in the Elderly. *World J. Surg.* **2018**, *42*, 4063–4069. [CrossRef]
97. Kim, J.M.; Kim, S.; Rhu, J.; Choi, G.-S.; Kwon, C.H.D.; Joh, J.-W. Elderly Hepatocellular Carcinoma Patients: Open or Laparoscopic Approach? *Cancers* **2020**, *12*, 2281. [CrossRef]
98. Mohamedahmed, A.Y.Y.; Zaman, S.; Albendary, M.; Wright, J.; Abdalla, H.; Patel, K.; Mankotia, R.; Sillah, A.K. Laparoscopic versus open hepatectomy for malignant liver tumours in the elderly: Systematic review and meta-analysis. *Updat. Surg.* **2021**, *73*, 1623–1641. [CrossRef]
99. Cho, S.W.; Steel, J.; Tsung, A.; Marsh, J.W.; Geller, D.A.; Gamblin, T.C. Safety of Liver Resection in the Elderly: How Important Is Age? *Ann. Surg. Oncol.* **2010**, *18*, 1088–1095. [CrossRef]
100. Tanaka, S.; Ueno, M.; Iida, H.; Kaibori, M.; Nomi, T.; Hirokawa, F.; Ikoma, H.; Nakai, T.; Eguchi, H.; Kubo, S. Preoperative assessment of frailty predicts age-related events after hepatic resection: A prospective multicenter study. *J. Hepato-Biliary-Pancreat. Sci.* **2018**, *25*, 377–387. [CrossRef]
101. Tanaka, S.; Iida, H.; Ueno, M.; Hirokawa, F.; Nomi, T.; Nakai, T.; Kaibori, M.; Ikoma, H.; Eguchi, H.; Shinkawa, H.; et al. Preoperative Risk Assessment for Loss of Independence Following Hepatic Resection in Elderly Patients. *Ann. Surg.* **2019**, *274*, e253–e261. [CrossRef] [PubMed]
102. Tanaka, S.; Iida, H.; Ueno, M.; Hirokawa, F.; Yoshida, H.; Ishii, H.; Nomi, T.; Nakai, T.; Kaibori, M.; Ikoma, H.; et al. Postoperative loss of independence 1 year after liver resection: Prospective multicentre study. *Br. J. Surg.* **2022**, *109*, e54–e55. [CrossRef] [PubMed]
103. Hales, C.M.; Fryar, C.D.; Carroll, M.D.; Freedman, D.S.; Ogden, C.L. Trends in Obesity and Severe Obesity Prevalence in US Youth and Adults by Sex and Age, 2007-2008 to 2015-2016. *JAMA* **2018**, *319*, 1723–1725. [CrossRef]
104. World Health Organization. Obesity and Overweight. Available online: https://www.who.int/news-room/fact-sheets/detail/obesity-and-overweight (accessed on 18 October 2022).
105. McCurry, J. Japan battles with obesity. *Lancet* **2007**, *369*, 451–452. [CrossRef]
106. Ministry of Health, Labour and Welfare of Japan. Report of national health and nutrition 2018. Available online: https://www.mhlw.go.jp/content/10900000/000688863.pdf (accessed on 1 March 2020).

107. Berentzen, T.L.; Gamborg, M.; Holst, C.; Sørensen, T.I.; Baker, J.L. Body mass index in childhood and adult risk of primary liver cancer. *J. Hepatol.* **2014**, *60*, 325–330. [CrossRef]
108. Larsson, S.C.; Wolk, A. Overweight, obesity and risk of liver cancer: A meta-analysis of cohort studies. *Br. J. Cancer* **2007**, *97*, 1005–1008. [CrossRef]
109. Mullen, J.T.; Davenport, D.L.; Hutter, M.M.; Hosokawa, P.W.; Henderson, W.G.; Khuri, S.F.; Moorman, D.W. Impact of Body Mass Index on Perioperative Outcomes in Patients Undergoing Major Intra-abdominal Cancer Surgery. *Ann. Surg. Oncol.* **2008**, *15*, 2164–2172. [CrossRef]
110. Dindo, D.; Muller, M.K.; Weber, M.; Clavien, P.-A. Obesity in general elective surgery. *Lancet* **2003**, *361*, 2032–2035. [CrossRef]
111. Yu, X.; Yu, H.; Fang, X. The impact of body mass index on short-term surgical outcomes after laparoscopic hepatectomy, a retrospective study. *BMC Anesthesiol.* **2015**, *16*, 29. [CrossRef]
112. WHO Expert Consultation. Appropriate body-mass index for Asian populations and its implications for policy and intervention strategies. *Lancet* **2004**, *363*, 157–163. [CrossRef]
113. Ishihara, A.; Tanaka, S.; Shinkawa, H.; Yoshida, H.; Takemura, S.; Amano, R.; Kimura, K.; Ohira, G.; Nishio, K.; Kubo, S. Superiority of laparoscopic liver resection to open liver resection in obese individuals with hepatocellular carcinoma: A retrospective study. *Ann. Gastroenterol. Surg.* **2021**, *6*, 135–148. [CrossRef] [PubMed]
114. Cucchetti, A.; Cescon, M.; Ercolani, G.; Di Gioia, P.; Peri, E.; Pinna, A.D. Safety of hepatic resection in overweight and obese patients with cirrhosis. *Br. J. Surg.* **2011**, *98*, 1147–1154. [CrossRef] [PubMed]
115. Tanaka, S.; Iimuro, Y.; Hirano, T.; Hai, S.; Suzumura, K.; Nakamura, I.; Kondo, Y.; Fujimoto, J. Safety of hepatic resection for hepatocellular carcinoma in obese patients with cirrhosis. *Surg. Today* **2013**, *43*, 1290–1297. [CrossRef]
116. Gedaly, R.; McHugh, P.P.; Johnston, T.D.; Jeon, H.; Ranjan, D.; Davenport, D.L. Obesity, Diabetes, and Smoking are Important Determinants of Resource Utilization in Liver Resection: A Multicenter Analysis of 1029 Patients. *Ann. Surg.* **2009**, *249*, 414–419. [CrossRef] [PubMed]
117. Balzan, S.; Nagarajan, G.; Farges, O.; Galleano, C.Z.; Dokmak, S.; Paugam-Burtz, C.; Belghiti, J. Safety of Liver Resections in Obese and Overweight Patients. *World J. Surg.* **2010**, *34*, 2960–2968. [CrossRef]
118. Uchida, H.; Iwashita, Y.; Saga, K.; Takayama, H.; Watanabe, K.; Endo, Y.; Yada, K.; Ohta, M.; Inomata, M. Benefit of laparoscopic liver resection in high body mass index patients. *World J. Gastroenterol.* **2016**, *22*, 3015–3022. [CrossRef]
119. Soubrane, O.; Schwarz, L.; Cauchy, F.; Perotto, L.O.; Brustia, R.; Bernard, D.; Scatton, O. A Conceptual Technique for Laparoscopic Right Hepatectomy Based on Facts and Oncologic Principles. *Ann. Surg.* **2015**, *261*, 1226–1231. [CrossRef]
120. Tomishige, H.; Morise, Z.; Kawabe, N.; Nagata, H.; Ohshima, H.; Kawase, J.; Arakawa, S.; Yoshida, R.; Isetani, M. Caudal approach to pure laparoscopic posterior sectionectomy under the laparoscopy-specific view. *World J. Gastrointest. Surg.* **2013**, *5*, 173–177. [CrossRef]
121. Kwan, B.; Waters, P.S.; Keogh, C.; Cavallucci, D.J.; O'Rourke, N.; Bryant, R.D. Body mass index and surgical outcomes in laparoscopic liver resections: A systematic review. *ANZ J. Surg.* **2021**, *91*, 2296–2307. [CrossRef]
122. Nomi, T.; Fuks, D.; Ferraz, J.-M.; Kawaguchi, Y.; Nakajima, Y.; Gayet, B. Influence of body mass index on postoperative outcomes after laparoscopic liver resection. *Surg. Endosc.* **2015**, *29*, 3647–3654. [CrossRef]
123. Ome, Y.; Hashida, K.; Yokota, M.; Nagahisa, Y.; Okabe, M.; Kawamoto, K. The safety and efficacy of laparoscopic hepatectomy in obese patients. *Asian J. Surg.* **2019**, *42*, 180–188. [CrossRef]
124. Toriguchi, K.; Hatano, E.; Sakurai, T.; Seo, S.; Taura, K.; Uemoto, S. Laparoscopic Liver Resection in Obese Patients. *World J. Surg.* **2015**, *39*, 1210–1215. [CrossRef] [PubMed]
125. Giulianotti, P.C. Robotics in General Surgery. *Arch. Surg.* **2003**, *138*, 777–784. [CrossRef] [PubMed]
126. Patriti, A.; Ceccarelli, G.; Bartoli, A.; Spaziani, A.; Lapalorcia, L.M.; Casciola, L. Laparoscopic and robot-assisted one-stage resection of colorectal cancer with synchronous liver metastases: A pilot study. *J. Hepato-Biliary-Pancreat. Surg.* **2009**, *16*, 450–457. [CrossRef] [PubMed]
127. Liu, R.; Wakabayashi, G.; Kim, H.-J.; Choi, G.-H.; Yiengpruksawan, A.; Fong, Y.; He, J.; Boggi, U.; Troisi, R.I.; Efanov, M.; et al. International consensus statement on robotic hepatectomy surgery in 2018. *World J. Gastroenterol.* **2019**, *25*, 1432–1444. [CrossRef] [PubMed]
128. Ayabe, R.I.; Azimuddin, A.; Cao, H.S.T. Robot-assisted liver resection: The real benefit so far. *Langenbeck's Arch. Surg.* **2022**, 1–9. [CrossRef]
129. Troisi, R.I.; Pegoraro, F.; Giglio, M.C.; Rompianesi, G.; Berardi, G.; Tomassini, F.; De Simone, G.; Aprea, G.; Montalti, R.; De Palma, G.D. Robotic approach to the liver: Open surgery in a closed abdomen or laparoscopic surgery with technical constraints? *Surg. Oncol.* **2019**, *33*, 239–248. [CrossRef]
130. Vigano, L.; Laurent, A.; Tayar, C.; Tomatis, M.; Ponti, A.; Cherqui, D. The Learning Curve in Laparoscopic Liver Resection. *Ann. Surg.* **2009**, *250*, 772–782. [CrossRef]
131. Nomi, T.; Fuks, D.; Kawaguchi, Y.; Mal, F.; Nakajima, Y.; Gayet, B. Learning curve for laparoscopic major hepatectomy. *Br. J. Surg.* **2015**, *102*, 796–804. [CrossRef]
132. Lee, W.; Woo, J.-W.; Lee, J.-K.; Park, J.-H.; Kim, J.-Y.; Kwag, S.-J.; Park, T.; Jeong, S.-H.; Ju, Y.-T.; Jeong, E.-J.; et al. Comparison of Learning Curves for Major and Minor Laparoscopic Liver Resection. *J. Laparoendosc. Adv. Surg. Tech.* **2016**, *26*, 457–464. [CrossRef]

133. Navarro, J.G.; Kang, I.; Rho, S.Y.; Choi, G.H.; Han, D.H.; Kim, K.S.; Choi, J.S. Major Laparoscopic Versus Open Resection for Hepatocellular Carcinoma: A Propensity Score-Matched Analysis Based on Surgeons' Learning Curve. *Ann. Surg. Oncol.* **2020**, *28*, 447–458. [CrossRef] [PubMed]
134. Lanfranco, A.R.; Castellanos, A.E.; Desai, J.P.; Meyers, W.C. Robotic Surgery. *Ann. Surg.* **2004**, *239*, 14–21. [CrossRef] [PubMed]
135. Moore, L.; Wilson, M.; Waine, E.; Masters, R.S.W.; McGrath, J.S.; Vine, S.J. Robotic technology results in faster and more robust surgical skill acquisition than traditional laparoscopy. *J. Robot. Surg.* **2014**, *9*, 67–73. [CrossRef] [PubMed]
136. Stewart, C.L.; Fong, A.; Payyavula, G.; DiMaio, S.; Lafaro, K.; Tallmon, K.; Wren, S.; Sorger, J.; Fong, Y. Study on augmented reality for robotic surgery bedside assistants. *J. Robot. Surg.* **2021**, 1–8. [CrossRef]
137. Chen, P.-D.; Wu, C.-Y.; Hu, R.-H.; Chen, C.-N.; Yuan, R.-H.; Liang, J.-T.; Lai, H.-S.; Wu, Y.-M. Robotic major hepatectomy: Is there a learning curve? *Surgery* **2017**, *161*, 642–649. [CrossRef]
138. Efanov, M.; Alikhanov, R.; Tsvirkun, V.; Kazakov, I.; Melekhina, O.; Kim, P.; Vankovich, A.; Grendal, K.; Berelavichus, S.; Khatkov, I. Comparative analysis of learning curve in complex robot-assisted and laparoscopic liver resection. *HPB* **2017**, *19*, 818–824. [CrossRef]
139. Zhu, P.; Liao, W.; Ding, Z.-Y.; Chen, L.; Zhang, W.-G.; Zhang, B.-X.; Chen, X.-P. Learning Curve in Robot-Assisted Laparoscopic Liver Resection. *J. Gastrointest. Surg.* **2018**, *23*, 1778–1787. [CrossRef]
140. Chong, C.C.; Fuks, D.; Lee, K.-F.; Zhao, J.J.; Choi, G.H.; Sucandy, I.; Chiow, A.K.H.; Marino, M.V.; Gastaca, M.; Wang, X.; et al. Propensity Score–Matched Analysis Comparing Robotic and Laparoscopic Right and Extended Right Hepatectomy. *JAMA Surg.* **2022**, *157*, 436. [CrossRef]
141. Chong, C.C.N.; Lok, H.T.; Fung, A.K.Y.; Fong, A.K.W.; Cheung, Y.S.; Wong, J.; Lee, K.F.; Lai, P.B.S. Robotic versus laparoscopic hepatectomy: Application of the difficulty scoring system. *Surg. Endosc.* **2019**, *34*, 2000–2006. [CrossRef]
142. Lorenz, E.; Arend, J.; Franz, M.; Rahimli, M.; Perrakis, A.; Negrini, V.; Gumbs, A.A.; Croner, R.S. Robotic and laparoscopic liver resection—Comparative experiences at a high-volume German academic center. *Langenbeck's Arch. Surg.* **2021**, *406*, 753–761. [CrossRef]
143. Jiang, B.; Yan, X.-F.; Zhang, J.-H. Meta-analysis of laparoscopic versus open liver resection for hepatocellular carcinoma. *Hepatol. Res.* **2018**, *48*, 635–663. [CrossRef] [PubMed]
144. Machairas, N.; Papaconstantinou, D.; Tsilimigras, D.I.; Moris, D.; Prodromidou, A.; Paspala, A.; Spartalis, E.; Kostakis, I.D. Comparison between robotic and open liver resection: A systematic review and meta-analysis of short-term outcomes. *Updat. Surg.* **2019**, *71*, 39–48. [CrossRef]
145. Wong, D.J.; Wong, M.J.; Choi, G.H.; Wu, Y.M.; Lai, P.B.; Goh, B.K.P. Systematic review and meta-analysis of robotic versus open hepatectomy. *ANZ J. Surg.* **2018**, *89*, 165–170. [CrossRef] [PubMed]
146. Kamarajah, S.K.; Bundred, J.; Manas, D.; Jiao, L.R.; Abu Hilal, M.; White, S.A. Robotic versus conventional laparoscopic liver resections: A systematic review and meta-analysis. *Scand. J. Surg.* **2020**, *110*, 290–300. [CrossRef] [PubMed]
147. Coletta, D.; Sandri, G.B.L.; Giuliani, G.; Guerra, F. Robot-assisted versus conventional laparoscopic major hepatectomies: Systematic review with meta-analysis. *Int. J. Med. Robot. Comput. Assist. Surg.* **2020**, *17*, e2218. [CrossRef]
148. Zhu, P.; Liao, W.; Zhang, W.-G.; Chen, L.; Shu, C.; Zhang, Z.-W.; Huang, Z.-Y.; Chen, Y.-F.; Lau, W.Y.; Zhang, B.-X.M.; et al. A Prospective Study Using Propensity Score Matching to Compare Long-term Survival Outcomes After Robotic-assisted, Laparoscopic, or Open Liver Resection for Patients with BCLC Stage 0-A Hepatocellular Carcinoma. *Ann. Surg.* **2022**, *277*, e103–e111. [CrossRef]
149. Lee, K.-F.; Chong, C.; Cheung, S.; Wong, J.; Fung, A.; Lok, H.-T.; Lo, E.; Lai, P. Robotic versus open hemihepatectomy: A propensity score-matched study. *Surg. Endosc.* **2020**, *35*, 2316–2323. [CrossRef]
150. Magistri, P.; Tarantino, G.; Guidetti, C.; Assirati, G.; Olivieri, T.; Ballarin, R.; Coratti, A.; Di Benedetto, F. Laparoscopic versus robotic surgery for hepatocellular carcinoma: The first 46 consecutive cases. *J. Surg. Res.* **2017**, *217*, 92–99. [CrossRef]
151. Schmelzle, M.; Feldbrügge, L.; Galindo, S.A.O.; Moosburner, S.; Kästner, A.; Krenzien, F.; Benzing, C.; Biebl, M.; Öllinger, R.; Malinka, T.; et al. Robotic vs. laparoscopic liver surgery: A single-center analysis of 600 consecutive patients in 6 years. *Surg. Endosc.* **2022**, *36*, 5854–5862. [CrossRef]

Disclaimer/Publisher's Note: The statements, opinions and data contained in all publications are solely those of the individual author(s) and contributor(s) and not of MDPI and/or the editor(s). MDPI and/or the editor(s) disclaim responsibility for any injury to people or property resulting from any ideas, methods, instructions or products referred to in the content.

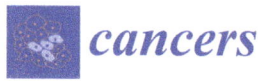

Article

An International Retrospective Observational Study of Liver Functional Deterioration after Repeat Liver Resection for Patients with Hepatocellular Carcinoma

Zenichi Morise [1,*], Luca Aldrighetti [2], Giulio Belli [3], Francesca Ratti [2], Tan To Cheung [4], Chung Mau Lo [4], Shogo Tanaka [5], Shoji Kubo [5], Yukiyasu Okamura [6], Katsuhiko Uesaka [6], Kazuteru Monden [7], Hiroshi Sadamori [7], Kazuki Hashida [8], Kazuyuki Kawamoto [8], Naoto Gotohda [9], KuoHsin Chen [10,11], Akishige Kanazawa [12], Yutaka Takeda [13], Yoshiaki Ohmura [13], Masaki Ueno [14], Toshiro Ogura [15], Kyung Suk Suh [16], Yutaro Kato [17], Atsushi Sugioka [17], Andrea Belli [18], Hiroyuki Nitta [19], Masafumi Yasunaga [20], Daniel Cherqui [21,22], Nasser Abdul Halim [21], Alexis Laurent [22], Hironori Kaneko [23], Yuichiro Otsuka [23], Ki Hun Kim [24], Hwui-Dong Cho [24], Charles Chung-Wei Lin [25,26], Yusuke Ome [27], Yasuji Seyama [27], Roberto I. Troisi [28], Giammauro Berardi [29], Fernando Rotellar [30], Gregory C. Wilson [31], David A. Geller [31], Olivier Soubrane [32], Tomoaki Yoh [32], Takashi Kaizu [33], Yusuke Kumamoto [33], Ho-Seong Han [34], Ela Ekmekcigil [34], Ibrahim Dagher [35], David Fuks [36], Brice Gayet [36], Joseph F. Buell [37], Ruben Ciria [38], Javier Briceno [38], Nicholas O'Rourke [39], Joel Lewin [39], Bjorn Edwin [40], Masahiro Shinoda [41], Yuta Abe [41], Mohammed Abu Hilal [42,43], Mohammad Alzoubi [43,44], Minoru Tanabe [15] and Go Wakabayashi [45]

Citation: Morise, Z.; Aldrighetti, L.; Belli, G.; Ratti, F.; Cheung, T.T.; Lo, C.M.; Tanaka, S.; Kubo, S.; Okamura, Y.; Uesaka, K.; et al. An International Retrospective Observational Study of Liver Functional Deterioration after Repeat Liver Resection for Patients with Hepatocellular Carcinoma. *Cancers* 2022, 14, 2598. https://doi.org/10.3390/cancers14112598

Academic Editor: Patrizia Pontisso

Received: 24 April 2022
Accepted: 11 May 2022
Published: 24 May 2022

Publisher's Note: MDPI stays neutral with regard to jurisdictional claims in published maps and institutional affiliations.

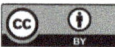

Copyright: © 2022 by the authors. Licensee MDPI, Basel, Switzerland. This article is an open access article distributed under the terms and conditions of the Creative Commons Attribution (CC BY) license (https://creativecommons.org/licenses/by/4.0/).

1 Department of General Surgery, Fujita Health University School of Medicine Okazaki Medical Center, Okazaki 444-0827, Japan
2 Hepatobiliary Division in Department of Surgery, San Raffaele Hospital, 20132 Milano, Italy; aldrighetti.luca@hsr.it (L.A.); ratti.francesca@hsr.it (F.R.)
3 Department of General and HPB Surgery, Loreto Nuovo Hospital, 80127 Naples, Italy; chirurgia.loretonuovo@tin.it
4 Division of HBP and Liver Transplant, University of Hong Kong Queen Mary Hospital, Hong Kong, China; tantocheung@hotmail.com (T.T.C.); chungmlo@hku.hk (C.M.L.)
5 Department of Hepato-Biliary-Pancreatic Surgery, Osaka City University Graduate School of Medicine, Osaka 545-8586, Japan; m8827074@msic.med.osaka-cu.ac.jp (S.T.); m7696493@msic.med.osaka-cu.ac.jp (S.K.)
6 Division of Hepato-Biliary-Pancreatic Surgery, Shizuoka Cancer Center Hospital, Sunto, Shizuoka 411-8777, Japan; yu.okamura@scchr.jp (Y.O.); k.uesaka@scchr.jp (K.U.)
7 Departments of Surgery, Fukuyama City Hospital, Fukuyama 721-8511, Japan; monden0319@yahoo.co.jp (K.M.); shimin-byouin@city.fukuyama.hiroshima.jp (H.S.)
8 Department of Surgery, Kurashiki Central Hospital, Kurashiki 710-8602, Japan; kh14813@kchnet.or.jp (K.H.); kk7159@kchnet.or.jp (K.K.)
9 Division of Hepatobiliary and Pancreatic Surgery, National Cancer Center Hospital East, Kashiwa 277-8577, Japan; ngotohda@east.ncc.go.jp
10 Division of General Surgery, Department of Surgery, Far-Eastern Memorial Hospital, New Taipei City 220, Taiwan; chen.kuohsin@gmail.com
11 Department of Electrical Engineering, Yuan Ze University, Taoyuan City 320, Taiwan
12 Department of Hepato-Biliary-Pancreatic Surgery, Osaka City General Hospital, Osaka 534-0021, Japan; kanazawaaki@mac.com
13 Department of Surgery, Kansai Rosai Hospital, Amagasaki 660-8511, Japan; takeda-yutaka@kansaih.johas.go.jp (Y.T.); ohmura-yoshiaki@kansaih.johas.go.jp (Y.O.)
14 Second Department of Surgery, Wakayama Medical University, Wakayama 641-8509, Japan; ma@wakayama-med.ac.jp
15 Department of Hepatobiliary and Pancreatic Surgery, Graduate School of Medicine, Tokyo Medical and Dental University, Tokyo 113-8510, Japan; ogumsrg@tmd.ac.jp (T.O.); tana.msrg@tmd.ac.jp (M.T.)
16 Department of Hepatobiliary and Pancreatic Surgery, Seoul National University Hospital, Seoul 03080, Korea; kssuh2000@gmail.com
17 Department of Gastrointestinal Surgery, Fujita Health University School of Medicine, Toyoake 470-1192, Japan; y-kato@fujita-hu.ac.jp (Y.K.); sugioka@fujita-hu.ac.jp (A.S.)
18 Department of Abdominal Surgical Oncology, Fondazione G.Pascale-IRCCS, National Cancer Institute of Naples, 80131 Napoli, Italy; a.belli@istitutotumori.na.it
19 Department of Surgery, Iwate Medical University, Morioka 028-3695, Japan; hnitta@iwate-med.ac.jp
20 Department of Surgery, Kurume University School of Medicine, Kurume 830-0011, Japan; m-yasunaga@saiseikai-futsukaichi.org

21 Paul Brousse Hospital, 94800 Villejuif, France; daniel.cherqui@aphp.fr (D.C.); nasserah@clalit.org.il (N.A.H.)
22 Paris-Sud University, 91190 Gif-sur-Yvette, France; alexis.laurent@aphp.fr
23 Division of General and Gastroenterological Surgery, Department of Surgery, Toho University Faculty of Medicine, Tokyo 143-8540, Japan; hironori@med.toho-u.ac.jp (H.K.); yotsuka@med.toho-u.ac.jp (Y.O.)
24 Division of Hepatobiliary Surgery and Liver Transplantation, Department of Surgery, Ulsan University and Asan Medical Center, Seoul 05505, Korea; khkim620@amc.seoul.kr (K.H.K.); hwuidongcho@gmail.com (H.-D.C.)
25 Department of Surgery and Surgical Oncology, Koo Foundation Sun Yat-Sen Cancer Center, Taipei 112, Taiwan; charleslin@ircadtaiwan.com.tw
26 IRCAD-AITS, Changhua 505, Taiwan
27 Department of Surgery, Tokyo Metropolitan Cancer and Infectious Diseases Center Komagome Hospital, Tokyo 113-8677, Japan; yusuke_omen@yahoo.co.jp (Y.O.); seyamaysur-tky@umin.ac.jp (Y.S.)
28 Department of Clinical Medicine and Surgery, University of Naples Federico II, 80138 Napoli, Italy; roberto.troisi@unina.it
29 General Hepato-Biliary and Liver Transplantation Surgery, Ghent University Hospital Medical School, 9000 Gent, Belgium; gberardi1@gmail.com
30 Hepato-Bilio-Pancreatic Unit of Clinica Universitaria de Navarra, 31008 Pamplona, Spain; frotellar@gmail.com
31 Department of Surgery, University of Pittsburgh, Pittsburgh, PA 15213, USA; wilsongc@upmc.edu (G.C.W.); gellerda@upmc.edu (D.A.G.)
32 Department of HPB Surgery and Liver Transplant, Beaujon Hospital, Clichy 92110, France; olivier.soubrane@gmail.com (O.S.); tomyoh@kuhp.kyoto-u.ac.jp (T.Y.)
33 Department of Surgery, Kitasato University School of Medicine, Sagamihara 252-0374, Japan; t-kaizu@kitasato-u.ac.jp (T.K.); kumamoto@kitasato-u.ac.jp (Y.K.)
34 Seoul National University College of Medicine, Bundang Hospital, Seongnam-si 13620, Korea; hanhs@snubh.org (H.-S.H.); eekmekcigil@gmail.com (E.E.)
35 Antoine Beclere Hospital, 92140 Clamart, France; ibrahim.dagher@aphp.fr
36 Department of Digestive Diseases, Institute Mutualiste Montsouris, University of Paris Descartes, 75014 Paris, France; davidfuks80@gmail.com (D.F.); brice.gayet@imm.fr (B.G.)
37 Tulane Transplant Abdominal Institute, Tulane University, New Orleans, LA 70112, USA; joseph.buell@hcahealthcare.com
38 Unit of Hepatobiliary Surgery and Liver Transplantation, University Hospital Reina Sofia, 30003 Murcia, Spain; rubenciria@gmail.com (R.C.); javibriceno@hotmail.com (J.B.)
39 Department of General Surgery and HPB Surgery, Royal Brisbane Hospital, The University of Queensland, St Lucia, QLD 4072, Australia; orourke.nick@gmail.com (N.O.); joel.lewin@uqconnect.edu.au (J.L.)
40 Department of Hepatopancreatobiliary Surgery, Oslo University Hospital-Rikshospitalet, 0372 Oslo, Norway; bjoedw@ous-hf.no
41 Department of Surgery, Keio University School of Medicine, Tokyo 160-8582, Japan; masa02114@yahoo.co.jp (M.S.); abey3666@gmail.com (Y.A.)
42 Istituto Ospedaliero—Fondazione Poliambulanza, 25124 Brescia, BS, Italy; abuhilal9@gmail.com
43 University Hospital Southampton, Hampshire SO16 6YD, UK; mhm0001900@yahoo.com
44 General Surgery Department, The University of Jordan, Amman 11972, Jordan
45 Department of Surgery, Ageo Central General Hospital, Ageo 362-8588, Japan; go324@mac.com
* Correspondence: zmorise@fujita-hu.ac.jp

Simple Summary: For 657 cases of segment or less repeat liver resection with results of plasma albumin and bilirubin levels and platelet counts before and 3 months after surgery, the indicators were compared before and after surgery. There were 268 open repeat after open and 224 cases laparoscopic repeat after laparoscopic liver resection. The background factors and liver functional indicators before and after surgery, and the changes were compared between both groups. Plasma levels of albumin ($p = 0.006$) and total bilirubin ($p = 0.01$) were decreased, and ALBI score ($p = 0.001$) indicated worse liver function after surgery. Though laparoscopic group had poorer performance status and liver function, changes of the values and overall survivals were similar between both groups. Plasma levels of albumin and bilirubin and ALBI score could be the liver functional indicators for liver functional deterioration after liver resection. The laparoscopic group with poorer conditions showed a similar deterioration of liver function and overall survival to the open group.

Abstract: Whether albumin and bilirubin levels, platelet counts, ALBI, and ALPlat scores could be useful for the assessment of permanent liver functional deterioration after repeat liver resection was examined, and the deterioration after laparoscopic procedure was evaluated. For 657 patients with liver resection of segment or less in whom results of plasma albumin and bilirubin levels and platelet counts before and 3 months after surgery could be retrieved, liver functional indicators were compared before and after surgery. There were 268 patients who underwent open repeat after previous open liver resection, and 224 patients who underwent laparoscopic repeat after laparoscopic liver resection. The background factors, liver functional indicators before and after surgery and their changes were compared between both groups. Plasma levels of albumin ($p = 0.006$) and total bilirubin ($p = 0.01$) were decreased, and ALBI score ($p = 0.001$) indicated worse liver function after surgery. Laparoscopic group had poorer preoperative performance status and liver function. Changes of liver functional values before and after surgery and overall survivals were similar between laparoscopic and open groups. Plasma levels of albumin and bilirubin and ALBI score could be the indicators for permanent liver functional deterioration after liver resection. Laparoscopic group with poorer conditions showed the similar deterioration of liver function and overall survivals to open group.

Keywords: laparoscopic liver resection; repeat liver resection; liver function; liver functional deterioration; overall survival

1. Introduction

The treatment options for hepatocellular carcinoma (HCC) are liver resection (LR) [1], liver transplantation [2], transarterial chemoembolization, local ablation therapy [3], and currently emerging systemic (immune-) chemotherapy using kinase inhibitors and immune checkpoint inhibitor [4,5]. Although some treatments provide the hope for a cure of the current HCC [3,6–8], most patients of HCC with underlying chronic liver disease (CLD) are developing metachronous multicentric HCCs from its preoplastic background. When considering treatments for the patients, not only the oncological therapeutic effects to the current tumor, but also the post-treatment residual liver function for the future HCC treatments should be taken into account. The strategy of combination therapy during the long treatment history of HCC patients, depending on each patient's tumor condition and liver function at each time, is needed [9,10]. Although the strategy should be planned with liver functional assessments of the deterioration after treatments, there is currently no good tool for the assessment.

We (ILLS-Tokyo collaborator group) conducted international multi-institutional propensity score-based studies for laparoscopic repeat LR (LRLR) with patients with HCC, comparing to open repeat LR (ORLR) [11,12]. In the study [11], the overall survival curves after LRLR and ORLR were clearly separated with the better tendency in LRLR (not significant with p-value of 0.086), although the disease-free survival curves were identical and overlapped. We speculated that overall survival after LRLR was better since less liver functional damage of LRLR [13] made the repeat treatments more accessible and the number of deceased patients due to liver insufficiency decreased.

Recently, ALBI score [14,15] calculated with plasma albumin and total bilirubin levels and ALPlat score [16] calculated with plasma albumin level and blood platelet counts were proposed as the indicators of liver functional reserve for the preoperative evaluation of LR. In this study, we examined whether plasma albumin level, total bilirubin level, blood platelet counts, ALBI score, and ALPlat score could be useful as liver functional indicators for the assessment of permanently settled liver functional deterioration 3 months after repeat LR (RLR) and, using the indicators, evaluated that the extent of liver functional deterioration after LRLR compared to ORLR.

2. Methods

2.1. Participating Centers and Registered Patients

The present study involved 42 high-volume liver surgery centers around the world that provided data from patients who underwent RLR for HCC between January 2007 and December 2017. Institutional Review Board (IRB) approval was obtained from the coordinating center, with a data transfer agreement and IRB approval having been provided by all centers.

The centers registered 1582 patients, including 934 and 648 treated by ORLR and LRLR. Each case was discussed under a multidisciplinary setting in each center, and each patient provided informed consent for the procedure. The detail of registered patients' number from each center in original patient group was described in a previous study [10].

This study conformed to the ethical guidelines of Declaration of Helsinki and was retrospective in nature. Approval from the ethics committee of each institution was obtained (HM20-094 for primary investigator's institution, FHU).

2.2. Selection of Patients and Data Collection

For 1582 registered patients, the results of usual laboratory blood examination were examined. A total of 875 patients, in whom the results of plasma albumin level, total bilirubin level, and blood platelet counts before and 3 months after surgery could be retrieved, were extracted. Background factors of the patients with ORLR or LRLR are described in Table 1. Then, 657 patients, who underwent segment or less resection, were selected for the first study searching indicators for liver functional change 3 months after RLR in order to eliminate the impact of decreased liver volume after LR.

Table 1. Background factors of all patients (n = 875) with ORLR or LRLR before RLR.

	ORLR, n = 450	LRLR, n = 425	p Value
Age (years old)	66.07 ± 10.77	68.03 ± 10.60	0.007 *
Sex (male:female)	355:95	322:103	0.270
BMI	22.98 ± 3.43	23.98 ± 3.96	<0.001 *
Performance status (0:1:2)	411:37:1	365:55:5	0.016 *
Size of tumor (mm)	23.59 ± 17.52	20.49 ± 10.74	0.002 *
Number of tumors (1:2:3:>4)	315:87:23:25	335:70:13:7	0.003 *
Tumor location (AL:PS)	159:107	145:77	0.223
Extent of resection (Segment or less: Section: 2 or more sections)	329:72:49	382:33:10	<0.001 *
Albumin (g/dL)	4.09 ± 0.41	4.01 ± 0.48	0.006 *
Total Bilirubin (mg/dL)	0.73 ± 0.32	0.76 ± 0.35	0.095
Platelet (X10^4/microL)	14.77 ± 6.11	13.93 ± 5.10	0.026 *
Presence of fibrosis (NL:CH:LF:LC)	73:56:114:202 [#]	49:39:120:213 [##]	0.056
Child–Pugh score (5:6:7:>8)	393:46:9:2	322:84:14:5	<0.001 *

RLR: repeat liver resection, ORLR: open repeat liver resection, LRLR: laparoscopic repeat liver resection. Data are shown as mean ± SD or number of cases. *: statistically significant. [#]: There are 5 missing data, [##]: There are 4 missing data.

The following data were obtained as background factors: patient characteristics (age, sex, body mass index (BMI), and preoperative performance status (PS)); indicators of preoperative liver function (presence of liver fibrosis, plasma total bilirubin level (mg/dL), plasma albumin level (g/dL), blood platelet count (/microL), Child–Pugh score)); tumor characteristics (number, size (mm), and location (anterolateral or posterosuperior segments)); surgical procedures (ORLR or LRLR) and the previous LR procedure (open or laparoscopic).

In addition, the results 3 months after RLR of plasma albumin level, total bilirubin level, and blood platelet counts were obtained.

2.3. Analysis of the Indicators of Liver Function before and 3 Months after RLR

The results before and 3 months after RLR of plasma albumin level, total bilirubin level, and blood platelet counts were compared in the selected 657 patients. Furthermore, calculated ALBI scores [14,15] and ALPlat scores [16] before and after RLR were compared (Table 2).

Table 2. Analysis of the indicators of liver function before and 3 months after repeat liver resection.

	Pre-Operative Data	Post-Operative Data	p Value
Albumin (g/dL)	4.04 ± 0.45	3.97 ± 0.53	0.006 *
Total Bilirubin (mg/dL)	0.76 ± 0.33	0.81 ± 0.40	0.010 *
Platelet ($\times 10^4$/microL)	14.07 ± 5.02	14.12 ± 5.20	0.862
ALBI score	−2.73 ± 0.40	−2.65 ± 0.48	0.001 *
AlPlat score	504.49 ± 70.46	498.24 ± 77.05	0.125

Data are shown as mean ± SD. *: statistically significant.

2.4. Comparison between the Patients Who Underwent ORLR after Previous Open LR (OO group) and LRLR after Previous Laparoscopic LR (LL Group): Background Factors, Indicators for Liver Function before RLR, Their Changes after RLR, and Overall Survival after RLR

There were 268 patients who underwent ORLR after previous open LR (OO group) and 224 patients who underwent LRLR after previous laparoscopic LR (LL group) among selected 657 patients with segment or less RLR. Selected patients' numbers for the final analysis, comparing ORLR and LRLR in the present study, from each center are in the description of Table 3

Table 3. Comparison between OO group and LL group: Background factors, indicators for liver function before RLR, and after RLR.

Before LR	OO	LL	p Value
Age (years old)	67.37 ± 10.36	68.62 ± 9.96	0.176
Sex (male:female)	214:54	167:57	0.194
BMI	22.94 ± 3.44	23.96 ± 3.98	0.002 *
Performance status (1:2:3)	250:17:1	194:29:1	0.043 *
Number of tumors (1:2:3:>4)	188:58:14:8	176:38:6:4	0.209
Size of tumor (mm)	20.93 ± 15.21	19.00 ± 9.52	0.089
Tumor location (AL:PS)	159:107	145:77	0.223
Albumin (g/dL)	4.09 ± 0.39	3.94 ± 0.49	<0.001 *
Total Bilirubin (mg/dL)	0.73 ± 0.31	0.75 ± 0.35	0.698
Platelet ($\times 10^4$/microL)	14.58 ± 4.89	13.57 ± 5.41	0.031 *
ALBI score	−2.78 ± 0.34	−2.65 ± 0.46	<0.001 *
AlPlat score	514.32 ± 61.09	490.43 ± 79.95	<0.001 *
Presence of fibrosis (NL:CH:LF:LC)	48:41:70:106	21:23:63:114	0.006 *
Child-Pugh score (5:6:7:>8)	239:25:4:0	160:53:7:4	<0.001 *
3 months after LR			
Albumin (g/dL)	4.03 ± 0.47	3.89 ± 0.55	0.003 *
Total Bilirubin (mg/dL)	0.77 ± 0.36	0.80 ± 0.39	0.461
Platelet (X10^4/microL)	14.77 ± 5.09	13.68 ± 5.56	0.025 *
ALBI score	−2.71 ± 0.42	−2.59 ± 0.52	0.003 *
AlPlat score	510.10 ± 69.08	486.70 ± 83.60	0.001 *

Data are shown as mean ± SD or number of cases. *: statistically significant. OO group: Cases who underwent open repeat liver resection after previous open liver resection. LL group: Cases who underwent laparoscopic repeat liver resection after previous laparoscopic liver resection. RLR: repeat liver resection, LR; liver resection, BMI: body mass index, AL: tumors located anterolateral segments (segments 2–6), PS: tumors located posterosuperior segments (segments1,7,8), NL: normal liver, CH:chronic hepatitis, LF: liver fibrosis, LC: liver cirrhosis.

The factors listed before (background factors, indicators for liver function, ALBI score, and ALPlat score) RLR; plasma albumin level, total bilirubin level, blood platelet counts, ALBI score, and ALPlat score 3 months after RLR were compared between LL and OO groups.

Changes of the values before and after RLR in albumin, bilirubin, platelet, ALBI score, and ALPlat score were compared between LL and OO groups.

Overall survival after RLR was compared between LL and OO groups.

2.5. Statistical Analyses

Data are expressed as mean ± standard deviation or as the number of patients. Between-group differences in categorical variables were analyzed by Pearson's Chi-squared test or Fisher's exact test with Yates correction, as appropriate. Between group differences in continuous parametric variables were analyzed by un-paired Student's *t*-test or ANOVA, and between-group differences in continuous non-parametric variables were analyzed by Mann–Whitney or Kruskal–Wallis test. Survival was plotted by the Kaplan–Meier method, and between-group differences were analyzed by log-rank test. Statistical analyses were performed with the use of SPSS Statistics 25 (IBM Corp., Armonk, NY, USA) or R 3.3.4 (R Foundation for Statistical Computing, Vienna, Austria). $p < 0.05$ was considered statistically significant.

3. Results

3.1. Analyses of the Indicators for Liver Function before and 3 Months after RLR

Plasma levels of albumin (4.04 ± 0.45 vs. 3.97 ± 0.53 g/dL, $p = 0.006$) was significantly decreased and total bilirubin (0.76 ± 0.33 vs. 0.81 ± 0.40 mg/dL, $p = 0.01$) was significantly increased 3 months after RLR compared to those values before RLR. The difference in blood platelet counts was not significant (14.07 ± 5.02 vs. $14.12 \pm 5.20 \times 10^4$/microL, $p = 0.862$). Consequently, ALBI score (-2.73 ± 0.40 vs. -2.65 ± 0.48, $p = 0.001$) indicated significantly worse liver function 3 months after RLR, but not ALPlat score (504.49 ± 70.46 vs. 498.24 ± 77.05, $p = 0.125$).

3.2. Comparison between OO Group and LL Group: Background Factors, Indicators for Liver Function before RLR, and Those, Their Changes, and Overall Survivals after RLR

There was significantly higher BMI and poorer PS in the LL group. The LL group had significantly higher incidence of liver fibrosis and Child–Pugh score before RLR, although there were no significant differences between OO and LL groups in tumor-related factors, such as tumor number, size, and location. In addition, there were significant differences before and also after RLR in plasma level of albumin (OO vs. LL before RLR: 4.09 ± 0.39 vs. 3.94 ± 0.49 g/dL, $p < 0.001$; OO vs. LL after RLR: 4.03 ± 0.47 vs. 3.89 ± 0.55 g/dL, $p = 0.003$), blood platelet count (14.58 ± 4.89 vs. $13.57 \pm 5.41 \times 10^4$/microL, $p = 0.031$; 14.77 ± 5.09 vs. $13.68 \pm 5.56 \times 10^4$/microL, $p = 0.025$), ALBI score (-2.78 ± 0.34 vs. -2.65 ± 0.46, $p < 0.001$; -2.71 ± 0.42 vs. -2.59 ± 0.52, $p = 0.003$), and ALPlat score (514.32 ± 61.09 vs. 490.43 ± 79.95, $p < 0.001$; 510.10 ± 69.08 vs. 486.70 ± 83.60, $p = 0.001$) between LL vs. OO groups. (Table 3)

All the changes of values before and after RLR in albumin, bilirubin, platelet, ALBI score, and ALPlat score were similar without significant differences between LL and OO groups. (Table 4)

There was no significant difference in overall survival after RLR between LL and OO groups. (Figure 1, $p = 0.576$).

OO patients were registered from Clinica Universitaria de Navarra = 2 (number of patients), Wakayama Medical University Hospital = 13, Osaka City University = 30, Queen Mary Hospital = 34, Shizuoka Cancer Center = 47, University of Pittsburgh = 2, University Hospital Reina Sofia = 1, Kitazato University = 7, Komagome Hospital = 5, Osaka City General Hospital = 5, Kurume University = 18, Kurashiki Central Hospital = 18, National Cancer Center Hospital East = 37, Kansai Rosai Hospital = 4, Tokyo Medical and Dental University = 22, Toho University = 6, Fujita Health University Hospital = 4, Keio University = 3 and LL from Seoul National University Bundang Hospital = 2, Clinica Universitaria de Navarra = 2, Wakayama Medical University Hospital = 4, Osaka City University = 15, Queen Mary Hospital = 5, Fujita Health University Bantane Hospital = 15, Shizuoka Cancer Center = 3, Kitazato University = 1, Komagome Hospital = 4, Koo Foundation Sun Yat-Sen Cancer Center = 2, Far-Eastern Memorial Hospital = 20, Osaka City General Hospital = 32, Kurume University = 1, Kurashiki Central Hospital = 23, National Cancer Center Hospital East = 4, Tulane University = 1, Institute Mutualiste Montsouris = 10, Kansai Rosai Hospital = 33, Tokyo Medical and Dental University = 1, Toho University = 4, Asan Medical Center = 3, Fujita Health University Hospital = 22, and Keio University = 17.

Table 4. Comparison between OO group and LL group: Changes in indicators for liver function before and after RLR.

	OO	LL	p Value
Change of Alb (g/dL)	0.068 ± 0.40	0.054 ± 0.42	0.710
Change of Total Bilirubin (mg/dL)	−0.036 ± 0.34	−0.049 ± 0.33	0.653
Change of Platelet ($\times 10^4$/microL)	−0.19 ± 4.26	−0.11 ± 3.34	0.830
Change of ALBI score	−0.064 ± 0.35	−0.063 ± 0.38	0.969
Change of ALPlat score	4.23 ± 53.46	3.73 ± 53.59	0.919

Data are shown as mean ± SD. OO group: Cases who underwent open repeat liver resection after previous open liver resection. LL group: Cases who underwent laparoscopic repeat liver resection after previous laparoscopic liver resection.

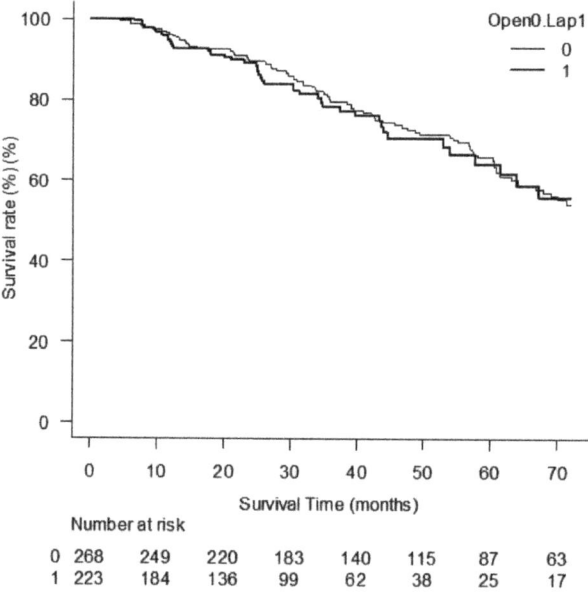

Figure 1. Overall survival after RLR between LL and OO groups.

4. Discussion

The present study showed that the plasma level of albumin, that of total bilirubin, and ALBI score indicated significantly worsened liver function 3 months after RLR comparing to the preoperative values. Although ALBI [14,15] and ALPlat [16] scores are advocated for liver functional evaluation before HCC treatments including LR, there are no established assessment indicators for the permanent deterioration of liver function settled stable 3 months after treatments. These factors, plasma level of albumin, that of total bilirubin, and ALBI score, could be the candidate indicators for the assessments of liver functional permanent deterioration after LR. Using these indicators, evaluation for the extent of liver functional deterioration after LRLR compared to ORLR were also performed in present study.

With the original patient group for the present study, we conducted international multi-institutional studies for LRLR to HCC patients, compared to ORLR [11,12]. The studies showed that LRLR is feasible and has short-term advantages of less intraoperative blood loss and less morbidity for selected patients. In the first study [11], the overall survival curves after LRLR and ORLR were clearly separated with the better tendency in LRLR, although the disease-free survival curves were identical. Overall survival of HCC patients with CLD after LR is determined not only by the recurrence of the resected HCC, but also by metachronous multicentric HCCs and liver insufficiency [8,9]. During the long and repeated treatment history of patients with HCC, they should have enough residual liver function after each treatment which makes them possible to undergo repeat combination treatments. We hypothesized that overall survival after LRLR was better since less deterioration of liver function after LRLR [12], in addition to less adhesion, made the repeat treatments more accessible and the number of deceased patients due to liver insufficiency decreased.

The main advantages of LLR for repeat treatments are thought to be less adhesion after LR and less damage to the liver and surrounding structures, such as collateral vessels [17], using the laparoscopic direct approach to the surgical area [18–20], sometimes without complete dissection of adhesion. Those could work not only on the technical aspects during LR, but also on the liver function after treatments resulting in less deterioration. Both possible advantages were verified by simple comparison of OO (open repeat LR after open LR) and LL (laparoscopic repeat LR after laparoscopic LR) groups, excluding the patients who underwent both open and laparoscopic procedures, in the present study. Selecting the resections of segmentectomy or less were for minimizing the impact on the deterioration from the decreased functional liver volume. There was no difference in tumor number, size, and location (in anterolateral segments or posterosuperior segments) between OO and LL groups. Thereafter, tumor and surgical factors are similar in both groups compared. On the other hand, the LL group had patients with poorer general (poorer PS and higher BMI) and liver condition (more fibrosis, lower albumin and platelet, worse ALBI/ALPLat/Child–Pugh scores) compared to the OO group. LL group patients with poorer liver and general conditions and similar tumor and surgical factors showed similar deterioration of liver function and resulted in similar overall survival to OO group patients. It could be translated that LL group patients could have gone through repeat LR well, despite the fact that they were allocated to LRLR due to the fear of liver decompensation and morbidity after ORLR. It may show the advantage of LLR, that it could prolong the overall survival of the HCC patients with CLD as a powerful local therapy which can be applied repeatedly with minimal deterioration of liver function.

The deterioration of liver function by each HCC treatment is usually smaller and more difficult to detect than years-long deterioration by CLD, except major hepatectomies which remove a large volume of functional liver. The present study showed that plasma level of albumin, that of total bilirubin, and ALBI score are the possible indicators for the assessment of liver functional permanent deterioration after LR. However, LR should have heaviest damage on liver function among the treatment options and, also, the evaluation of each individual case in different condition should be more difficult. Therefore, further investigations are needed for the assessment of liver functional change after each treatment during repeated treatments for the patients with metachronous multicentric HCCs and CLD.

Author Contributions: Z.M., L.A., G.B. (Giulio Belli), F.R. (Francesca Ratti), T.T.C., C.M.L., S.T., S.K., Y.O. (Yukiyasu Okamura), K.U., K.M., H.S., K.H., K.K., N.G., K.C., A.K., Y.T., Y.O. (Yoshiaki Ohmura), M.U., T.O., K.S.S., Y.K. (Yutaro Kato), A.S., A.B., H.N., M.Y., D.C., N.A.H., A.L., H.K., Y.O. (Yuichiro Otsuka), K.H.K., H.-D.C., C.C.-W.L., Y.O. (Yusuke Ome), Y.S., R.I.T., G.B. (Giammauro Berardi), F.R.

(Fernando Rotellar), G.C.W., D.A.G., O.S., T.Y., T.K., Y.K. (Yusuke Kumamoto)., H.-S.H., E.E., I.D., D.F., B.G., J.F.B., R.C., J.B., N.O., J.L., B.E., M.S., Y.A., M.A.H., M.A., M.T. and G.W. collected the data at their various institutions and discussed results. Z.M., L.A. and G.B. (Giammauro Berardi) designed this study, collected the data, and drafted this paper. D.C., G.W. and M.T. co-organized the international study and discussed results during the drafting of this paper. All authors have read and agreed to the published version of the manuscript.

Funding: This study has no related funding.

Institutional Review Board Statement: This study conformed to the ethical guidelines of Declaration of Helsinki and was retrospective in nature. Approval from the ethics committee of each institution was obtained (HM20-094 for primary investigator's institution, FHU). Informed consent was obtained from all subjects.

Informed Consent Statement: Informed consent was obtained from all subjects involved in the study.

Data Availability Statement: The data presented in this study are available on request from the corresponding author.

Conflicts of Interest: All authors declare no conflict of interest nor sources of funding related to this study.

References

1. Capussotti, L.; Ferrero, A.; Viganò, L.; Polastri, R.; Tabone, M. Liver resection for HCC with cirrhosis: Surgical perspectives out of EASL/AASLD guidelines. *Eur. J. Surg. Oncol.* **2009**, *35*, 11–15. [CrossRef] [PubMed]
2. Hwang, S.; Lee, S.G.; Belghiti, J. Liver transplantation for HCC: Its role: Eastern and Western perspectives. *J. Hepatobiliary Pancreat. Sci.* **2010**, *17*, 443–448. [CrossRef] [PubMed]
3. Lau, W.Y.; Leung, T.W.; Yu, S.C.; Ho, S.K. Percutaneous local ablative therapy for hepatocellular carcinoma: A review and look into the future. *Ann. Surg.* **2003**, *237*, 171–179. [CrossRef] [PubMed]
4. Kudo, M.; Finn, R.S.; Qin, S.; Han, K.H.; Ikeda, K.; Piscaglia, F.; Cheng, A.L.; Baron, A.; Han, G.; Lopez, C.; et al. Lenvatinib versus sorafenib in first-line treatment of patients with unresectable hepatocellular carcinoma: A randomised phase 3 non-inferiority trial. *Lancet* **2018**, *391*, 1163–1173. [CrossRef]
5. Finn, R.S.; Qin, S.; Ikeda, M.; Galle, P.R.; Ducreux, M.; Kim, T.Y.; Cheng, A.L.; Kudo, M.; Merle, P.; Li, D.; et al. Atezolizumab plus Bevacizumab in Unresectable Hepatocellular Carcinoma. *N. Engl. J. Med.* **2020**, *382*, 1894–1905. [CrossRef] [PubMed]
6. Mazzaferro, V.; Regalia, E.; Doci, R.; Andreola, S.; Pulvirenti, A.; Bozzetti, F.; Gennari, L.; Montalto, F.; Ammatuna, M.; Morabito, A. Liver transplantation for the treatment of small hepatocellular carcinomas in patients with cirrhosis. *N. Engl. J. Med.* **1996**, *334*, 693–699. [CrossRef] [PubMed]
7. Ryder, S.D. Guidelines for the diagnosis and treatment of hepatocellular carcinoma (HCC) in adults. *Gut* **2003**, *52*, 1–8. [CrossRef] [PubMed]
8. Rahbari, N.N.; Mehrabi, A.; Mollberg, N.M.; Müller, S.A.; Koch, M.; Büchler, M.W.; Weitz, J. Hepatocellular carcinoma: Current management and perspectives for the future. *Ann. Surg.* **2011**, *253*, 453–469. [CrossRef] [PubMed]
9. El-Serag, H.B.; Marrero, J.A.; Rudolph, L.; Reddy, K.R. Diagnosis and treatment of hepatocellular carcinoma. *Gastroenterology* **2008**, *134*, 1752–1763. [CrossRef] [PubMed]
10. Llovet, J.M.; Fuster, J.; Bruix, J. The Barcelona approach: Diagnosis, staging, and treatment of hepatocellular carcinoma. *Liver Transpl.* **2004**, *10*, S115–S120. [CrossRef] [PubMed]
11. Morise, Z.; Aldrighetti, L.; Belli, G.; Ratti, F.; Belli, A.; Cherqui, D.; Alzoubi, M.; Lo, M.; Kubo, S.; Monden, K.; et al. ILLS-Tokyo Collaborator group. Laparoscopic repeat liver resection for hepatocellular carcinoma: A multicentre propensity score-based study. *Br. J. Surg.* **2020**, *107*, 889–895. [CrossRef] [PubMed]
12. 3Miyama, A.; Morise, Z.; Aldrighetti, L.; Belli, G.; Ratti, F.; Cheung, T.-T.; Lo, C.-M.; Tanaka, S.; Kubo, S.; Okamura, Y.; et al. Multicenter Propensity Score-Based Study of Laparoscopic Repeat Liver Resection for Hepatocellular Carcinoma: A Subgroup Analysis of Cases with Tumors Far from Major Vessels. *Cancers* **2021**, *13*, 3187.
13. Morise, Z.; Ciria, R.; Cherqui, D.; Chen, K.H.; Belli, G.; Wakabayashi, G. Can we expand the indications for laparoscopic liver resection? A systematic review and meta-analysis of laparoscopic liver resection for patients with hepatocellular carcinoma and chronic liver disease. *J. Hepatobiliary Pancreat. Sci.* **2015**, *22*, 342–352. [CrossRef] [PubMed]
14. Johnson, P.J.; Berhane, S.; Kagebayashi, C.; Satomura, S.; Teng, M.; Reeves, H.L.; Toyoda, H.; Fox, R.; Palmer, D.; Lai, P.; et al. Assessment of liver function in patients with hepatocellular carcinoma: A new evidence-based approach-the ALBI grade. *J. Clin. Oncol.* **2015**, *33*, 550–558. [CrossRef] [PubMed]
15. Pinato, D.J.; Sharma, R.; Allara, E.; Yen, C.; Arizumi, T.; Kubota, K.; Carr, B.I.; Kim, Y.-W.; Kudo, M.; Guerra, V.; et al. The ALBI grade provides objective hepatic reserve estimation across each BCLC stage of hepatocellular carcinoma. *J. Hepatol.* **2017**, *66*, 338–346. [CrossRef] [PubMed]

16. Yamamoto, G.; Taura, K.; Ikai, I.; Fujikawa, T.; Nishitai, R.; Kaihara, S.; Uemoto, S.; Okuda, Y.; Tanabe, K.; Nishio, T.; et al. ALPlat criterion for the resection of hepatocellular carcinoma based on a predictive model of posthepatectomy liver failure. *Surgery* **2020**, *167*, 410–416. [CrossRef] [PubMed]
17. Kanazawa, A.; Tsukamoto, T.; Shimizu, S.; Kodai, S.; Yamamoto, S.; Yamazoe, S.; Ohira, G.; Nakajima, T. Laparoscopic liver resection for treating recurrent hepatocellular carcinoma. *J. Hepatobiliary Pancreat. Sci.* **2013**, *20*, 512–517. [CrossRef] [PubMed]
18. Tomishige, H.; Morise, Z.; Kawabe, N.; Nagata, H.; Ohshima, H.; Kawase, J.; Arawaka, S.; Isetani, M.; Yoshida, R. Caudal approach to pure laparoscopic posterior sectionectomy under the laparoscopy-specific view. *World J. Gastrointest. Surg.* **2013**, *5*, 173–177. [CrossRef] [PubMed]
19. Wakabayashi, G.; Cherqui, D.; Geller, D.A.; Han, H.S.; Kaneko, H.; Buell, J.F. Laparoscopic hepatectomy is theoretically better than open hepatectomy: Preparing for the 2nd International Consensus Conference on Laparoscopic Liver Resection. *J. Hepatobiliary Pancreat. Sci.* **2014**, *21*, 723–731. [CrossRef] [PubMed]
20. Soubrane, O.; Schwarz, L.; Cauchy, F.; Perotto, L.O.; Brustia, R.; Bernard, D.; Scatton, O. A conceptual technique for laparoscopic right hepatectomybased on facts and oncologic principles: The caudal approach. *Ann. Surg.* **2015**, *261*, 1226–1231. [CrossRef] [PubMed]

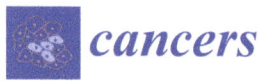

Article

Safety and Feasibility of Laparoscopic Parenchymal-Sparing Hepatectomy for Lesions with Proximity to Major Vessels in Posterosuperior Liver Segments 7 and 8

Hirokatsu Katagiri *, Hiroyuki Nitta, Syoji Kanno, Akira Umemura, Daiki Takeda, Taro Ando, Satoshi Amano and Akira Sasaki

Department of Surgery, Iwate Medical University School of Medicine, 2-1-1 Idai-dori, Yahaba 028-3609, Iwate, Japan; hnitta@iwate-med.ac.jp (H.N.); kannos@iwate-med.ac.jp (S.K.); aumemura@iwate-med.ac.jp (A.U.); dtakeda@iwate-med.ac.jp (D.T.); antaro@iwate-med.ac.jp (T.A.); satoshia@iwate-med.ac.jp (S.A.); sakira@iwate-med.ac.jp (A.S.)
* Correspondence: hkatagi@iwate-med.ac.jp; Tel.: +81-196-13-7111; Fax: +81-199-07-7344

Simple Summary: Improvements in perioperative management and surgical techniques have enabled laparoscopic liver resection for posterosuperior liver segments. Recent studies have reported the safety and feasibility of selected posterosuperior lesions; however, laparoscopic parenchymal-sparing hepatectomy for lesions with proximity to major vessels in posterosuperior segments has not yet been examined. The aim of this study is to examine the safety and feasibility of laparoscopic parenchymal-sparing hepatectomy for lesions with proximity to major vessels in posterosuperior segments 7 and 8. The present study demonstrated that laparoscopic parenchymal-sparing hepatectomy for lesions with proximity to major vessels in posterosuperior segments 7 and 8 is safe and feasible in a specialized center with a team experienced in laparoscopic liver surgery, and the HALS technique still plays an important role as minimally invasive liver resection. These findings suggest the possibility of taking steps to perform more advanced minimally invasive liver resections.

Citation: Katagiri, H.; Nitta, H.; Kanno, S.; Umemura, A.; Takeda, D.; Ando, T.; Amano, S.; Sasaki, A. Safety and Feasibility of Laparoscopic Parenchymal-Sparing Hepatectomy for Lesions with Proximity to Major Vessels in Posterosuperior Liver Segments 7 and 8. *Cancers* 2023, 15, 2078. https://doi.org/10.3390/cancers15072078

Academic Editor: Matteo Donadon

Received: 19 March 2023
Revised: 29 March 2023
Accepted: 30 March 2023
Published: 30 March 2023

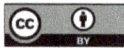

Copyright: © 2023 by the authors. Licensee MDPI, Basel, Switzerland. This article is an open access article distributed under the terms and conditions of the Creative Commons Attribution (CC BY) license (https://creativecommons.org/licenses/by/4.0/).

Abstract: Laparoscopic parenchymal-sparing hepatectomy (PSH) for lesions with proximity to major vessels (PMV) in posterosuperior segments (PSS) has not yet been sufficiently examined. The aim of this study is to examine the safety and feasibility of laparoscopic PSH for lesions with PMV in PSS 7 and 8. We retrospectively reviewed the outcomes of laparoscopic liver resection (LLR) and open liver resection (OLR) for PSS lesions and focused on patients who underwent laparoscopic PSH for lesions with PMV in PSS. Blood loss was lower in the LLR group ($n = 110$) than the OLR group ($n = 16$) ($p = 0.009$), and no other short-term outcomes were significantly different. Compared to the pure LLR group ($n = 93$), there were no positive surgical margins or complications in hand-assisted laparoscopic surgery (HALS) ($n = 17$), despite more tumors with PMV ($p = 0.009$). Regarding pure LLR for one tumor lesion, any short-term outcomes in addition to the operative time were not significantly different between the PMV ($n = 23$) and no-PMV ($n = 48$) groups. The present findings indicate that laparoscopic PSH for lesions with PMV in PSS is safe and feasible in a matured team, and the HALS technique still plays an important role.

Keywords: laparoscopic; hepatectomy; liver resection; posterosuperior; parenchymal sparing

1. Introduction

Since laparoscopic liver resection (LLR) was first reported in the early 1990s, it has gradually spread as a minimally invasive surgery [1]. Previous studies have demonstrated that LLR results in improved short-term outcomes and comparable oncological outcomes compared with open liver resection (OLR). Currently, LLR is one of the standard treatments for anterolateral segments and left lateral sectionectomy [2–5]. However, LLR for posterosuperior liver segments (PSS; segments 1, 4b, 7, and 8) remains the most challenging procedure. According to the European Consensus Conference held in Southampton in 2017, a technically demanding resection for lesions located in PSS has yet to be fully standardized and should only be performed in specialized centers [6].

In recent years, appropriate anesthetic respiratory and circulatory management and the development of surgical techniques have enabled LLR to be performed safely at many hospitals, and recent studies have indicated that LLR is technically feasible and safe for selected patients with lesions in PSS [7–14]. Nevertheless, laparoscopic parenchymal-sparing hepatectomy (PSH) for liver lesions with proximity to major vessels (PMV) in PSS has not yet been examined. Due to the variation in the degree of difficulty of LLR, depending on the procedure of the hepatectomy and tumor conditions, a difficulty scoring system that assigns increasing values to tumors in close proximity to major vessels was proposed [15]. In PSS, especially segments 7 and 8, this factor is likely to have a greater impact on surgical outcomes.

The aim of the present study is to examine the safety and feasibility of laparoscopic PSH for lesions with PMV in PSS, especially segments 7 and 8, and to explore the possibility of taking further steps to perform minimally invasive liver resections.

2. Materials and Methods
2.1. Selection of Patients and Data Collection

A prospective database of the patients treated at our institution was retrospectively reviewed. Between January 2011 and December 2021, 1041 patients underwent liver resections at our institution. Consistently, 80–90% of cases had been treated with laparoscopic surgery during the inclusion period. During this study period, 165 patients underwent PSH for liver tumors (hepatocellular cell carcinoma, metastatic liver cancer, cholangiocellular carcinoma, and benign tumors) located in PSS 7 or 8. From this subset, we excluded 39 patients who underwent hepatectomies for four or more lesions, combined resection of other organs, hybrid technique, or resections concomitant with laparoscopic major hepatectomy. The exclusion criteria for LLR were 4 or more lesions resected, lesions spreading to other organs needed reconstruction, patients needing regional lymph node dissection, and the need for bile ducts and/or vessels resection with reconstruction. These are indicated for open surgery. Neither the size of the lesions nor cirrhosis were exclusion criteria.

A total of 126 patients (110 patients in the LLR group and 16 patients in the OLR group) who underwent PSH for lesions located in PSS 7 or 8 were retrospectively reviewed. To assess safety and feasibility within the LLR group, we divided the 110 patients in the LLR group into two groups: a group of 35 patients with lesions with PMV and a group of 75 patients with lesions with no PMV (no-PMV). To clarify the role of the hand-assisted laparoscopic surgery (HALS) technique, we reviewed 93 patients in the pure LLR group and 17 patients in the HALS group. Finally, to account for some discrepancies in the background factors, we further analyzed patients who underwent pure LLR for one tumor lesion, including 71 patients (23 patients in the PMV group and 48 patients in the no-PMV group).

The following variables were examined in our analysis: patient characteristics (age, sex, and body mass index (BMI); histories of preoperative chemotherapy, upper abdominal surgery, and hepatectomy; Child–Pugh score, and physical status score by the American Society of Anesthesiologists physical status classification (ASA-PS)); preoperative laboratory data (plasma aspartate aminotransferase (AST), plasma alanine aminotransferase (ALT), plasma total bilirubin, plasma albumin level, prothrombin time international normalized ratio (PT-INR), blood platelet count, and indocyanine green retention rate at 15 min); pathological factors (presence of liver cirrhosis, tumor number, tumor size, and location); intraoperative factors (surgical procedures, Pringle's maneuver, operation time, volume of blood loss, blood transfusion rate, sacrifice of major hepatic veins, and positive surgical margin); and postoperative information (length of hospital stay, morbidity, and mortality).

The present study protocol was approved by the Institutional Review Board of Iwate Medical University. All patients were informed about this study, and consent was obtained.

2.2. Definitions

Laparoscopic liver resection was defined as a pure laparoscopic surgery or a HALS technique. Proximity to major vessels was defined as the main or second branches of Glisson's tree, major hepatic vein, and inferior vena cava [15] (Figure 1a,b). Postoperative morbidity was graded according to the Clavien–Dindo classification [16]. Postoperative mortality was defined as any death occurring within 90 days of liver resection. The surgical margin was defined as microscopically positive if tumor cells were identified along the periphery of the resected specimen.

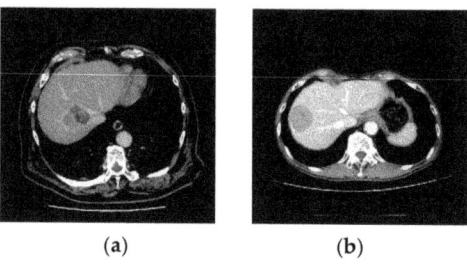

(a)   (b)

Figure 1. (a) A lesion with proximity to major vessels. (b) A lesion with no proximity to major vessels.

2.3. Surgical Procedure

For segment 7 resections, the patients were treated in the left half-lateral decubitus position. For segment 8 resections, the patients were treated in the supine position. An anti-Trendelenburg position was used in all cases. The operator stood to the right of the patient, while the assistant and scopist were on the patient's left. The anesthesiologist maintained a low central vein pressure of ≤ 3 mmHg and a low airway pressure ≤ 15 cm H_2O to reduce bleeding from the hepatic vein [17]. A carbon dioxide pneumoperitoneum was maintained at 10 mmHg. Visual exploration of the abdominal cavity was conducted with a flexible endoscope. Intraoperative ultrasonography was routinely used to identify the location of the tumors and surgical boundaries and to confirm hepatic blood flow. In the HALS technique, a hand-assisted device (Wound Retractor^{TM}, Applied Medical, Rancho Santa Margarita, CA, USA) was placed in the right abdominal horizontal incision (7–9 cm). The intermittent Pringle's maneuver was continuously repeated during parenchymal transection. Trocar placement is shown in Figure 2a,b.

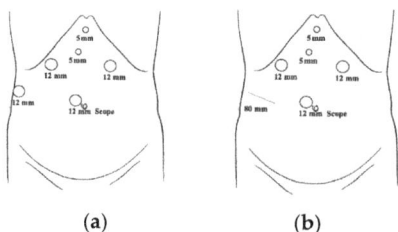

(a)   (b)

Figure 2. (a) Trocar placement for pure LLR. (b) Trocar placement for HALS. The blue line is the incision placed by a hand-assisted device.

We mobilized the right liver from the lateral and posterior abdominal walls and created a space on the right side of the inferior vena cava for dorsal retraction during parenchymal transection. This procedure is a crucial preparation for bleeding control. Following these preparatory steps, the liver parenchyma of segments 7 and 8 were transected using the clamp crush method and a sealing device. Bleeding from small branches of the hepatic veins was controlled by a saline dripping monopolar soft-coagulation system. Instances of bleeding caused by tearing in the small crotch of vessels branches, which we call a hangnail injury, were treated by making a clean cut while the initial tear was small (Figure 3a–c). After making a clean cut, a saline dripping monopolar soft-coagulation system was used to achieve hemostasis (Figure 3d). In case of bleeding from the branches of major hepatic veins, compression of the liver parenchyma from the dorsal side, which we call dorsal compression, enabled a safe operation with controlled bleeding (Figure 4). If necessary, the hepatic vein was divided using a stapler with a 60 mm cartridge. After resection of the targeted liver tissue was performed, the specimen was extracted through an incision using a protective bag.

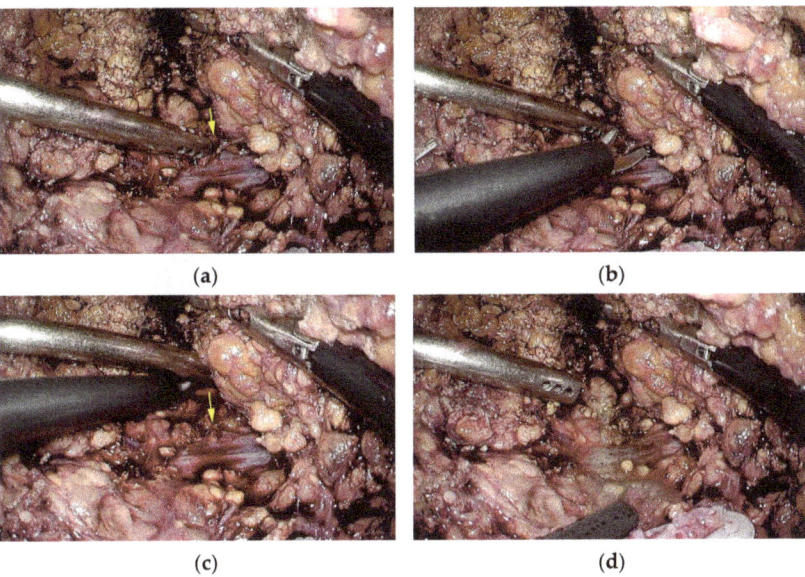

Figure 3. (a) The small crotch formed teared from vessels. The yellow arrow is the hangnail injury. (b) Sharply cutting the small branch teared from vessels. (c) Releasing the tension against the vessels. The yellow arrow is the hangnail injury. (d) The hemostasis using a saline dripping monopolar soft-coagulation system.

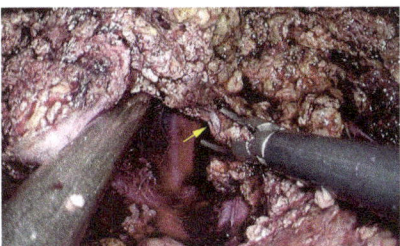

Figure 4. Dorsal compression, compressing the liver parenchyma from the dorsal side, enables control of bleeding from a branch of the hepatic vein. The yellow arrow is the bleeding point from the hepatic vein.

2.4. Statistical Analysis

The continuous variables are described as medians with interquartile ranges, whereas the categorical variables are described as totals and frequencies. Differences in groups were assessed through Student's *t*-test or ANOVA for the continuous parametric variables,

Mann–Whitney U test for the continuous non-parametric variables, and Pearson's chi-squared test or Fisher's exact test (for expected counts of <5) for the categorical variables. Survival was estimated using the Kaplan–Meier method and compared between the groups using the log-rank test. Statistical analysis was performed using JMP software (version 13.2.0, SAS Institute, Cary, NC, USA). Variables with a p-value < 0.05 were considered statistically significant.

3. Results

3.1. Analysis of 126 Patients

We analyzed the data of 126 patients, of which 110 underwent LLR and 16 underwent OLR. Male patients were more common in the OLR group (LLR vs. OLR: 68.2% vs. 93.7%, $p = 0.034$). Histories of upper abdominal surgery and hepatectomy were more common in the OLR group (LLR vs. OLR: 24.5% vs. 68.7%, $p < 0.001$ and 12.7% vs. 43.7%, $p = 0.002$, respectively). Patients with liver cirrhosis were more frequent in the LLR group (LLR vs. OLR: 13.6% vs. 0.0%, $p = 0.010$). Except for the indocyanine green retention rates at 15 min (LLR vs. OLR: 13% vs. 15%, $p = 0.030$), there was no significant difference in the laboratory data. The patient characteristics are shown in Table 1.

Table 1. Characteristics of all patients that underwent PSH for lesions in PSS 7 and 8.

	LLR (n = 110)	OLR (n = 16)	p-Value
Sex (male)	75 (68.2%)	15 (93.7%)	0.034 *
Age (years)	68 (25–85)	72 (61–83)	0.065
ASA-PS			0.254
1	26 (23.6%)	1 (6.2%)	
2	66 (60.0%)	11 (68.8%)	
3	18 (16.4%)	4 (25.0%)	
BMI (kg/m^2)	23.7 (16.1–35.2)	23.2 (17.1–29.7)	0.371
Histories of upper abdominal surgery	27 (24.5%)	11 (68.7%)	<0.001 *
Histories of hepatectomy	14 (12.7%)	7 (43.7%)	0.002 *
Preoperative chemotherapy	28 (25.5%)	3 (18.7%)	0.561
Child–Pugh B	2 (1.8%)	0 (0.0%)	0.586
Cirrhosis	15 (13.6%)	0 (0.0%)	0.010 *
Laboratory data			
Albumin (g/dL)	4.1 (3.1–5.0)	4.1 (3.5–4.6)	0.788
AST (IU/L)	24 (12–146)	26 (12–174)	0.447
ALT (IU/L)	22 (6–218)	23 (8–184)	0.303
Total bilirubin (mg/dL)	0.6 (0.2–1.9)	0.6 (0.3–1.1)	0.697
PT-INR	1.03 (0.85–1.43)	1.02 (0.94–1.24)	0.897
Platelet count (10^3/μL)	180 (64–702)	170 (95–325)	0.885
ICG-R15 (%)	13 (2–53)	15 (3–44)	0.030 *

Data are shown as median (range) or number of cases (percentage). *: statistically significant. LLR, laparoscopic liver resection; OLR, open liver resection; ASA-PS, American Society of Anesthesiologists physical status; BMI, body mass index; AST, aspartate aminotransferase; ALT, alanine aminotransferase; PT-INR, prothrombin time international normalized ratio; ICG-R15, indocyanine green retention rates at 15 min.

The perioperative outcomes are shown in Table 2. Patients who underwent PSH for lesions with PMV in PSS 7 and 8 were 31.8% in the LLR group and 31.3% in the OLR group ($p = 0.963$). The major hepatic vein of four patients in the LLR group was sacrificed to remove malignant tumors (LLR vs. OLR: 3.6% vs. 0.0%, $p = 0.438$). No patients were converted to open surgery in the LLR group. Median blood loss was significantly lower in the LLR group (LLR vs. OLR: 54 mL vs. 226 mL, $p = 0.009$). Pringle's maneuver was performed less frequently in the OLR group (LLR vs. OLR: 84.6% vs. 37.5%, $p < 0.001$). The median maximum tumor diameter and surgical margin were larger in the LLR group (LLR vs. OLR: 25.5 mm vs. 22.5 mm, $p = 0.016$, and 3.5 mm vs. 2.0 mm, $p = 0.010$, respectively). The positive surgical margin rate was higher in the OLR group (LLR vs. OLR: 4.5% vs. 18.7%, $p = 0.030$). There was no significant difference between the two groups in the median operative time (LLR vs. OLR: 205 min vs. 195 min, $p = 0.557$), median number of tumors (LLR vs. OLR: 1 vs. 1, $p = 0.205$), and morbidity rate (LLR vs. OLR: 8.1% vs. 18.7%, $p = 0.178$). Clavien–Dindo $\geq$ 3 morbidities were due to two surgical site infections (SSIs) and one bile leakage in the OLR group, and three SSIs, three bile leakages, two pleural fluids, and one portal vein thrombosis in the LLR group. There was no mortality within 90 days after the hepatectomy.

Table 2. Perioperative outcomes of LLR and OLR groups.

	LLR (n = 110)	OLR (n = 16)	p-Value
Pathological Diagnosis			0.029 *
HCC	44 (40.0%)	5 (31.2%)	
CRLM	49 (44.6%)	1 (6.3%)	
CCC	0 (0.0%)	8 (50.0%)	
Other malignancy	11 (10.0%)	2 (12.5%)	
Benign	6 (5.4%)	0 (0.0%)	
Surgical procedure of LLR			NA
Pure	93 (84.5%)	NA	
HALS	17 (15.5%)	NA	
Operative time (minutes)	205 (66–710)	195 (131–338)	0.557
Blood loss (mL)	54 (1–3026)	226 (90–2880)	0.009 *
Blood transfusion	2 (1.8%)	1 (6.3%)	0.277
Pringle's maneuver	93 (84.6%)	6 (37.5%)	<0.001 *
Lesions with proximity to major vessels	35 (31.8%)	5 (31.3%)	0.963
Sacrifice of major hepatic veins	4 (3.6%)	0 (0.0%)	0.438
Largest tumor diameter (mm)	25.5 (7.0–110.0)	22.5 (10.0–170.0)	0.016 *
Number of tumors	1 (1–3)	1 (1–3)	0.205
Surgical margin (mm)	3.5 (0.0–25.0)	2.0 (0.0–9.0)	0.010 *
Positive surgical margin	5 (4.5%)	3 (18.7%)	0.030 *
Length of hospital stay (days)	10 (4–158)	13 (7–110)	0.129
Morbidity (Clavien–Dindo $\geq$ 3)	9 (8.1%)	3 (18.7%)	0.178
Mortality	0 (0.0%)	0 (0.0%)	NA

Data are shown as median (range) or number of cases (percentage). *: statistically significant. LLR, laparoscopic liver resection; OLR, open liver resection; HCC, hepatocellular carcinoma; CRLM, colorectal liver metastases; CCC, cholangiocellular carcinoma; LLR, laparoscopic liver resection; HALS, hand-assisted laparoscopic surgery; NA, not applicable.

The median follow-up period was 780 (7–4018) days in the LLR group and 1310 (50–2869) days in the OLR group. Although the primary source of malignancy may have differed, there was no significant difference in the 5-year overall survival rate between the two groups (LLR vs. OLR: 73.9% vs. 74.3%, $p = 0.943$; Figure 5).

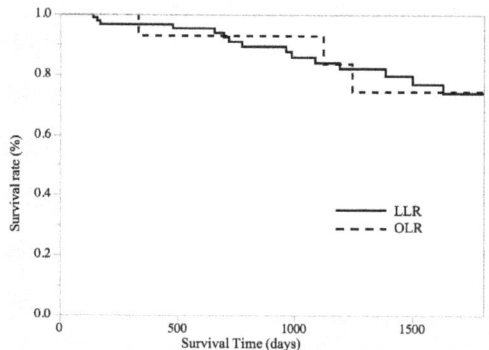

Figure 5. Overall survival after LLR and OLR groups.

3.2. Analysis of 110 Patients Who Underwent Laparoscopic PSH for Lesions in PSS 7 and 8 with and with No PMV

To assess safety and feasibility within the LLR group, the 110 LLR patients were divided into two groups—35 patients in the PMV group and 75 patients in the no-PMV group—and reviewed. The patient characteristics are shown in Table 3. Both of the patients with Child–Pugh B score were included in the PMV group. Statistically, plasma levels of albumin, AST, and PT-INR were significantly different between the two groups.

Table 3. Characteristics of patients that underwent laparoscopic PSH for lesions in PSS 7 and 8.

	PMV (*n* = 35)	No-PMV (*n* = 75)	*p*-Value
Sex (male)	24 (68.6%)	51 (68.0%)	0.952
Age (years)	70 (25–83)	68 (27–85)	0.879
ASA-PS			0.828
1	7 (20.0%)	19 (25.3%)	
2	22 (62.9%)	44 (58.7%)	
3	6 (17.1%)	12 (16.0%)	
BMI (kg/m^2)	25.3 (19.2–35.1)	23.5 (16.1–35.2)	0.064
Histories of upper abdominal surgery	8 (22.8%)	19 (25.3%)	0.878
Histories of hepatectomy	4 (11.4%)	10 (13.3%)	0.78
Preoperative chemotherapy	5 (14.3%)	23 (30.7%)	0.066
Child–Pugh B	2 (5.7%)	0 (0.0%)	0.036 *
Cirrhosis	6 (17.1%)	9 (12.0%)	0.464
Laboratory data			
Albumin (g/dL)	4.0 (3.1–4.6)	4.1 (3.4–5.0)	0.006 *
AST (IU/L)	30 (13–146)	22 (12–141)	0.023 *
ALT (IU/L)	26 (8–102)	20 (6–218)	0.264
Total bilirubin (mg/dL)	0.6 (0.2–1.9)	0.5 (0.3–1.6)	0.344
PT-INR	1.04 (0.90–1.34)	1.02 (0.85–1.43)	0.018 *
Platelet count (10^3/μL)	163 (73–339)	186 (64–702)	0.238
ICG-R15 (%)	13 (3–33)	13 (2–53)	0.143

Data are shown as median (range) or number of cases (percentage). *: statistically significant. PMV, lesions with proximity to major vessels; no-PMV, lesions with no proximity to major vessels; ASA-PS, American Society of Anesthesiologists physical status; BMI, body mass index; AST, aspartate aminotransferase; ALT, alanine aminotransferase; PT-INR, prothrombin time international normalized ratio; ICG-R15, indocyanine green retention rates at 15 min.

The perioperative outcomes are shown in Table 4. In the PMV group, the HALS technique was performed more often (PMV vs. no-PMV: 28.6% vs. 9.3%, $p = 0.009$). The median operative time was significantly longer in the PMV group (PMV vs. no-PMV: 237 min vs. 185 min, $p = 0.030$). All four patients whose major hepatic veins were sacrificed were included in the PMV group. The median tumor diameter was larger in the PMV group (PMV vs. no-PMV: 36.0 mm vs. 24.0 mm, $p < 0.001$). The median surgical margin of the specimens was smaller in the PMV group (PMV vs. no-PMV: 3.0 mm vs. 5.0 mm, $p = 0.010$); however, there was no significant difference in the rate of positive surgical margin between the two groups.

Table 4. Surgical outcomes of PMV and no-PMV groups.

	PMV (*n* = 35)	No-PMV (*n* = 75)	*p*-Value
Pathological Diagnosis			0.146
HCC	20 (57.1%)	24 (32.0%)	
CRLM	10 (28.6%)	39 (52.0%)	
Other malignancy	2 (5.7%)	9 (12.0%)	
Benign	3 (8.6%)	3 (4.0%)	
Surgical procedure of LLR			0.009 *
Pure	25 (71.4%)	68 (90.7%)	
HALS	10 (28.6%)	7 (9.3%)	
Operative time (minutes)	237 (105–397)	185 (66–710)	0.030 *
Blood loss (mL)	121 (10–1942)	50 (1–3026)	0.116
Blood transfusion	1 (2.9%)	1 (1.3%)	0.577
Pringle's maneuver	31 (88.6%)	62 (82.7%)	0.425
Sacrifice of major hepatic veins	4 (11.4%)	0 (0.0%)	0.003 *
Largest tumor diameter (mm)	36.0 (7.0–110.0)	24.0 (8.0–80.0)	<0.001 *
Number of tumors	1 (1–3)	1 (1–3)	0.033 *
Surgical margin (mm)	3.0 (0.0–13.0)	5.0 (0.0–25.0)	0.010 *
Positive surgical margin	2 (5.7%)	3 (4.0%)	0.687
Length of hospital stay (days)	10 (5–50)	9 (4–158)	0.721
Morbidity (Clavien–Dindo ≥ 3)	4 (11.4%)	5 (6.7%)	0.396

Data are shown as median (range) or number of cases (percentage). *: statistically significant. PMV, lesions with proximity to major vessels; no-PMV, lesions with no proximity to major vessels; HCC, hepatocellular carcinoma; CRLM, colorectal liver metastases; HALS, hand-assisted laparoscopic surgery.

3.3. Analysis of Patients Who Underwent Pure Laparoscopic and HALS PSH in PSS 7 and 8 for Lesions with and with No PMV

To clarify the role of the HALS technique, we reviewed 93 patients in the pure LLR group and 17 patients in the HALS group. The patient characteristics are shown in Table 5. Histories of upper abdominal surgery and hepatectomy were significantly higher in the HALS group (pure LLR vs. HALS: 21.5% vs. 41.2%, $p = 0.039$, and 9.7% vs. 29.4%, $p = 0.025$, respectively). Statistically, plasma levels of albumin and the indocyanine green retention rates at 15 min were significantly different between the two groups.

As shown in Table 6, there were no significant differences in short-term outcomes, although lesions with PMV were significantly more resected using the HALS technique ($p = 0.009$). Moreover, there were no positive surgical margins or complications in the HALS group, and there were no significant differences (pure LLR vs. HALS: 5.4% vs. 0.0%, $p = 0.328$, and 9.7% vs. 0.0%, $p = 0.181$, respectively).

Table 5. Characteristics of patients that underwent pure laparoscopic and HALS PSH for lesions in PSS 7 and 8.

	Pure LLR (n = 93)	HALS (n = 17)	p-Value
Sex (male)	61 (65.6%)	14 (82.4%)	0.173
Age (years)	69 (25–85)	65 (48–83)	0.729
ASA-PS			0.987
1	22 (23.7%)	4 (23.5%)	
2	56 (60.2%)	10 (58.8%)	
3	15 (16.1%)	3 (17.7%)	
BMI (kg/m^2)	23.5 (16.1–35.2)	24.5 (19.9–35.1)	0.099
Histories of upper abdominal surgery	20 (21.5%)	7 (41.2%)	0.039 *
Histories of hepatectomy	9 (9.7%)	5 (29.4%)	0.025 *
Preoperative chemotherapy	25 (26.9%)	3 (17.7%)	0.422
Child–Pugh B	2 (2.2%)	0 (0.0%)	0.542
Cirrhosis	13 (14.0%)	2 (11.8%)	0.807
Laboratory data			
Albumin (g/dL)	4.1 (3.1–5.0)	3.9 (3.4–4.3)	0.018 *
AST (IU/L)	25 (12–146)	23 (17–141)	0.537
ALT (IU/L)	21 (6–102)	22 (8–218)	0.367
Total bilirubin (mg/dL)	0.6 (0.2–1.6)	0.6 (0.3–1.9)	0.163
PT-INR	1.03 (0.85–1.34)	1.04 (0.90–1.43)	0.187
Platelet count (10^3/μL)	180 (64–702)	160 (73–339)	0.648
ICG-R15 (%)	12 (2–53)	16 (6–33)	0.008 *

Data are shown as median (range) or number of cases (percentage). *: statistically significant. LLR, laparoscopic liver resection; HALS, hand-assisted laparoscopic surgery; ASA-PS, American Society of Anesthesiologists physical status; BMI, body mass index; AST, aspartate aminotransferase; ALT, alanine aminotransferase; PT-INR, prothrombin time international normalized ratio; ICG-R15, indocyanine green retention rates at 15 min.

Table 6. Surgical outcomes of pure LLR and HALS.

	Pure LLR (n = 93)	HALS (n = 17)	p-Value
Pathological Diagnosis			0.891
HCC	36 (38.7%)	8 (47.1%)	
CRLM	43 (46.2%)	6 (35.3%)	
Other malignancy	9 (9.7%)	2 (11.7%)	
Benign	5 (5.4%)	1 (5.9%)	
Lesions with proximity to major vessels	25 (26.9%)	10 (58.8%)	0.009 *
Operative time (minutes)	203 (66–710)	211 (138–339)	0.831
Blood loss (mL)	52 (1–3026)	110 (28–881)	0.667
Blood transfusion	2 (2.2%)	0 (0.0%)	0.542
Pringle's maneuver	81 (87.1%)	12 (70.6%)	0.083
Sacrifice of major hepatic veins	3 (3.2%)	1 (5.9%)	0.591
Number of tumors	1 (1–3)	1 (1–3)	0.678
Largest tumor diameter (mm)	25.0 (7.0–110.0)	33.0 (8.0–80.0)	0.135
Surgical margin (mm)	4.0 (0.0–25.0)	3.0 (1.0–10.0)	0.237
Positive surgical margin	5 (5.4%)	0 (0.0%)	0.328
Length of hospital stay (days)	9 (4–158)	10 (6–18)	0.452
Morbidity (Clavien–Dindo ≥ 3)	9 (9.7%)	0 (0.0%)	0.181

Data are shown as median (range) or number of cases (percentage). *: statistically significant. LLR, laparoscopic liver resection; HALS, hand-assisted laparoscopic surgery; HCC, hepatocellular carcinoma; CRLM, colorectal liver metastases.

3.4. Analysis of 71 Patients Who Underwent Pure Laparoscopic PSH for One Tumor Lesion with PMV in PSS 7 and 8

To account for some background factors, we performed a further analysis of patients who underwent pure laparoscopic PSH (pPSH) for one tumor lesion with PMV in PSS 7 and 8, including 71 patients (23 patients in the pPSH-PMV group and 48 patients in the pPSH-no-PMV group). The patient characteristics are shown in Table 7. Child–Pugh B patients were included only in the pPSH-PMV group. Statistically, the plasma levels of albumin, AST, ALT, and PT-INR were significantly different between the two groups. There were no significant differences in any other variables between the two groups.

Table 7. Characteristics of patients that underwent pure laparoscopic PSH for one tumor lesion with PMV in PSS 7 and 8.

	pPSH-PMV (n = 23)	pPSH-no-PMV (n = 48)	p-Value
Sex (male)	15 (65.2%)	29 (60.4%)	0.696
Age (years)	72 (25–83)	69 (27–85)	0.567
ASA-PS			0.853
1	4 (17.4%)	10 (20.8%)	
2	14 (60.9%)	30 (62.5%)	
3	5 (21.7%)	8 (16.7%)	
BMI (kg/m^2)	24.5 (19.2–31.4)	23.6 (16.1–35.2)	0.588
Histories of upper abdominal surgery	6 (26.1%)	11 (22.9%)	0.847
Histories of hepatectomy	2 (8.7%)	5 (10.4%)	0.82
Preoperative chemotherapy	2 (8.7%)	12 (25.0%)	0.106
Child–Pugh B	2 (8.7%)	0 (0.0%)	0.038 *
Cirrhosis	5 (21.7%)	8 (16.7%)	0.605
Laboratory data			
Albumin (g/dL)	4.0 (3.1–4.4)	4.2 (3.6–5.0)	0.001 *
AST (IU/L)	36 (13–146)	22 (13–80)	0.024 *
ALT (IU/L)	27 (9–102)	20 (9–100)	0.029 *
Total bilirubin (mg/dL)	0.6 (0.2–1.1)	0.6 (0.3–1.6)	0.593
PT-INR	1.05 (0.98–1.34)	1.02 (0.85–1.28)	0.006 *
Platelet count (10^3/μL)	167 (73–331)	181 (64–702)	0.167
ICG-R15 (%)	11 (3–26)	12 (3–53)	0.829

Data are shown as median (range) or number of cases (percentage). *: statistically significant. pPSH, pure laparoscopic parenchymal-sparing hepatectomy; PMV, lesions with proximity to a major vessel; no-PMV, lesions with no proximity to a major vessel; ASA-PS, American Society of Anesthesiologists physical status; BMI, body mass index; AST, aspartate aminotransferase; ALT, alanine aminotransferase; PT-INR, prothrombin time international normalized ratio; ICG-R15, indocyanine green retention rates at 15 min.

As shown in Table 8, the perioperative outcomes were compared between the two groups. All of the three patients whose major hepatic veins were sacrificed were included in the pPSH-PMV group. The median tumor diameter was significantly larger in the pPSH-PMV group (pPSH-PMV vs. pPSH-no-PMV: 36.0 mm vs. 23.0 mm, $p < 0.001$). The median operative time was significantly different between the two groups (pPSH-PMV vs. pPSH-no-PMV: 240 min vs. 163 min, $p = 0.002$). The median surgical margin of the specimens was smaller in the pPSH-PMV group (pPSH-PMV vs. pPSH-no-PMV: 3.0 mm vs. 5.0 mm, $p = 0.008$); however, there was no significant difference in the rate of positive surgical margin between the two groups (pPSH-PMV vs. pPSH-no-PMV: 8.3% mm vs. 3.8%, $p = 0.310$). The median blood loss, length of hospital stay, and Clavien–Dindo $\geq$ 3 morbidities were not significantly different between the two groups (pPSH-PMV vs. pPSH-no-PMV: 98 mL vs. 50 mL, $p = 0.364$; 10 days vs. 9 days, $p = 0.654$, and 11.1% vs. 6.4%, $p = 0.387$, respectively).

Table 8. Surgical outcomes of pPSH-PMV and pPSH-no-PMV groups.

	pPSH-PMV (n = 23)	pPSH-no-PMV (n = 48)	p-Value
Pathological Diagnosis			0.283
HCC	15 (65.2%)	18 (37.5%)	
CRLM	5 (21.7%)	20 (41.7%)	
Other malignancy	1 (4.4%)	7 (14.6%)	
Benign	2 (8.7%)	3 (6.2%)	
Operative time (minutes) *	240 (105–397)	163 (66–710)	0.002 *
Blood loss (mL) *	98 (10–1942)	50 (90–3026)	0.364
Blood transfusion	1 (4.4%)	1 (2.1%)	0.589
Pringle's maneuver	22 (95.6%)	38 (79.2%)	0.072
Sacrifice of major hepatic veins	3 (13.0%)	0 (0.0%)	0.011 *
Largest tumor diameter (mm) *	36.0 (10.0–110.0)	23.0 (8.0–55.0)	<0.001 *
Surgical margin (mm) *	3.0 (0.0–13.0)	5.0 (0.0–25.0)	0.008 *
Positive surgical margin	3 (8.3%)	3 (3.8%)	0.31
Length of hospital stay (days) *	10 (5–50)	9 (7–110)	0.654
Morbidity (Clavien–Dindo $\geq$ 3)	4 (11.1%)	5 (6.4%)	0.387

Data are shown as median (range) or number of cases (percentage). *: statistically significant. pPSH, pure laparoscopic parenchymal-sparing hepatectomy; PMV, lesions with proximity to a major vessel; no-PMV, lesions with no proximity to a major vessel; HCC, hepatocellular carcinoma; CRLM.

4. Discussion

The lesions located in PSS 7 and 8 were considered difficult to address using LLR due to limited visualization, restrictions on surgical manipulation, and their proximity to major hepatic veins. At the Consensus Conference held at Morioka in 2014, the jury concluded that PSH for PSS was not a minor operation and was still considered an innovative procedure [5]. According to expert recommendations, LLR for lesions with PMV is not contraindicated to be performed in a specialized center [18]. Recent international consensus meetings held in Southampton recommended that PSH for PSS be performed by experienced surgeons in select patients in high-volume centers [6]. Some comparative studies have reported that, for tumors in PSS, LLR is superior to OLR in terms of intraoperative blood loss, postoperative hospital stay, and major complication rates [7–13]. In the present study, we showed that LLR for lesions in PSS resulted in lower intraoperative blood loss than OLR and that there was no difference in short-term and long-term outcomes between the two groups. However, these results should be carefully interpreted because some selection biases possibly exist in both groups despite our criteria for open or laparoscopic surgery. Moreover, we cannot assert that there are no differences in the long-term results because various types of tumors were included in this study. With regards to the cholangiocellular carcinoma in this study in PSS 7 and 8, a regional hepatic hilum lymphadenectomy was not performed because the main legion was located far from the hepatic hilum.

Some tumors in PSS 7 and 8 can be closer in proximity to major hepatic veins than others. Laparoscopic major hepatectomies have frequently been performed for lesions with PMV in PSS [19]. A previous report demonstrated that PSH for colorectal liver metastases (CRLM) has been associated with decreased mortality and equivalent survival compared to major hepatectomies [20]. Another report showed that laparoscopic minor hepatectomies for lesions in PSS showed no statistical difference in blood loss or operation time [21]. We examined the safety and feasibility of laparoscopic PSH for lesions with PMV in PSS because the proximity to the major hepatic veins is likely to have a greater impact on short-term surgical outcomes. This study shows that laparoscopic PSH for lesions with PMV in PSS 7 and 8 remains safe and feasible in terms of short-term outcomes. The operative time in the pPSH-PMV group was longer than in the pPSH-no-PMV group. However, there was no difference in intraoperative blood loss, complication rates, or postoperative hospital stay between the two groups, despite the larger tumor diameters in the pPSH-PMV group compared to the pPSH-no-PMV group. Although an appropriate surgical margin might not be adequately guaranteed when performing PSH for lesions with PMV in PSS, our results demonstrated that there was no difference in the positive surgical margin rate between the two groups. Frequent intraoperative ultrasound may contribute to securing the margin [13].

A previous study that compared the HALS technique to OLR for CRLM in PSS demonstrated that the HALS technique is a safe, feasible, and preferable approach because it leads to a lower complication rate and shorter hospital stays without compromising survival and disease recurrence [7]. We adopted the HALS technique for patients with tumors located in close proximity to major hepatic veins in PSS that would likely have required sacrificing the major hepatic veins in preoperative estimations. Although various types of tumors were included, there were tendencies toward lower positive surgical margins and lower complication rates in the HALS group. The HALS technique for lesions with PMV in PSS is useful because it permits a good view of the operation field during parenchymal transection and controls bleeding when performing continuous dorsal compression. In addition, it is oncologically useful to detect multiple small superficial lesions and ensure safe surgical margins, especially for borderline invasive tumors, such as CRLMs, using tactile sensation. Currently, we consider that the HALS technique still plays an important role as a minimally invasive form of liver resection and not simply a bridge between open and laparoscopic surgeries.

Good visibility, adequate preparation for bleeding control, and effective management in the event of bleeding are important factors in safely performing LLR for tumors in PSS [22]. Some successive approaches to overcoming poor surgical manipulation or operating views in PSS have been reported [23–28]. We believe that full mobilization of the right side of the liver is essential for obtaining a better view of the operating field, controlling bleeding, and performing LLR for lesions with PMV in PSS. Fortunately, we were able to obtain a good visualization of the operation field and perform LLR without stress by using a flexible scope with almost the same port placement for lesions in any segment (Figure 2a,b). It should be emphasized that the experience and skill of a scopist is as important as the operator's proficiency. Moreover, full mobilization of the right side of the liver becomes a crucial preparation for bleeding control. We propose that creating a space on the right side of the inferior vena cava and compressing the liver parenchyma from the dorsal side (dorsal compression) enable a safe operation with controlled bleeding [29] (Figure 4). In addition to pneumoperitoneum and anesthesia management, it is highly beneficial that the force of gravity can be used for hemostasis by positioning the main blood vessels on the dorsal side of the resection plane (left half-lateral decubitus position l for segment 7 and supine position for segment 8) [30]. Dorsal compression also enables subtle adjustment to maintain a bleeding point ventral to such major vessels as the right hepatic vein and the inferior vena cava. The most important hemostatic management is probably the hangnail injury described above. Attempting to treat blindly or applying too much tension for visualization could result in tearing of the major vessels, leading to hemorrhage and irreparable damage. It is crucial to cleanly cut away a hangnail injury, rather than tearing it away while the initial tear is small. After making a clean cut, a saline dripping monopolar soft-coagulation system facilitates hemostasis using many of the aforementioned management methods (Figure 3a–d). The application of our useful surgical procedures and techniques may enable the achievement of a good view of the operation field, preparation for controlling bleeding, and management in the event of bleeding, while providing significant benefits for safety and feasibility.

Although pneumoperitoneal pressure is highly beneficial for bleeding control when performing laparoscopic PSH with PMV in PSS, caution regarding paradoxical carbon dioxide embolism should always be exercised [31]. Operating close to the major vessels carries the risk of damaging the major hepatic vein. Even if the bleeding is controlled successfully, it is important to keep in mind the possibility of cerebral infarction by paradoxical gas embolism and to be prepared for treatment by methods such as discontinuing pneumoperitoneum, changing the patient's position from head-up to head-down, or closure of the injured vein either directly or by dorsal compression.

This study has certain limitations. First, this study was not a prospective or a randomized study but a retrospective design. Second, we could not perform effective statistical analyses due to the small sample size. Third, we were unable to sufficiently examine the long-term results of pure LLR for each type of cancer disease due to the short follow-up period. Fourth, this study did not show any differences in hospital stays, which may be explained by Japan's national health insurance. Although the lengths of hospital stays are mainly determined by physicians' clinical judgment, patients and their family members often participate in determining discharge dates. It may be difficult to compare the lengths of hospital stays in Japan with those in other countries. Finally, a few patients underwent open PSH for liver tumors located in PSS 7 or 8 because most of the single-tumor lesions in these segments were resected laparoscopically in our institution.

5. Conclusions

The present findings indicate that laparoscopic PSH for lesions with PMV in PSS, especially segments 7 and 8, is safe and feasible in high-volume specialized centers with a team experienced in laparoscopic liver surgery. Nevertheless, it will be necessary to consider and estimate the surgeon's experience and well-selected indications in the future. Furthermore, the HALS technique still plays an important role as a minimally invasive liver resection method, beyond being a mere bridge between open and laparoscopic surgeries.

Author Contributions: H.K., H.N. and A.S. designed this study. H.K. drafted this paper. H.K., H.N., S.K., A.U., D.T., T.A. and S.A. collected the data. H.K. analyzed and interpreted the data. H.K., H.N., S.K., A.U., D.T., T.A., S.A. and A.S. discussed the results. H.N. and A.S. critically revised the manuscript. All authors have read and agreed to the published version of the manuscript.

Funding: This research received no external funding.

Institutional Review Board Statement: The study was conducted according to the guidelines of the Declaration of Helsinki, and approved by the Institutional Review Board of Iwate Medical University (MH2019-122, 23 October 2019).

Informed Consent Statement: Informed consent was obtained from all subjects involved in the study.

Data Availability Statement: The data presented in this study are available on request from the corresponding author.

Conflicts of Interest: The authors declare no conflict of interest.

References

1. Reich, H.; McGlynn, F.; DeCaprio, J.; Budin, R. Laparoscopic excision of benign liver lesions. *Obstet. Gynecol.* **1991**, *78*, 956–958. [PubMed]
2. Ciria, R.; Cherqui, D.; Geller, D.A.; Briceno, J.; Wakabayashi, G. Comparative Short-term Benefits of Laparoscopic Liver Resection: 9000 Cases and Climbing. *Ann. Surg.* **2016**, *263*, 761–777. [CrossRef]
3. Haber, P.K.; Wabitsch, S.; Krenzien, F.; Benzing, C.; Andreou, A.; Schöning, W.; Öllinger, R.; Pratschke, J.; Schmelzle, M. Laparoscopic liver surgery in cirrhosis–Addressing lesions in posterosuperior segments. *Surg. Oncol.* **2019**, *28*, 140–144. [CrossRef] [PubMed]
4. Kasai, M.; Cipriani, F.; Gayet, B.; Aldrighetti, L.; Ratti, F.; Sarmiento, J.M.; Scatton, O.; Kim, K.-H.; Dagher, I.; Topal, B.; et al. Laparoscopic versus open major hepatectomy: A systematic review and meta-analysis of individual patient data. *Surgery* **2018**, *163*, 985–995. [CrossRef] [PubMed]

5. Wakabayashi, G.; Cherqui, D.; Geller, D.A.; Buell, J.F.; Kaneko, H.; Han, H.S.; Asbun, H.; O'rourke, N.; Tanabe, M.; Koffron, A.J.; et al. Recommendations for laparoscopic liver resection: A report from the second international consensus conference held in Morioka. *Ann. Surg.* **2015**, *261*, 619–629. [CrossRef]
6. Abu Hilal, M.; Aldrighetti, L.; Dagher, I.; Edwin, B.; Troisi, R.I.; Alikhanov, R.; Aroori, S.; Belli, G.; Besselink, M.; Briceno, J.; et al. The Southampton Consensus Guidelines for Laparoscopic Liver Surgery: From Indication to Implementation. *Ann. Surg.* **2018**, *268*, 11–18. [CrossRef] [PubMed]
7. Abu-Zaydeh, O.; Sawaied, M.; Berger, Y.; Mahamid, A.; Goldberg, N.; Sadot, E.; Haddad, R. Hand-Assisted Laparoscopic Surgery Is Superior to Open Liver Resection for Colorectal Liver Metastases in the Posterosuperior Segments. *Front. Surg.* **2021**, *8*, 746427. [CrossRef]
8. Efanov, M.; Granov, D.; Alikhanov, R.; Rutkin, I.; Tsvirkun, V.; Kazakov, I.; Vankovich, A.; Koroleva, A.; Kovalenko, D. Expanding indications for laparoscopic parenchyma-sparing resection of posterosuperior liver segments in patients with colorectal metastases: Comparison with open hepatectomy for immediate and long-term outcomes. *Surg. Endosc.* **2021**, *35*, 96–103. [CrossRef]
9. Kwon, Y.; Cho, J.Y.; Han, H.-S.; Yoon, Y.-S.; Lee, H.W.; Lee, J.S.; Lee, B.; Kim, M. Improved Outcomes of Laparoscopic Liver Resection for Hepatocellular Carcinoma Located in Posterosuperior Segments of the Liver. *World J. Surg.* **2021**, *45*, 1178–1185. [CrossRef]
10. Lopez-Lopez, V.; Ome, Y.; Kawamoto, Y.; Ruiz, A.G.; Campos, R.R.; Honda, G. Laparoscopic Liver Resection of Segments 7 and 8: From the Initial Restrictions to the Current Indications. *J. Minim. Invasive Surg.* **2020**, *23*, 5–16. [CrossRef]
11. Morikawa, T.; Ishida, M.; Takadate, T.; Aoki, T.; Ohtsuka, H.; Mizuma, M.; Hayashi, H.; Nakagawa, K.; Motoi, F.; Naitoh, T.; et al. Laparoscopic partial liver resection improves the short-term outcomes compared to open surgery for liver tumors in the posterosuperior segments. *Surg. Today* **2019**, *49*, 214–223. [CrossRef] [PubMed]
12. Xiao, L.; Xiang, L.-J.; Li, J.-W.; Chen, J.; Fan, Y.-D.; Zheng, S.-G. Laparoscopic versus open liver resection for hepatocellular carcinoma in posterosuperior segments. *Surg. Endosc.* **2015**, *29*, 2994–3001. [CrossRef] [PubMed]
13. Zheng, H.; Huang, S.G.; Qin, S.M.; Xiang, F. Comparison of laparoscopic versus open liver resection for lesions located in posterosuperior segments: A meta-analysis of short-term and oncological outcomes. *Surg. Endosc.* **2019**, *33*, 3910–3918. [CrossRef]
14. Yoon, Y.-S.; Han, H.-S.; Cho, J.Y.; Ahn, K.S. Total laparoscopic liver resection for hepatocellular carcinoma located in all segments of the liver. *Surg. Endosc.* **2010**, *24*, 1630–1637. [CrossRef] [PubMed]
15. Ban, D.; Tanabe, M.; Ito, H.; Otsuka, Y.; Nitta, H.; Abe, Y.; Hasegawa, Y.; Katagiri, T.; Takagi, C.; Itano, O.; et al. A novel difficulty scoring system for laparoscopic liver resection. *J. Hepato-Biliary-Pancreat. Sci.* **2014**, *21*, 745–753. [CrossRef]
16. Dindo, D.; Demartines, N.; Clavien, P.-A. Classification of Surgical Complications: A new proposal with evaluation in a cohort of 6336 patients and results of a survey. *Ann. Surg.* **2004**, *240*, 205–213. [CrossRef]
17. Kobayashi, S.; Honda, G.; Kurata, M.; Tadano, S.; Sakamoto, K.; Okuda, Y.; Abe, K. An Experimental Study on the Relationship Among Airway Pressure, Pneumoperitoneum Pressure, and Central Venous Pressure in Pure Laparoscopic Hepatectomy. *Ann. Surg.* **2016**, *263*, 1159–1163. [CrossRef]
18. Abu Hilal, M.; Van Der Poel, M.J.; Samim, M.; Besselink, M.G.H.; Flowers, D.; Stedman, B.; Pearce, N.W. Laparoscopic Liver Resection for Lesions Adjacent to Major Vasculature: Feasibility, Safety and Oncological Efficiency. *J. Gastrointest. Surg.* **2015**, *19*, 692–698. [CrossRef]
19. Cho, J.Y.; Han, H.-S.; Yoon, Y.-S.; Shin, S.-H. Feasibility of laparoscopic liver resection for tumors located in the posterosuperior segments of the liver, with a special reference to overcoming current limitations on tumor location. *Surgery* **2008**, *144*, 32–38. [CrossRef]
20. Gold, J.S.; Are, C.; Kornprat, P.; Jarnagin, W.R.; Gönen, M.; Fong, Y.; DeMatteo, R.P.; Blumgart, L.H.; D'Angelica, M. Increased Use of Parenchymal-Sparing Surgery for Bilateral Liver Metastases From Colorectal Cancer Is Associated With Improved Mortality Without Change in Oncologic Outcome: Trends in treatment over time in 440 patients. *Ann. Surg.* **2008**, *247*, 109–117. [CrossRef]
21. Cho, J.Y.; Han, H.S.; Yoon, Y.S.; Shin, S.H. Outcomes of Laparoscopic Liver Resection for Lesions Located in the Right Side of the Liver. *Arch. Surg.* **2009**, *144*, 25–29. [CrossRef]
22. Morise, Z.; Aldrighetti, L.; Belli, G.; Ratti, F.; Cheung, T.T.; Lo, C.M.; Tanaka, S.; Kubo, S.; Okamura, Y.; Uesaka, K.; et al. An International Retrospective Observational Study of Liver Functional Deterioration after Repeat Liver Resection for Patients with Hepatocellular Carcinoma. *Cancers* **2022**, *14*, 2598. [CrossRef]
23. Cipriani, F.; Shelat, V.G.; Rawashdeh, M.; Francone, E.; Aldrighetti, L.; Takhar, A.; Armstrong, T.; Pearce, N.W.; Abu Hilal, M. Laparoscopic Parenchymal-Sparing Resections for Nonperipheral Liver Lesions, the Diamond Technique: Technical Aspects, Clinical Outcomes, and Oncologic Efficiency. *J. Am. Coll. Surg.* **2015**, *221*, 265–272. [CrossRef]
24. Lee, W.; Han, H.-S.; Yoon, Y.-S.; Cho, J.Y.; Choi, Y.; Shin, H.K. Role of intercostal trocars on laparoscopic liver resection for tumors in segments 7 and 8. *J. Hepato-Biliary-Pancreat. Sci.* **2014**, *21*, E65–E68. [CrossRef] [PubMed]
25. Morise, Z. Laparoscopic liver resection for posterosuperior tumors using caudal approach and postural changes: A new technical approach. *World J. Gastroenterol.* **2016**, *22*, 10267–10274. [CrossRef] [PubMed]
26. Morise, Z.; Wakabayashi, G. First quarter century of laparoscopic liver resection. *World J. Gastroenterol.* **2017**, *23*, 3581–3588. [CrossRef] [PubMed]
27. Ogiso, S.; Conrad, C.; Araki, K.; Nomi, T.; Anil, Z.; Gayet, B. Laparoscopic Transabdominal with Transdiaphragmatic Access Improves Resection of Difficult Posterosuperior Liver Lesions. *Ann. Surg.* **2015**, *262*, 358–365. [CrossRef]

28. Okuda, Y.; Honda, G.; Kobayashi, S.; Sakamoto, K.; Homma, Y.; Honjo, M.; Doi, M. Intrahepatic Glissonean Pedicle Approach to Segment 7 from the Dorsal Side During Laparoscopic Anatomic Hepatectomy of the Cranial Part of the Right Liver. *J. Am. Coll. Surg.* **2018**, *226*, e1–e6. [CrossRef]
29. Nitta, H.; Sasaki, A.; Katagiri, H.; Kanno, S.; Umemura, A. Is Laparoscopic Hepatectomy Safe for Giant Liver Tumors? Proposal from a Single Institution for Totally Laparoscopic Hemihepatectomy Using an Anterior Approach for Giant Liver Tumors Larger Than 10 cm in Diameter. *Curr. Oncol.* **2022**, *29*, 8261–8268. [CrossRef]
30. Lee, W.; Han, H.-S.; Yoon, Y.-S.; Cho, J.Y.; Choi, Y.; Shin, H.K.; Jang, J.Y.; Choi, H.; Kwon, S.U. Comparison of laparoscopic liver resection for hepatocellular carcinoma located in the posterosuperior segments or anterolateral segments: A case-matched analysis. *Surgery* **2016**, *160*, 1219–1226. [CrossRef]
31. Kawahara, T.; Hagiwara, M.; Takahashi, H.; Tanaka, M.; Imai, K.; Sawada, J.; Kunisawa, T.; Furukawa, H. Cerebral Infarction by Paradoxical Gas Embolism During Laparoscopic Liver Resection with Injury of the Hepatic Vessels in a Patient without a Right-to-Left Systemic Shunt. *Am. J. Case Rep.* **2017**, *18*, 687–691. [CrossRef] [PubMed]

Disclaimer/Publisher's Note: The statements, opinions and data contained in all publications are solely those of the individual author(s) and contributor(s) and not of MDPI and/or the editor(s). MDPI and/or the editor(s) disclaim responsibility for any injury to people or property resulting from any ideas, methods, instructions or products referred to in the content.

Article

Minimally Invasive Anatomic Liver Resection for Hepatocellular Carcinoma Using the Extrahepatic Glissonian Approach: Surgical Techniques and Comparison of Outcomes with the Open Approach and between the Laparoscopic and Robotic Approaches

Yutaro Kato [1,*], Atsushi Sugioka [2], Masayuki Kojima [3], Satoshi Mii [3], Yuichiro Uchida [3], Hideaki Iwama [3], Takuya Mizumoto [3], Takeshi Takahara [3] and Ichiro Uyama [1]

1 Department of Advanced Robotic and Endoscopic Surgery, Fujita Health University, Toyoake 470-1192, Japan; iuyama@fujita-hu.ac.jp
2 International Medical Center, Fujita Health University Hospital, Toyoake 470-1192, Japan; sugioka@fujita-hu.ac.jp
3 Department of Surgery, Fujita Health University, Toyoake 470-1192, Japan; kojima@fujita-hu.ac.jp (M.K.); smii@fujita-hu.ac.jp (S.M.); yuichiro.uchida@fujita-hu.ac.jp (Y.U.); hideaki.iwama@fujita-hu.ac.jp (H.I.); takuya.mizumoto@fujita-hu.ac.jp (T.M.); takeshi.takahara@fujita-hu.ac.jp (T.T.)
* Correspondence: y-kato@fujita-hu.ac.jp; Tel.: +81-562-939-965

Simple Summary: Surgical techniques and outcomes of minimally invasive anatomic liver resection (AR) for hepatocellular carcinoma (HCC) are undefined. In 327 HCC patients undergoing 185 open (OAR) and 142 minimally invasive (MIAR; 102 laparoscopic and 40 robotic) ARs, perioperative and long-term outcomes were compared, using propensity score matching. After matching (91:91), compared to OAR, MIAR was significantly associated with longer operative time; less blood loss; a lower transfusion rate; lower rates of 90-day major morbidity, bile leak or collection, and 90-day mortality; and shorter hospital stay. On the other hand, laparoscopic and robotic AR cohorts after matching (31:31) had comparable perioperative outcomes. Postoperative overall and recurrence-free survivals of newly developed HCC were comparable between OAR and MIAR or between laparoscopic and robotic cases. MIAR was technically standardized using the extrahepatic Glissonian approach. MIAR was safe, feasible, and oncologically acceptable and would be the first choice of AR in selected HCC patients.

Abstract: Surgical techniques and outcomes of minimally invasive anatomic liver resection (AR) using the extrahepatic Glissonian approach for hepatocellular carcinoma (HCC) are undefined. In 327 HCC cases undergoing 185 open (OAR) and 142 minimally invasive (MIAR; 102 laparoscopic and 40 robotic) ARs, perioperative and long-term outcomes were compared between the approaches, using propensity score matching. After matching (91:91), compared to OAR, MIAR was significantly associated with longer operative time (643 vs. 579 min, $p = 0.028$); less blood loss (274 vs. 955 g, $p < 0.0001$); a lower transfusion rate (17.6% vs. 47.3%, $p < 0.0001$); lower rates of major 90-day morbidity (4.4% vs. 20.9%, $p = 0.0008$), bile leak or collection (1.1% vs. 11.0%, $p = 0.005$), and 90-day mortality (0% vs. 4.4%, $p = 0.043$); and shorter hospital stay (15 vs. 29 days, $p < 0.0001$). On the other hand, laparoscopic and robotic AR cohorts after matching (31:31) had comparable perioperative outcomes. Overall and recurrence-free survivals after AR for newly developed HCC were comparable between OAR and MIAR, with potentially improved survivals in MIAR. The survivals were comparable between laparoscopic and robotic AR. MIAR was technically standardized using the extrahepatic Glissonian approach. MIAR was safe, feasible, and oncologically acceptable and would be the first choice of AR in selected HCC patients.

Keywords: minimally invasive liver resection; anatomic liver resection; robotic liver resection; laparoscopic liver resection; Glissonian approach; hepatocellular carcinoma

1. Introduction

Anatomic liver resection (AR) is a hepatectomy procedure, where an anatomically determined liver territory that is supplied by the arbitrary Glissonian or portal pedicles (GPs) is completely and optimally resected. Therefore, AR includes both major liver resection of three or more Couinaud's segments as well as parenchyma-preserving resection represented by mono- or bi- (sub)segmentectomy and monosectionectomy, and their combinatory resection. AR is expected to achieve both high curability and functional safety in liver resection for malignancy. In particular, parenchyma-sparing AR (PSAR), such as isolated segmentectomy and sectionectomy, is considered to confer benefits for resection of hepatocellular carcinoma (HCC), which is characterized by intra-portal vein tumor spread and accompanying impaired hepatic functional reserve [1–3].

The safety and feasibility of minimally invasive AR (MIAR) has been partly established in previous studies [4–9], though MIAR, particularly PSAR, is still not technically standardized and is regarded as a group of procedures suitable for expert hands or for high volume centers [5,6,8]. Furthermore, perioperative and long-term outcomes of MIAR have not been fully studied nor have they been compared to those of open AR (OAR) in detail. Surgical HCC patients have been shown to obtain oncological benefits from AR, if technically and functionally applicable, compared to non-anatomic liver resection (NAR) [2,3,9]. Therefore, technical standardization of MIAR and evaluation of its surgical results in HCC patients in comparison to those of OAR, can serve to reinforce or revise surgical strategies for HCC.

In this single-center study on 327 consecutive AR cases of HCC, including 185 OAR and 142 MIAR cases, we present our standardized surgical techniques for MIAR and compare perioperative outcomes between OAR and MIAR, as well as between laparoscopic and robotic AR, using propensity score matching (PSM) analyses. In addition, long-term outcomes after AR for newly developed HCC were compared between OAR and MIAR, as well as between laparoscopic and robotic AR. Based on the results, we discuss the technical, surgical, and oncologic aspects of MIAR in surgical management of HCC.

2. Materials and Methods

2.1. Terminology and Definition of AR

The terminology for liver anatomy and procedures of hepatectomy was primarily based on the Brisbane 2000 Terminology of Liver Anatomy and Resections [10] and Couinaud's classification [11]. Additionally, the anatomic subsegmentectomy was determined according to the PAM-meeting classification [12]. Thus, AR included trisectionectomy, bisectionectomy including right or left hemihepatectomy and central bisectionectomy, monosectionectomy, (sub)segmentectomy, and their continuous combination. Anatomic subsegmentectomy was defined as the resection of an isolated liver territory that is supplied by the third (or fourth) order division GPs or by its combination with the adjacent GPs smaller than sectional GPs. Isolated total caudate lobectomy was included in the segmentectomy and resection of the Spiegel lobe by dividing the left caudate GP at its root and was defined as subsegmentectomy [13]. Left lateral sectionectomy was included in sectionectomy because it was performed using the extrahepatic Glissonian approach, where GPs to Sg2 and Sg3 were isolated and divided extrahepatically before starting parenchymal dissection. In this study, we excluded AR cases with biliary or vascular reconstruction, those with concomitant extrahepatic procedures, and live donor hepatectomy.

2.2. Surgical Indications for MIAR for HCC

At our institution, AR was the first choice of hepatectomy procedure for HCC, if appropriate and applicable, irrespective of the surgical approaches; open, laparoscopic, or robotic. Selection of AR and the type of hepatectomy were based on the location, number, and size of tumors as well as patients' hepatic functional reserve, mostly according to the so-called Makuuchi criteria, and physical status [14].

Selection of OAR or MIAR was based on the operative difficulties depending on the tumor and patient characteristics (Ban's criteria) [15] and the surgeons' capability. It was also dependent on the chronological era, social background, and surgeons' preference. Basic indications for MIAR were in accordance with the following conditions: (1) tumors with a diameter ≤15 cm, without limitation of tumor location; (2) five or fewer excision sites; and (3) no need for biliary or vascular reconstruction. Several carefully selected cases with reconstructive procedures were performed on a clinical-study-based practice.

Selection of the surgical approaches was greatly affected by the medical paying system. Until 2015, before the start of national insurance coverage of MIAR in our country, the open approach was the first choice for AR in most patients, while from 2016, the laparoscopic approach had the priority, if indicated. Until March 2022, robotic liver resection was a practice at patients' own expense in Japan, which significantly affected selection of the laparoscopic or robotic approach. After starting reimbursement of robotic liver resection from April 2022, robotic AR was selected at the surgeons' or patients' preferences as well as depending on the machine availability in the hospital.

2.3. Baseline Data Collection

Patient, tumor, and surgical baseline data were retrospectively collected from the patients' medical charts. The patient baseline data included age, sex, body mass index (BMI), American Society of Anesthesiology—Performance Status (ASA) score, presence of diabetes, serum biomarkers, etiology of background liver disease (hepatitis B (HBV), hepatitis C (HCV) or non-B and non-C (NBNC)), indocyanine green (ICG) retention rate at 15 min (ICGR15), Child–Pugh grade, and histologically proven cirrhosis (postoperative evaluation). Tumor characteristics included location, number and size of the tumors, tumor stages according to the classification of the Liver Cancer Study Group of Japan [16], and serum tumor markers (alpha-fetoprotein (AFP); des-gamma-carboxy prothrombin (DCP)). Posterosuperior (PS) segments were defined as segments Sg1, Sg4a, Sg7, and Sg8 and were regarded as "locally difficult segments". The other segments were classified as anterolateral (AL) segments. Pathologic tumor stages and differentiation grades were determined postoperatively. The surgical baseline data included types of AR (left lateral sectionectomy, segmentectomy, sectionectomy, hemihepatectomy, or trisectionectomy) and repeat hepatectomy.

2.4. Surgical Techniques for AR

The surgical techniques of AR described below were consistently used either in OAR or MIAR and in any types of AR, irrespective of location of the target anatomic liver territory [5,6,17–19]. Inflow control was based on the extrahepatic Glissonian approach, where GPs to the target territory to be resected were first isolated and clamped or divided extrahepatically before parenchymal dissection was started.

Then, the optimal amount of parenchyma was resected along the demarcation line or the intersegmental plane that was visualized by macroscopic discoloration or by the ICG negative staining method [5,6,17]. During parenchymal dissection, the landmark hepatic veins (HVs) were exposed from their root side in the cranial-to-caudal direction (HV root-at first one-way parenchymal dissection). The extrahepatic Glissonian approach and HV root-at first one-way parenchymal dissection were facilitated by the anatomical background of Laennec's capsule at the hilum and major hepatic veins, as well as the hilar 'Gate theory', as described previously [6,13,18,19].

Several examples of the extrahepatic Glissonian approach to isolate the target GPs for MIAR are described in Figure 1. In left hemihepatectomy (Figure 1A), extrahepatic isolation of the left Glissonian pedicle above the hilar plate (G-UP) was facilitated by dissecting Gates I and III and passing forceps and a tape between the gates (Figure 1Aa). In isolated segmentectomy 8 (Figure 1B), to isolate the target GP of Sg8 (G8) extrahepatically (Figure 1Ba), the right anterior section GP (G-ant) was first isolated after cystic plate cholecystectomy in which the cystic plate was resected along with the gall bladder.

By exerting traction of G-ant downward, we isolated Sg5 GP (G5) extrahepatically, and finally, G8 was isolated extrahepatically, using the tape switching method (subtraction method) [6,13,19]. In right posterior sectionectomy (Figure 1C), the GP of the posterior section (G-post) was isolated extrahepatically by passing a tape between Gates V and VI (Figure 1Cg). Through selective occlusion of these target pedicles, the isolated ischemic anatomic territories were identified macroscopically as discolored areas or by using an ICG negative staining technique (Figure 1A(b),B(e),C(h)).

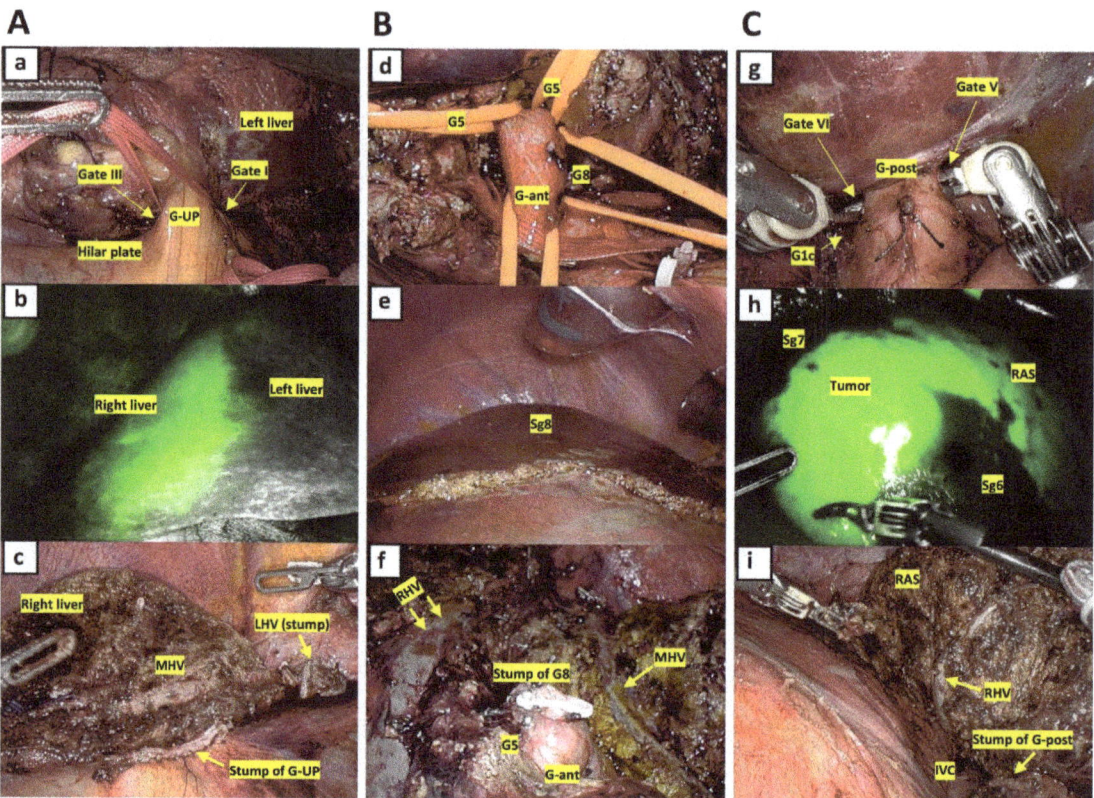

Figure 1. Anatomic liver resection using the extrahepatic Glissonian approach. (**A**) robotic left hemihepatectomy: (**a**) extrahepatic isolation of left Glissonian pedicle above the hilar plate (G-UP) by passing a tape between Gates I and III; (**b**) demarcation line between the right and left liver, using Firefly mode; (**c**) completion of left hemihepatectomy showing the exposed middle hepatic vein (MHV) and resected stumps of G-UP and left hepatic vein (LHV); (**B**) laparoscopic segmentectomy 8; (**d**) extrahepatic isolation of Glissonian pedicles of right anterior section (G-ant), Sg5 (G5), and Sg8 (G8); (**e**): selective isolated ischemia of Sg8; (**f**) completion of segmentectomy 8 showing the exposed MHV and right hepatic vein (RHV) and resected stump of G8; (**C**) robotic right posterior sectionectomy; (**g**) extrahepatic isolation of Glissonian pedicle of right posterior section (G-post); note Gates V and VI and caudate process pedicle (G1c); (**h**): Firefly mode after clamping G-post and intravenous ICG injection; note positive staining of the tumor and right anterior section (RAS) and negative staining of Sg6 and Sg7; (**i**) completion of right posterior sectionectomy showing the exposed RHV, inferior vena cava (IVC), and the resected stump of G-post.

Selective occlusion of inflow to the anatomic territory to be resected was followed by HV root-at first one-way parenchymal dissection, during which the already clamped target pedicles were exposed and divided on the liver dissecting plane. For parenchymal dissection, Cavitron Ultrasonic Surgical Aspirator (CUSA®) was used in open and laparoscopic cases, and a clamp-crushing method and ultrasonic coagulating shears were used in robotic cases. Pringle maneuver was not used routinely but was applied on demand. Parenchyma was dissected in the cranial-to-caudal direction, and AR was completed (Figure 1A(c),B(f),C(i)).

2.5. Perioperative Data

Intraoperative outcomes were evaluated by operative time, blood loss, liver parenchymal dissection time, transfusion (of any blood elements), use of the Pringle maneuver, and open conversion (in MIAR). Postoperative outcomes were evaluated by the serum maximum levels of maximum total bilirubin (TB), aspartate aminotransferase (AST) and C-reactive protein (CRP), the serum minimum level of prothrombin time (PT), morbidity graded according to the Clavien–Dindo (C–D) classification [20], mortality, R0 resection, and the length of postoperative hospital stay (LOS). Overall and major complications were defined as those within 90 postoperative days of any C–D grades and those of $\geq$C–D grade IIIa, respectively.

2.6. Statistical Analysis

Continuous data were expressed as median with range (baseline data) or interquartile range (perioperative data) and compared using the Kruskal–Wallis test. Categorical data were compared using the Pearson's chi-square test. In some comparative studies, 1:1 PSM was conducted to reduce biases. In comparison of perioperative outcomes between the OAR and MIAR cohorts, the following 11 variables were matched for PSM: age, sex, ASA class (I or II/$\geq$III), ICGR15 (<13.0%/$\geq$13.0%), etiology of underlying liver disease (HBV/HCV/NBNC), tumor number (single/multiple), tumor size (<4.0/$\geq$4.0, cm), tumor location (AL/PS), tumor stage (I or II/$\geq$III), types of resection (left lateral sectionectomy/segmentectomy/sectionectomy/$\geq$hemihepatectomy), and previous hepatectomy (yes/no). In comparison of perioperative outcomes between the laparoscopic and robotic cohorts, age, sex, presence of cirrhosis (yes/no), tumor number (single/multiple), tumor size (<3.0/$\geq$3.0, cm), types of resection, and previous hepatectomy (yes/no) were matched. In analyses of long-term outcomes, we examined newly developed HCC cases only.

In comparison of long-term outcomes between the OAR and MIAR cohorts, 11 variables, including age, sex, ASA class, etiology, presence of cirrhosis, ICGR15 (<13.0%/$\geq$13.0%), tumor number (single/multiple), tumor size (<4.0/$\geq$4.0, cm), tumor stage, pathological tumor differentiation, and types of resection, were matched to reduce biases. Long-term outcomes were also compared between the unmatched and matched laparoscopic and robotic AR cohorts. In this analysis, age, sex, tumor size (<4.0/$\geq$4.0, cm), tumor number (single/multiple), and presence of histology-proven cirrhosis (yes/no) were matched.

The PSM method was the nearest neighborhood method with a caliper width of 0.20. The standard mean deviation (SMD) was calculated for all studied variables, and an SMD <0.20 was confirmed for all matched variables, which indicated appropriate matching. The postoperative overall survival (OS) and recurrence-free survival (RFS) were analyzed only in patients with newly developed HCC, using the Kaplan–Meier method. p <0.050 was considered statistically significant. Statistical analyses were performed using JMP® software ver. 14.0 (SAS Institute, Cary, NC, USA).

3. Results

Between 2010 and October 2022, we performed 667 liver resections for HCC, including 306 open, 279 laparoscopic, and 82 robotic resections, at our institution. Among these 667 cases, we retrospectively reviewed the consecutive 327 AR cases, consisting of 185 OAR and 142 MIAR (102 laparoscopic and 40 robotic) cases, where AR using the extrahepatic Glissonian approach was performed without biliary or vascular reconstruction or concomitant resection of extrahepatic organs.

3.1. Perioperative Outcomes

3.1.1. Comparison between OAR and MIAR

Patient and Tumor Baseline Data

Patient and tumor baseline data were compared between OAR and MIAR (Table 1). Before PSM (185 OAR and 142 MIAR cases), compared to OAR, MIAR was significantly associated with higher BMI, lower ASA class, lower ICGR15, lower Child–Pugh class, smaller tumor size, lower AFP and DCP levels, and more favorable tumor stage. Further, compared to OAR, MIAR was significantly associated with a lower rate of sectionectomy or more extensive procedures, a lower proportion of major resection, and a higher rate of the repeat hepatectomy setting. After 1:1 PSM (91:91), the OAR and MIAR groups were comparable in terms of all studied variables.

Table 1. Comparison of baseline data between open and minimally invasive AR for HCC.

	Before PSM			After PSM		
	OAR (N = 185)	MIAR (N = 142)	p	OAR (N = 91)	MIAR (N = 91)	p
Age, years	73 (31–91)	71 (11–86)	0.102	72 (43–91)	72 (29–86)	0.570
Sex, M/F	147/38	113/29	0.979	73/18	73/18	1.000
BMI, kg/m^2	23.0 (14.7–54.0)	23.6 (15.2–36.3)	**0.013**	23.1 (17.2–54.0)	23.8 (16.0–36.3)	0.456
ASA score, I or II/≥III	145/40	130/12	**0.001**	80/11	81/10	0.817
Diabetes, n (%)	71 (38.4)	53 (37.3)	0.846	38 (41.8)	36 (39.6)	0.763
Total bilirubin, mg/dL	0.7 (0.3–6.4)	0.8 (0.2–1.7)	0.097	0.7 (0.3–1.8)	0.7 (0.2–1.7)	0.782
Prothrombin time, %	98 (18–145)	96 (28–129)	0.386	97 (64–145)	95 (63–129)	0.319
Platelet count, ×10^4/mm^3	14.9 (1.2–47.2)	15.5 (4.0–42.2)	0.783	14.7 (1.2–47.2)	15.0 (4.6–29.5)	0.809
ICGR15, %	14.2 (0.6–52.6)	11.1 (0.0–68.3)	**0.0002**	14.1 (0.6–41.0)	12.1 (0.0–68.3)	0.072
≥13.0%, n (%)	100 (55.3)	49 (36.6)	**0.001**	49 (53.9)	42 (46.2)	0.299
Child-Pugh class, A/B	177/8	141/1	**0.047**	86/5	90/1	0.097
Etiology, HBV/HCV/NBNC	37/70/78	35/48/59	0.561	19/30/42	20/31/40	0.956
Cirrhosis (histology), n (%)	58 (31.4)	53 (37.3)	0.258	31 (34.1)	34 (37.4)	0.643
Tumor characteristics						
Location, PS (%)/AL	130 (70.3)/55	88 (62.0)/54	0.115	66 (72.5)/25	61 (67.0)/30	0.420
Number	1 (1–23)	1 (1–6)	0.053	1 (1–6)	1 (1–6)	0.254
Single/Multiple	122/63	107/35	0.066	70/21	63/28	0.242
Size, cm	5.0 (1.0–22.0)	3.2 (0.7–16.0)	**<0.0001**	4.0 (1.0–17.7)	3.8 (0.7–16.0)	0.143
≥4.0 cm, n (%)	114 (61.6)	53 (37.3)	**<0.0001**	47 (51.7)	44 (48.4)	0.657
Stage, I or II/≥III	94/91	108/34	**<0.0001**	63/28	59/32	0.528
AFP, ng/mL	15.1 (1.5–1,213,687.0)	6.4 (1.0–149,880.0)	**0.0005**	11.2 (1.5–636,200.0)	6.9 (1.0–149,880.0)	0.135
DCP, mAU/mL	287 (3–538,983)	67 (10–47,453)	**0.0003**	186 (10–159,600)	74 (10–47,453)	0.056
Types of resection, n (%)			**0.004**			0.976
Left lateral sectionectomy	5 (2.7)	8 (5.6)		4 (4.4)	4 (4.4)	
Segmentectomy	77 (41.6)	83 (58.5)		50 (55.0)	47 (51.7)	
Sectionectomy *	56 (30.3)	30 (21.1)		22 (24.2)	24 (26.4)	
≥Hemihepatectomy	47 (25.4)	21 (14.8)		15 (16.5)	16 (17.6)	
Major Hx (≥3 segs), n (%)	56 (30.3)	23 (16.2)	**0.003**	18 (19.8)	17 (18.7)	0.851
Repeat Hx, n (%)	21 (11.4)	29 (20.4)	**0.024**	13 (14.3)	12 (13.2)	0.830

AR: anatomic liver resection; PSM: propensity score matching; continuous variables: median (range); OAR and MIAR: open and minimally invasive anatomic liver resection, respectively; BMI: body mass index; ASA: American Society of Anesthesiology; ICGR15: the indocyanine green retention rate at 15 min; NBNC: non-B and non-C; PS: posterosuperior; AL: anterolateral; AFP: alpha-fetoprotein; DCP: des-gamma-carboxy prothrombin Sectionectomy *: mono- or central bisectionectomy except for left lateral sectionectomy; Hx: hepatectomy; Bold: statistically significant.

Perioperative Outcomes

Comparative perioperative outcomes are shown in Table 2. Before PSM, compared to OAR (n = 185), MIAR (n = 142) was significantly associated with less blood loss, a lower transfusion rate, lower postoperative serum maximum TB and CRP levels, higher maximum AST level, lower overall and major morbidity rates, a lower 90-day mortality rate, and shorter LOS.

After 1:1 PSM (91:91), compared to OAR, MIAR was significantly associated with longer operative time (643 vs. 579 min, p = 0.028), less blood loss (275 vs. 955 g, p < 0.0001), a lower transfusion rate (17.6% vs. 47.3%, p < 0.0001), a lower maximum TB (1.5 vs. 2.2 mg/dL, p < 0.0001), higher maximum AST (593 vs. 438 IU/L, p = 0.043), and lower maximum CRP (8.62 vs. 11.0 mg/dL, p = 0.017) levels. Furthermore, MIAR was significantly associated with lower rates of overall (36.3% vs. 57.1%, p = 0.005) and major (4.4% vs. 20.9%, p = 0.0008) morbidity, a lower rate of bile leak or collection (1.1% vs. 11.0%, p = 0.005), and shorter LOS (15 vs. 29 days, p < 0.0001).

Table 2. Comparison of perioperative outcomes between open and minimally invasive AR for HCC.

	Before PSM			After PSM		
	OAR (N = 185)	MIAR (N = 142)	p	OAR (N = 91)	MIAR (N = 91)	p
Operative time, min	591 (498–781)	637 (539–794)	0.128	579 (474–731)	643 (546–797)	**0.028**
Blood loss, g	1083 (575–2006)	244 (115–493)	**<0.0001**	955 (498–1753)	279 (121–524)	**<0.0001**
Transfusion*, n (%)	98 (53.0)	23 (16.2)	**<0.0001**	42 (47.3)	16 (17.6)	**<0.0001**
Pringle maneuver, n (%)	27 (14.6)	32 (22.5)	0.064	16 (17.6)	21 (23.1)	0.357
Open conversion, n (%)	NA	4 (2.8)	NA	NA	2 (2.2)	NA
Laboratory data						
Max TB, mg/dL	2.3 (1.6–3.4)	1.5 (1.2–2.0)	**<0.0001**	2.2 (1.6–3.1)	1.5 (1.2–1.9)	**<0.0001**
Max AST, IU/L	416 (291–808)	598 (315–1026)	**0.005**	438 (305–823)	593 (348–1016)	**0.043**
Min PT, %	63 (54–68)	63 (58–71)	0.093	64 (54–68)	62 (56–71)	0.810
Max CRP, mg/dL	10.40 (7.65–13.04)	9.00 (6.25–13.01)	**0.028**	11.10 (7.80–12.80)	8.62 (6.32–12.60)	**0.017**
Morbidity (≤90 days), n (%)						
Overall (≥CD-I)	97 (52.4)	50 (35.2)	**0.002**	52 (57.1)	33 (36.3)	**0.005**
Major (≥CD-IIIa)	33 (17.8)	12 (8.5)	**0.015**	19 (20.9)	4 (4.4)	**0.0008**
Bile leak or collection	14 (7.6)	6 (4.2)	0.211	10 (11.0)	1 (1.1)	**0.005**
Mortality, n (%)						
≤30 days	2 (1.1)	0 (0)	0.214	1 (1.1)	0 (0)	0.316
≤90 days	5 (2.7)	0 (0)	**0.048**	4 (4.4)	0 (0)	**0.043**
R0 resection, n (%)	179 (96.8)	141 (99.3)	0.116	88 (96.7)	90 (98.9)	0.312
Length of hospital stay, days	28 (20–40)	15 (12–19)	**<0.0001**	29 (21–43)	15 (13–19)	**<0.0001**

Continuous variables: median (interquartile range); AR: anatomic liver resection; PSM: propensity score matching; OAR and MIAR: open and minimally invasive anatomic liver resection, respectively; Transfusion*: any kinds of blood component or product; NA: not applicable; Max and Min: postoperative serum maximum and minimum levels, respectively, TB: total bilirubin; AST: aspartate aminotransferase; PT: prothrombin time; CRP: C-reactive protein, CD: Clavien–Dindo grade; Bold: statistically significant.

3.1.2. Comparison between Laparoscopic and Robotic AR for HCC

In the next set of analyses, we compared baseline data and perioperative outcomes between the two MIAR approaches: laparoscopic and robotic.

Patient and Tumor Baseline Data

Baseline data were compared between the laparoscopic and robotic AR groups (Table 3). Before PSM (102 laparoscopic vs. 40 robotic cases), compared to laparoscopic AR, robotic AR was significantly associated with a lower rate of cirrhosis, smaller tumor number and size, a lower AFP level, and a higher rate of repeat hepatectomy setting. After 1:1 PSM (31:31), all studied variables were comparable between the laparoscopic and robotic AR groups.

Perioperative Outcomes

Perioperative outcomes are shown in Table 4. Before PSM, laparoscopic and robotic AR groups had comparable outcomes, except for the significantly higher rate of Pringle maneuver application (35.0% vs. 17.7%, p = 0.026), the higher maximum AST level (767 vs. 546 IU/L, p = 0.026), and the lower minimum PT level (60% vs. 64%, p = 0.032) in the robotic AR group. After PSM, both groups had comparable perioperative outcomes.

Table 3. Comparison of baseline data between laparoscopic and robotic AR for HCC.

	Before PSM			After PSM		
	Laparoscopic AR (N = 102)	Robotic AR (N = 40)	p	Laparoscopic AR (N = 31)	Robotic AR (N = 31)	p
Age, years	70 (11–86)	72 (21–82)	0.353	70 (36–83)	72 (21–82)	0.989
Sex, M/F	80/22	33/7	0.589	25/6	25/6	1.000
BMI, kg/m^2	23.6 (15.2–36.3)	23.9 (17.9–30.3)	0.895	23.0 (18.0–33.9)	23.9 (17.9–30.3)	0.186
ASA score, I or II/≥III	94/8	36/4	0.678	29/2	28/3	0.641
Total bilirubin, mg/dL	0.8 (0.2–1.7)	0.7 (0.3–1.3)	0.479	0.7 (0.2–1.6))	0.7 (0.3–1.3)	0.854
Prothrombin time, %	96 (63–129)	97 (28–127)	0.701	96 (67–128)	97 (83–127)	0.849
Platelet count, x10^4/mm^3	15.7 (4.0–42.2)	15.3 (7.6–23.5)	0.665	15.5 (4.6–29.5)	15.1 (9.1–23.5)	0.961
ICGR15, %	11.1 (0.6–68.3)	10.9 (0.0–30.8)	0.284	10.5 (0.6–27.6)	11.8 (0.0–30.8)	0.554
≥13.0%, n (%)	35 (36.5)	14 (36.8)	0.967	6 (22.2)	13 (43.3)	0.091
Child-Pugh, A/B	101/1	40/0	0.530	31/0	31/0	1.000
Etiology, HBV/HCV/NBNC	24/36/42	11/12/17	0.805	7/11/13	9/8/14	0.247
Cirrhosis (histology), n (%)	46 (45.1)	7 (17.5)	**0.002**	6 (19.4)	7 (22.6)	0.755
Tumor characteristics						
Location, PS (%)/AL	65 (63.7)/37	23 (57.5)/17	0.492	20 (64.5)/11	16 (51.6)/15	0.303
Number	1 (1–4)	1 (1–6)	**0.047**	1 (1–3)	1 (1–6)	0.927
Single/Multiple	81/21	26/14	0.073	23/8	23/8	1.000
Size, cm	3.5 (0.7–16.0)	2.7 (1.2–12.5)	**0.027**	3.0 (1.5–16.0)	3.0 (1.2–12.5)	0.371
≥4.0 cm, n (%)	44 (43.1)	9 (22.5)	**0.022**	12 (38.7)	8 (25.8)	0.277
Stage, I or II/≥III	81/21	27/1	0.135	23/8	21/10	0.576
AFP, ng/mL	8.2 (1.9–149,880.0)	4.2 (1.0–5811.0)	**0.002**	7.1 (2.0–2708.5)	4.5 (1.0–5811.0)	0.113
DCP, mAU/mL	75 (10–47,453)	44 (11–30,899)	0.071	68 (11–47,032)	4.5 (1.0–5811.0)	0.251
Repeat Hx, n (%)	13 (12.8)	16 (40.0)	**0.0003**	6 (19.4)	7 (22.6)	0.755
Types of resection, n (%)			0.775			0.271
Left lateral sectionectomy	6 (5.9)	2 (5.0)		0 (0)	2 (6.5)	
Segmentectomy	58 (56.9)	25 (62.5)		18 (58.1)	20 (64.5)	
Sectionectomy*	21 (20.6)	9 (22.5)		10 (32.3)	5 (16.1)	
≥Hemihepatectomy	17 (16.7)	4 (10.0)		3 (9.7)	4 (12.9)	
Major Hx (≥3 segs), n (%)	19 (18.6)	4 (10.0)	0.838	31 (100)	4 (12.9)	0.719
Iwate criteria, level, n (%)			0.549			0.327
Intermediate	22 (21.6)	12 (30.0)		5 (16.1)	10 (32.3)	
Advanced	51 (50.0)	17 (42.5)		18 (58.1)	14 (45.2)	
Expert	29 (28.4)	11 (27.5)		8 (25.8)	7 (22.6)	
≥Advanced, n (%)	80 (78.4)	28 (70.0)	0.290	26 (83.9)	21 (67.7)	0.138

PSM: propensity score matching; AR: anatomic liver resection; continuous variables: median (range); BMI: body mass index; ASA: American Society of Anesthesiology; ICGR15: the indocyanine green retention rate at 15 min; NBNC: non-B and non-C; PS: posterosuperior; AL: anterolateral; AFP: alpha-fetoprotein; DCP: des-gamma-carboxy prothrombin; Sectionectomy*: mono- or central bisectionectomy except for left lateral sectionectomy; Hx: hepatectomy; Bold: statistically significant.

Table 4. Comparison of perioperative outcomes between laparoscopic and robotic AR for HCC.

	Before PSM			After PSM		
	Laparoscopic AR (N = 102)	Robotic AR (N = 40)	p	Laparoscopic AR (N = 31)	Robotic AR (N = 31)	p
Operative time, min	631 (525–774)	667 (566–893)	0.157	632 (569–732)	642 (564–891)	0.709
Parenchymal dissection time, min	240 (175–325)	273 (177–340)	0.548	248 (177–333)	227 (139–367)	0.906
Blood loss, g	245 (120–488)	200 (98–635)	0.890	227 (90–468)	170 (98–598)	0.989
Transfusion*, n (%)	16 (15.7)	7 (17.5)	0.792	3 (9.7)	6 (19.4)	0.279
Pringle maneuver, n (%)	18 (17.7)	14 (35.0)	**0.026**	5 (16.1)	10 (32.3)	0.138
Open conversion, n (%)	2 (2.0)	2 (5.0)	0.325	0 (0)	1 (3.2)	0.313
Laboratory data						
Max TB, mg/dL	1.5 (1.2–1.9)	1.5 (1.3–2.0)	0.701	1.4 (1.1–1.6)	1.5 (1.2–2.0)	0.073
Max AST, IU/L	546 (296–913)	767 (370–2,100)	**0.026**	593 (315–903)	707 (348–2,796)	0.275
Min PT, %	64 (59–72)	60 (49–71)	**0.032**	62 (58–73)	60 (51–72)	0.135
Max CRP, mg/dL	8.68 (6.32–12.72)	9.64 (5.97–12.18)	0.396	8.44 (6.32–12.6)	10.18 (5.45–14.11)	0.477

Table 4. Cont.

	Before PSM			After PSM		
	Laparoscopic AR (N = 102)	Robotic AR (N = 40)	p	Laparoscopic AR (N = 31)	Robotic AR (N = 31)	p
Morbidity (≤90 days), n (%)						
Overall (≥CD-I)	37 (36.3)	13 (32.5)	0.672	10 (32.3)	9 (29.0)	0.783
Major (≥CD-IIIa)	7 (6.9)	5 (12.5)	0.277	2 (6.5)	5 (16.1)	0.229
Bile leak or collection	5 (4.9)	1 (2.5)	0.522	2 (6.5)	1 (3.2)	0.554
Mortality, n (%)						
≤30 days	0 (0)	0 (0)	1.000	0 (0)	0 (0)	1.000
≤90 days	0 (0)	0 (0)	1.000	0 (0)	0 (0)	1.000
R0 resection, n (%)	101 (99.0)	40 (100)	0.530	31 (100)	31 (100)	1.000
Length of hospital stay, days	15 (12–19)	15 (11–18)	0.416	14 (11–18)	15 (11–18)	0.965

PSM: propensity score matching; AR: anatomic liver resection; continuous variables: median (interquartile range); Transfusion*: any kinds of blood component or product; Max and Min: postoperative serum maximum and minimum levels, respectively; TB: total bilirubin; AST: aspartate aminotransferase; PT: prothrombin time; CRP: C-reactive protein; CD: Clavien–Dindo grade; Bold: statistically significant.

3.2. Long-Term Outcomes after AR for Newly Developed HCC

In the next set of analyses, we studied long-term outcomes after AR in 276 patients with newly developed HCC, who underwent 163 OARs and 113 MIARs (89 laparoscopic and 24 robotic ARs), respectively, and compared OS and RFS between OAR and MIAR and between laparoscopic and robotic AR.

3.2.1. Comparison of Long-Term Outcomes between OAR and MIAR

Patient and Tumor Baseline Data

Baseline data were compared between 163 patients undergoing OAR and 113 patients undergoing MIAR for newly developed HCC (Table 5). Before PSM (163:113), compared to OAR, MIAR was significantly associated with higher BMI, a lower ASA class, lower ICGR 15, smaller tumor number and size, more favorable tumor stages, and higher AFP and DCP levels. In addition, types of resection were significantly more extensive, with a higher proportion of major resection in OAR than in MIAR. After 1:1 PSM (76:76), all studied variables were comparable between OAR and MIAR.

Table 5. Comparison of background data between open and minimally invasive AR for newly developed HCC.

	Before PSM			After PSM		
	OAR (N = 163)	MIAR (N = 113)	p	OAR (N = 76)	MIAR (N = 76)	p
Age, years	72 (31–91)	71 (21–86)	0.099	72 (43–86)	72 (29–85)	0.919
Sex, M/F	129/34	90/23	0.919	58/18	59/17	0.847
BMI, kg/m²	23.1 (14.7–54.0)	24.1 (16.0–36.3)	**0.011**	23.1 (14.7–54.0)	23.3 (16.0–36.3)	0.235
ASA score, I or II/≥III	125/38	103/10	**0.001**	64/12	67/9	0.481
Diabetes, n (%)	66 (40.5)	44 (38.9)	0.796	29 (38.2)	31 (40.8)	0.740
ICGR15, %	14.2 (0.6–52.6)	11.3 (0–39.4)	**0.0007**	12.6 (1.2–41.0)	12.1 (0–39.4)	0.227
≥13.0%, n (%)	89 (55.6)	40 (37.0)	**0.003**	35 (46.1)	36 (47.4)	0.871
Etiology, HBV/HCV/NBNC	32/56/75	23/37/53	0.961	16/27/33	14/25/37	0.803
Cirrhosis (histology), n (%)	49 (30.1)	41 (36.3)	0.278	31 (40.8)	31 (40.8)	1.000
Tumor characteristics						
Location, PS (%)/AL	119 (73.0)/44	71 (62.8)/42	0.073	53 (69.7)/23	55 (72.4)/21	0.721
Number	1 (1–23)	1 (1–4)	**0.049**	1 (1–23)	1 (1–4)	0.766
Single/Multiple	109/54	86/27	0.098	57/19	55/21	0.713
Size, cm	5.5 (1.2–22.0)	3.5 (0.7–16.0)	**<0.0001**	4.0 (1.2–22.0)	4.0 (0.7–16.0)	0.491
≥4.0 cm, n (%)	110 (67.5)	49 (43.4)	**<0.0001**	40 (52.6)	43 (56.6)	0.625
Stage, I/II/III/IVA/IVB	8/72/60/18/5	11/72/27/2/1	**0.0005**	6/42/24/3/1	8/42/23/2/1	0.973

Table 5. Cont.

	Before PSM			After PSM		
	OAR (N = 163)	MIAR (N = 113)	p	OAR (N = 76)	MIAR (N = 76)	p
AFP, ng/mL	15.9 (1.5–1,213,687.0)	7.3 (1.4–149,880.0)	**0.010**	13.7 (2.1–636,200.0)	9.8 (2.0–149,880.0)	0.340
DCP, mAU/mL	389 (3–538,983)	78 (10–47,453)	**0.002**	252 (3–538,983)	148 (10–47,453)	0.671
Differentiation			0.733			0.846
well	6	6		4	3	
moderate	150	102		70	69	
poor or sarcomatous	4	2		1	2	
combined	2	30		1	2	
necrosis	1	0		0	0	
Types of resection, n (%)			**0.0003**			0.905
Left lateral sectionectomy	5 (3.1)	7 (6.2)		4 (5.3)	3 (3.9)	
Segmentectomy	63 (38.7)	66 (58.4)		37 (48.7)	40 (52.6)	
Sectionectomy*	52 (31.9)	21 (18.6)		17 (22.4)	18 (23.7)	
≥Hemihepatectomy	43 (26.4)	19 (16.8)		18 (23.7)	15 (19.7)	
Major Hx (≥3 segs), n (%)	52 (31.9)	21 (18.6)	**0.014**	18 (23.7)	16 (21.1)	0.697

Continuous variables: median (range); PSM: propensity score matching; OAR and MIAR: open and minimally invasive anatomic liver resection, respectively; BMI: body mass index; ASA: American Society of Anesthesiology; ICGR15: the indocyanine green retention rate at 15 min; NBNC: non-B and non-C; PS: posterosuperior; AL: anterolateral; AFP: alpha-fetoprotein; DCP: des-gamma-carboxy prothrombin; Sectionectomy*: mono- or central bisectionectomy except for left lateral sectionectomy; Hx: hepatectomy; Bold: statistically significant.

Long-Term Outcomes

Comparing survival rates between the unmatched patients undergoing MIAR (n = 113) and OAR (n = 163), MIAR patients had statistically longer OS (Figure 2A, $p < 0.0001$; 5-year rate: 84.4% vs. 50.0%) and longer RFS (Figure 2B, $p < 0.0001$; 5-year rate: 47.1% vs. 25.1%) than OAR patients. For the matched cohorts after PSM, compared to OAR (n = 76), MIAR patients (n = 76) were associated with statistically longer OS (Figure 2C, $p = 0.005$; 5-year rate: 78.9% vs. 54.6%) and longer RFS (Figure 2D, $p = 0.010$; 5-year rate: 41.9% vs. 31.1%).

3.2.2. Comparison of Long-Term Outcomes between Laparoscopic and Robotic AR

Patient and Tumor Baseline Data

Patient and tumor baseline data were compared between the unmatched 89 laparoscopic AR and 24 robotic AR cases (Table 6). Before PSM, compared to laparoscopic AR, robotic AR was significantly associated with a lower rate of histology-proven cirrhosis (12.5% vs. 42.7%, $p = 0.006$) and a lower rate of tumors ≥4.0 cm (25.0% vs. 48.3%, $p = 0.041$). One-to-one PSM identified 22 laparoscopic and 22 robotic matched cases. After PSM, all evaluated patient and tumor characteristics were comparable between the laparoscopic and robotic AR cohorts.

Survival Data

Comparison between the unmatched cohorts of laparoscopic (n = 89) and robotic (n = 24) approaches showed comparable OS (Figure 3A) and RFS (Figure 3B). Similarly, OS (Figure 3C) and RFS (Figure 3D) were comparable between the matched laparoscopic AR (n = 22) and robotic AR (n = 22) cohorts.

Details of Postoperative Recurrence

In the study period, tumor recurrence was observed in 162 (58.7%) of the entire 276 patients, including 111 OAR and 51 MIAR patients; the recurrence rate was significantly lower in the unmatched MIAR than in the OAR cohorts (45.1% vs. 68.1%, $p < 0.0001$). Between the matched OAR and MIAR cohorts (76:76), the recurrence rate was still significantly higher in OAR (n = 50, 65.8%) than in MIAR (n = 37, 48.7%) ($p = 0.033$).

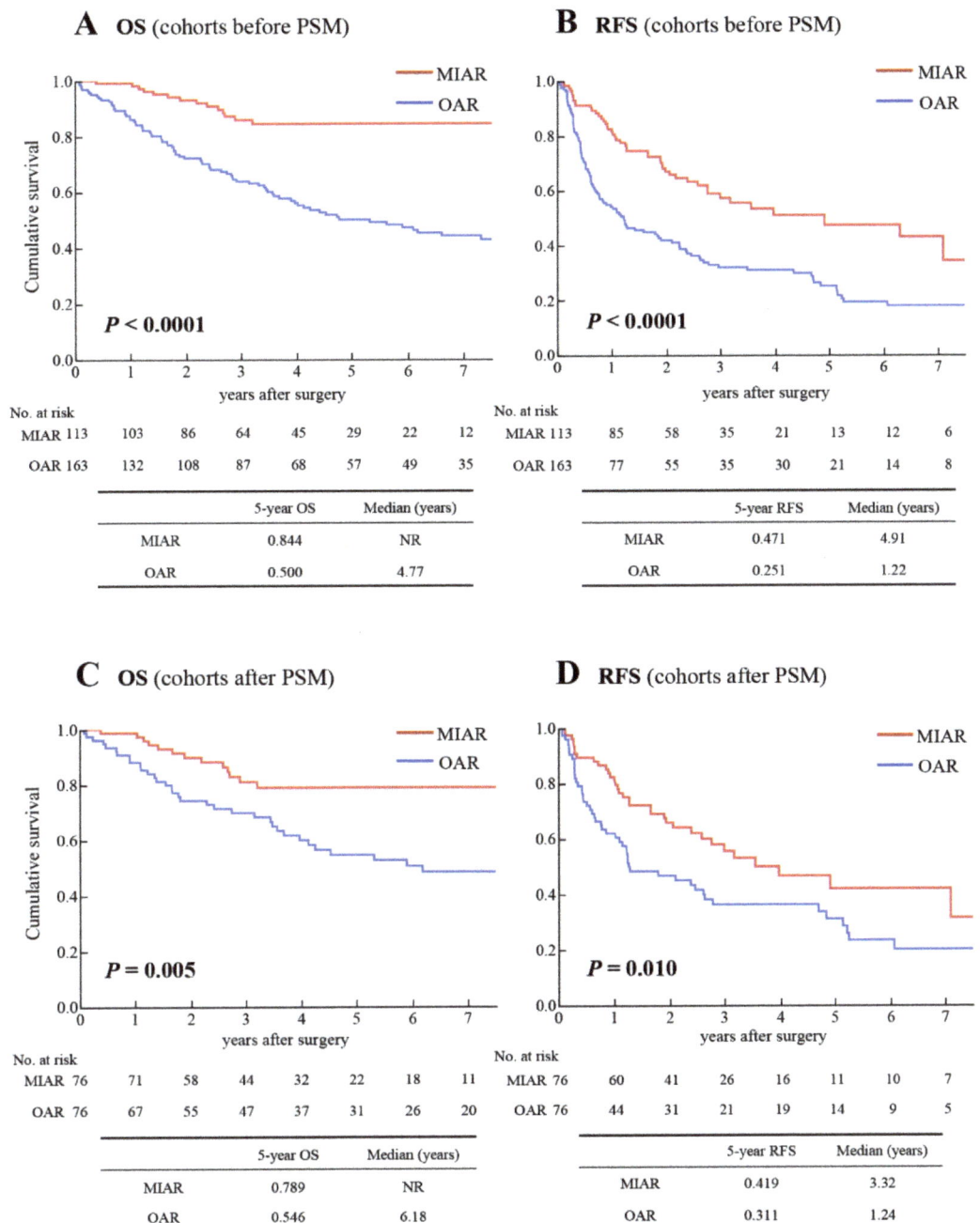

Figure 2. Overall (OS) and recurrence-free (RFS) survivals after OAR and MIAR: (**A**) OS in the comparative cohorts before PSM; (**B**). RFS in the comparative cohorts before PSM; (**C**) OS in the comparative cohorts after PSM; (**D**) RFS in the comparative cohorts after PSM; NR: not reached.

Table 6. Comparison of background data between laparoscopic and robotic AR for newly developed HCC.

	Before PSM			After PSM		
	Laparoscopic AR (N = 89)	Robotic AR (N = 24)	p	Laparoscopic AR (N = 22)	Robotic AR (N = 22)	p
Age, years	70 (29–86)	72 (21–82)	0.975	71 (53–83)	72 (48–82)	0.778
Sex, M/F	71/18	19/5	0.948	19/3	19/3	1.000
BMI, kg/m²	24.0 (16.0–36.3)	24.2 (17.9–30.3)	0.744	23.5 (18.0–33.2)	24.4 (17.9–30.3)	0.411
ASA score, I or II/≥III	81/8	22/2	0.920	21/1	20/2	0.550
Diabetes, n (%)	37 (41.6)	7 (29.2)	0.269	9 (40.9)	7 (31.8)	0.531
ICGR15, %	11.3 (0.6–39.4)	11.3 (0–17.5)	0.329	10.5 (4.3–20.9)	11.2 (0.0–16.0)	0.865
≥13.0%, n (%)	32 (37.7)	8 (34.8)	0.801	6 (28.6)	7 (31.8)	0.817
Etiology, HBV/HCV/NBNC	18/30/41	5/7/12	0.912	5/6/11	4/7/11	0.910
Cirrhosis (histology), n (%)	38 (42.7)	3 (12.5)	**0.006**	3 (13.6)	3 (13.6)	1.000
Child-Pugh class, A/B	88/1	24/0	0.602	22/0	22/0	1.000
Tumor characteristics						
Location, PS (%)/AL	57 (64.0)/32	14 (58.3)/10	0.607	10 (45.5)/12	13 (59.1)/9	0.365
Number	1 (1–4)	1 (1–4)	0.517	1 (1–2)	1 (1–4)	0.936
Single/Multiple	69/20	17/7	0.495	17/5	17/5	1.000
Size, cm	3.5 (0.7–16.0)	3.1 (1.5–12.5)	0.111	3.3 (1.5–6.0)	3.1 (1.5–6.0)	0.814
≥4.0 cm, n (%)	43 (48.3)	6 (25.0)	**0.041**	5 (22.7)	5 (22.7)	1.000
Stage, I/II/III/IVA/IVB	11/57/19/1/1	0/15/8/1/0	0.252	5/13/4/0	0/14/7/1	0.077
AFP, ng/mL	8.8 (2.0–14,980.0)	6.0 (1.4–5,811.0)	0.185	5.4 (2.0–2,708.5)	6.0 (1.4–1,372.0)	0.890
DCP, mAU/mL	95 (10–47,453)	43 (14–20,843)	0.073	40 (10–2,753)	43 (14–20,843)	0.576
Differentiation			0.471			0.178
well	6	0		2	0	
moderate	79	23		20	22	
poor or sarcomatous	2	1		0	0	
combined	2	0		0	0	
Types of resection, n (%)			0.950			0.731
Left lateral sectionetomy	6 (6.7)	1 (4.2)		1 (4.6)	0 (0)	
Segmentectomy	51 (57.3)	15 (62.5)		13 (59.1)	14 (63.6)	
Sectionectomy*	17 (19.1)	4 (16.7)		5 (22.7)	4 (18.2)	
≥Hemihepatectomy	15 (16.9)	15 (16.9)		3 (13.6)	4 (18.2)	

Continuous variables: median (range); AR: anatomic liver resection; BMI: body mass index; ASA: American Society of Anesthesiology; ICGR15: the indocyanine green retention rate at 15 min; NBNC: non-B and non-C; PS: posterosuperior; AL: anterolateral; AFP: alpha-fetoprotein; DCP: des-gamma-carboxy prothrombin; Sectionectomy*: mono- or central bisectionectomy except for left lateral sectionectomy; Hx: hepatectomy; Bold: statistically significant.

The details of recurrence and its treatments are shown in Table 7. In recurrent cases in the entire cohort, patterns of recurrence (intrahepatic and/or extrahepatic), the rate of extrahepatic recurrence, and recurrent organs were comparable between OAR and MIAR. Compared to OAR, MIAR was associated with significantly longer RFS (median: 15.4 vs. 7.6 months, $p = 0.007$) and a significantly lower rate of the first recurrence within 1 postoperative year (37.3% vs. 62.2%, $p = 0.003$). Pathologic tumor stages were more advanced in recurrent cases in the unmatched OAR cohort ($p = 0.008$), while they were comparable between the matched OAR and MIAR cohorts. Pathologic tumor differentiations were comparable between the recurrent cases in the unmatched and matched cohorts. Perioperative morbidity, which has been suggested to affect tumor recurrence in previous studies [21,22], was comparable between OAR and MIAR, both in the unmatched and matched cohorts.

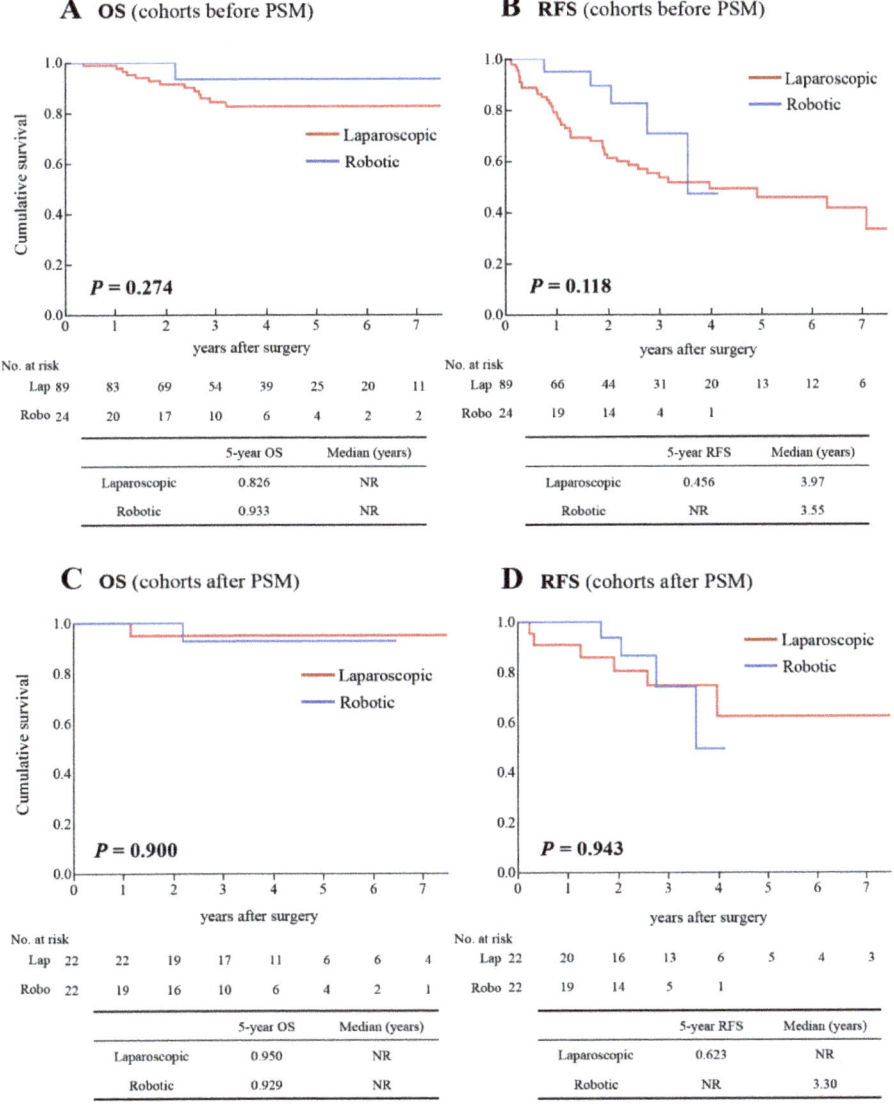

Figure 3. Overall (OS) and recurrence-free (RFS) survivals after laparoscopic and robotic anatomic resection: (**A**) OS in the unmatched cohorts; (**B**) RFS in the unmatched cohorts; (**C**) OS in the matched cohorts; (**D**) RFS in the matched cohorts; NR: not reached.

Table 7. Details of recurrence after OAR or MIAR for newly developed HCC.

	Recurrent Cases in the Unmatched Cohorts			Recurrent Cases in the Matched Cohorts		
	OAR (N = 111)	MIAR (N = 51)	p	OAR (N = 50)	MIAR (N = 37)	p
Patterns of recurrence, n (%)			0.463			0.715
Intrahepatic-only	84 (75.7)	43 (84.3)		37 (74.0)	30 (81.1)	
Extrahepatic-only	7 (6.3)	2 (3.9)		3 (6.0)	2 (5.4)	
Intra- and extra-hepatic	20 (18.0)	6 (11.8)		10 (20.0)	5 (13.5)	
Extrahepatic recurrence, n (%)	27 (24.3)	8 (15.7)	0.215	13 (26.0)	7 (18.9)	0.438
Lung	13 (11.7)	5 (9.8)	0.720	6 (12.0)	5 (13.5)	0.834
Bone	11 (9.9)	2 (3.9)	0.193	6 (12.0)	1 (2.7)	0.115
Lymph node	9 (8.2)	2 (3.9)	0.325	5 (10.0)	2 (5.4)	0.436
Hematogenous metastasis	22 (19.8)	6 (11.8)	0.208	9 (18.0)	5 (13.5)	0.573
Recurrence-free survival (mo), range	7.6 (0.5–73.9)	15.4 (1.4–86.3)	**0.007**	9.4 (0.8–73.9)	15.4 (1.4–86.3)	0.125
First recurrence <1 year, n (%)	69 (62.2)	19 (37.3)	**0.003**	27 (54.0)	13 (35.1)	0.081
First recurrence <2 years, n (%)	87 (78.4)	34 (66.7)	0.111	38 (76.0)	24 (64.9)	0.257
Pathologic tumor stage, n (%)			**0.008**			0.696
I or II	49 (44.1)	34 (66.7)		29 (58.0)	23 (62.2)	
≥III	62 (55.9)	17 (33.3)		21 (42.0)	14 (37.8)	
Pathologic differentiation, n (%)			0.557			0.830
well	3 (2.7)	2 (3.9)		2 (4.0)	1 (2.7)	
moderate	104 (93.7)	46 (88.5)		46 (92.0)	33 (89.2)	
poor or sarcomatous	2 (1.8)	1 (1.9)		1 (2.0)	1 (2.7)	
combined	2 (1.8)	3 (5.8)		1 (2.0)	2 (5.4)	
Perioperative morbidity, n (%)						
Any (C–D grade ≥I)	57 (51.4)	21 (41.2)	0.229	25 (50.0)	16 (43.2)	0.533
Major (C–D grade ≥III)	18 (16.2)	6 (11.8)	0.459	5 (10.0)	5 (13.5)	0.612
Bile leak/collection	9 (8.1)	3 (5.9)	0.615	2 (4.0)	2 (5.4)	0.757
Treatment for recurrent tumor, n (%)						
Resection						
Any organs	35 (31.5)	23 (45.1)	0.094	16 (32.0)	15 (40.5)	0.411
Liver (n/with liver recurrence)	32/104 (30.8)	23/49 (46.9)	0.052	14/50 (29.8)	15/35 (42.9)	0.221
Use of MTA* or immunotherapy**	19 (17.7)	9 (17.1)	0.934	11 (22.0)	9 (24.3)	0.799

OAR: open anatomic liver resection; MIAR: minimally invasive anatomic liver resection; C–D: Clavien–Dindo classification; *MTA: molecular targeted agent; immunotherapy**: immunotherapy using immune checkpoint inhibitors; Bold: statistically significant.

Regarding the treatments for cancer recurrence, in the unmatched cohorts, compared to OAR, MIAR tended to be associated with the higher rates of recurrent organ resection (45.1% vs. 31.5%, $p = 0.094$) and repeat hepatectomy (46.9% vs. 30.8%, $p = 0.052$). Systemic pharmacological treatment using molecular targeted agents (MTAs), such as sorafenib and lenvatinib, or immunotherapy using immune checkpoint inhibitors (ICIs), such as atezolizumab, were performed at a similar rate between the OAR and MIAR cohorts with recurrence (17.7% vs. 17.1%). On the other hand, in the matched cohorts, patterns of recurrence, RFS, timing of the first recurrence, and the rate of resection or systemic pharmacological treatment for recurrent tumors were comparable between OAR and MIAR (Table 7).

Times of Surgery and Associated Factors

To further investigate factors that potentially affect the long-term outcomes after resection of newly developed HCC, we studied the times or era of surgery because significant changes occurred socially in the strategies of HCC treatment as well as in the control of HCV using direct acting antivirals (DAAs) during the study period. We first examined the trends of application of OAR or MIAR throughout the study period (Figure 4). As shown, the ratio of OAR cases in all AR cases significantly decreased, and OAR was gradually replaced by MIAR over the years ($p < 0.0001$). Further, when the study period was divided into the early (2010–2015) and late (2016–2022) periods, MIAR was significantly more frequently performed than OAR in the late period in a comparison between the unmatched (n = 95 (84.1%) vs. n = 40 (24.5%), $p < 0.0001$) and matched (n = 61 (80.3%) vs. n = 14 (18.4%), $p < 0.0001$) cohorts.

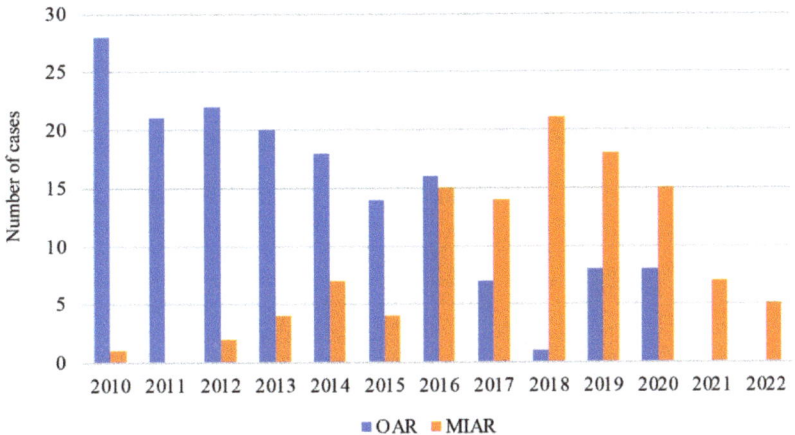

Figure 4. Annual number of cases undergoing OAR (blue bars) and MIAR (orange bars) for newly developed HCC.

At our institution, eradication of HCV using DAAs became active from around 2016, which was coincidental with a remarkable change in the surgical approach from OAR to MIAR. To exclude the impacts of HCV eradication on postoperative recurrence and hepatic functional status and to study the simple impact of different approaches on survival, we examined the long-term outcomes in 184 AR cases without associated HCV infection, i.e., 55 HBV and 129 NBNC cases. One-to-one PSM identified the 42 OAR and 42 MIAR matched cases from the 107 OAR and 77 MIAR unmatched cases. The survival data showed that OS in MIAR, with a 5-year rate of 85.2% and not-reached median survival, was significantly longer than OS in OAR, with a 5-year rate of 43.3% and the median survival time of 48.9 months ($p = 0.001$). Furthermore, RFS in MIAR, with a 5-year rate of 47.4% and the median time of 40.4 months, was significantly longer than RFS in OAR, with a 5-year rate of 21.8% and a median time of 7.6 months ($p = 0.004$).

4. Discussion

In this study, we described our surgical techniques of MIAR, including laparoscopic and robotic AR, and compared perioperative and long-term outcomes in HCC cases between OAR and MIAR as well as between laparoscopic and robotic AR, using PSM-based analyses. Our surgical techniques for AR in all studied cases were consistently based on the extrahepatic Glissonian approach and HV root-at first one-way parenchymal dissection, irrespective of the open, laparoscopic, or robotic approach. Furthermore, AR was primarily performed and managed only by surgeons with appropriate skills at our institution. These study settings may have reduced biases, such as surgical techniques and surgeons' experience, which were latent in previous comparative studies.

In the current study, we first audited perioperative outcomes in 142 MIAR cases and compared them to 185 OAR cases. A PSM (91:91)-based analyses showed that compared to OAR, MIAR was significantly associated with less blood loss, a lower transfusion rate, lower postoperative TB and CRP levels, lower rates of 90-day overall and major morbidity and bile leak or intraabdominal collection, a lower rate of 90-day mortality, and shorter LOS. On the other hand, a significantly higher postoperative AST level was observed in the MIAR compared to the OAR group. Next, we compared perioperative outcomes between matched laparoscopic and robotic AR cohorts (46:46), which showed comparable results. Finally, we studied the long-term outcomes after AR for newly developed HCC. PSM-based analyses matching patient and tumor characteristics and types of resection showed comparable or potentially superior OS and RFS in the MIAR cohort compared to those in the OAR cohort, as well as comparable outcomes between the laparoscopic and robotic approaches.

As for technical aspects of MIAR, we believe, from the current and previous results, that we can standardize MIAR by using the extrahepatic Glissonian approach and HV root-at first one-way parenchymal dissection [4–6,13,18,19,23]. Furthermore, the consistent usage of these standardized techniques, irrespective of OAR and MIAR, may reduce technical biases, being an advantage of this study setting. These techniques for AR, which were originally developed in OAR at our institution, have been safely and effectively translated into MIAR with acceptable curability, as shown by the favorable perioperative and long-term outcomes. In addition, as the most recent surgical platform, robotics was technically applicable to AR with surgical outcomes comparable to those of the laparoscopic approach. The most important advantage of the extrahepatic Glissonian approach for AR is accurate determination of the anatomic liver area to be resected before starting parenchymal dissection, which leads to accurate, safe, and optimal AR. On the other hand, one of the disadvantages of this approach is that although it is applicable in any type of AR for any liver segments, there are cases where extrahepatic isolation of peripheral subsegmental GPs is unsafe or impossible, depending on the liver anatomy. In this study, PSAR accounted for over 80% of OAR or MIAR cases. Although minimally invasive accurate PSARs are more demanding than standard right or left hemihepatectomy [6,24,25], they were technically standardized and performed safely in this series. Therefore, MIAR including PSAR can provide HCC patients with benefits of not only minimally invasiveness but also safety and curability.

Previous studies comparing open and minimally invasive liver resections have shown less blood loss, decreased morbidity, and shorter LOS in the latter [23,26–29]. Laparoscopic and robotic liver resections were shown to have comparable perioperative outcomes [23,30]. Results of the current study are in line with those of these studies, though the cohort setting was different; very few studies exclusively selected AR cases for the cohort. However, recent large studies have demonstrated advantages of the robotic approach on perioperative outcomes over the laparoscopic approach in selected types of AR [31–33].

Several studies have shown comparable long-term outcomes after resection of HCC between the open and minimally invasive approaches [26,28]. Only one study showed a survival advantage of the laparoscopic over the open approach, though significant biases were suggested in the study setting [29]. In our results, surprisingly, long-term outcomes after MIAR for newly developed HCC appeared to be more favorable than those after OAR (Figure 2). Both OS and RFS were statistically longer in the MIAR than in the OAR cohort, not only before, but also after PSM. The longer OS and RFS in the unmatched MIAR cohort could be largely explained by the more favorable tumor characteristics in this cohort represented by lower tumor stages, lower serum tumor markers, the need for less extensive hepatectomy, and a lower rate of early recurrence (Tables 5 and 7). Furthermore, the better patients' physical conditions in this cohort represented by the lower ASA scores and ICGR 15 (Table 5) might have beneficial impacts on postoperative survivals. Additionally, a higher rate of resection of recurrent tumors in the MIAR cohort (Table 7) could have contributed to the longer OS.

On the other hand, it is worth noting that even the matched MIAR cohort after PSM had significantly longer OS and RFS than the OAR cohort. To seek the scenarios behind such potentially better survivals in MIAR, we addressed several relevant points. First, we examined the details of recurrence and found that the patterns of recurrence, the incidence of extrahepatic metastasis and pathologic tumor differentiation, and stages were comparable between the cohorts (Table 7). Second, we examined the times or era of application of OAR or MIAR because the drastic changes in the surgical approach from OAR to MIAR at our institution (Figure 4) coincided with the changing trends in the pharmacological treatment for HCC recurrence toward MTAs or ICIs, along with significant success of HCV eradication by using DAAs. Our results showed, however, that these changes in non-surgical factors were comparable between the matched OAR and MIAR cohorts. Furthermore, OS and RFS in the HCC cohort excluding HCV-infected patients were still longer in MIAR than in OAR, suggesting that HCV eradication had minor impacts on the survival differences between MIAR and OAR in this study.

Other factors potentially contributing to the more favorable RFS in MIAR include theoretical immunological advantages conferred by its lower invasiveness. The advantages can stem from factors including less physical damage, less disturbance in the perioperative metabolic and nutritional status, and the resultant early recovery after surgery. In our results, such lower invasiveness in MIAR was evidenced by less blood loss, the lower levels of postoperative TB and CRP, and shorter LOS, compared to OAR (Table 2). Furthermore, lower rates of perioperative morbidity and blood transfusion in MIAR (Table 2) may have had beneficial impacts on its long-term outcomes, in line with previous studies on resected cancers including HCC [21,22,34,35].

Another point to be taken into consideration is that in most previous studies comparing open and minimally invasive hepatectomy, both AR and NAR were included. Since NAR tended to be performed for HCC patients with impaired hepatic functional reserve, inclusion of both AR and NAR cases in the study cohorts and the case number ratio of each cohort may have affected the entire comparative survival data on which both oncologic and hepatic functional factors had significant impacts.

Collectively, our data were not enough to explain the differences in the long-term outcomes between the matched OAR and MIAR cohorts, and in the first place, the relatively small sample size in each cohort precludes definite conclusions. Nonetheless, our results suggest that the long-term outcomes after AR for newly developed HCC were at least comparable between OAR and MIAR. Larger studies incorporating more evaluation facets, such as post-recurrence treatment modalities, patient nutritional status and immunity characteristics and tumor genetic information, are necessary to investigate the impact of a minimally invasive approach to AR on long-term outcomes of resected HCC.

In view of our results showing mostly better perioperative outcomes in MIAR than in OAR, as well as comparable or potentially more favorable long-term outcomes in MIAR, it is reasonable to suggest that MIAR would be the first choice for a surgical approach to HCC, at least by an expert. On the other hand, despite the expected functional merits of robotics providing surgical dexterity, the robotic approach did not show advantages in surgical outcomes over the laparoscopic approach to AR in this study. However, the sample size was small, particularly in the robotic group, and techniques of robotic liver surgery are still developing. Nonetheless, the robotic platform may have potential advantages in perioperative outcomes in complex anatomic resection, such as less blood loss, decreased open conversion rate, and decreased morbidity, as suggested in other study settings [31–33]. Larger studies are warranted to investigate the potential differences in outcomes between laparoscopic and robotic AR.

There are several limitations to this study. First, this is a retrospective, observational, single-center study, though PSM was conducted to reduce biases. Second, the sample sizes in each PSM-matched cohort are relatively small. Third, long-term outcomes should be carefully interpreted because of the abovementioned small sample size, small number of matched variables in PSM-based analyses, and potential biases from 'difficult-to-match' factors, including selection of approach, learning curve of techniques, patient immunological status, era-dependent development of DAAs for HCV eradication, and advances in post-recurrence pharmacological therapy for HCC.

5. Conclusions

Although MIAR is technically demanding, particularly for HCC, because of potential underlying liver dysfunction, it can be technically standardized by the extrahepatic Glissonian approach and HV root-at first one-way parenchymal dissection. Furthermore,

MIAR for HCC was safe, feasible, and oncologically acceptable, with perioperative outcomes mostly superior to those in OAR and with comparable or potentially more favorable long-term outcomes. A laparoscopic or robotic approach would be the first choice for AR in selected surgical HCC patients, at least by experts. Further larger studies are warranted to investigate potential advantages of MIAR for HCC in terms of long-term outcomes, as well as perioperative and long-term advantages of the robotic or laparoscopic approach over the counterpart.

Author Contributions: Conceptualization, Y.K. and A.S.; methodology, Y.K.; software, Y.K., M.K., and S.M.; validation, A.S. and I.U.; formal analysis, Y.K. and S.M.; investigation, Y.K., M.K. and S.M.; resources, Y.K. and A.S.; data curation, Y.K., M.K. and S.M.; writing—original draft preparation, Y.K.; writing—review and editing, A.S., M.K., Y.U., H.I., T.M., T.T. and I.U.; supervision, A.S. and I.U.; project administration, A.S. and I.U. All authors have read and agreed to the published version of the manuscript.

Funding: This research received no external funding.

Institutional Review Board Statement: The study was conducted under approval by the Institutional Regulation Board (approval number: HM19-064) and in accordance with the Declaration of Helsinki (2000).

Informed Consent Statement: Informed consent was obtained from all subjects involved in the study. Written informed consent has been obtained from the patient(s) to publish this paper.

Data Availability Statement: The datasets are not available for public access due to patient privacy concerns but are available from the corresponding author on reasonable request.

Acknowledgments: The authors thank Yoshinao Tanahashi, Akira Yasuda, Sanae Nakajima, Gozo Kiguchi, Junichi Yoshikawa, and Koichi Suda for their contributions to surgery.

Conflicts of Interest: The authors declare no conflict of interest.

References

1. Makuuchi, M.; Hasegawa, H.; Yamazaki, S. Ultrasonically guided subsegmentectomy. *Surg. Gynecol. Obstet.* **1985**, *161*, 346–350.
2. Hasegawa, K.; Kokudo, N.; Imamura, H.; Matsuyama, Y.; Aoki, T.; Minagawa, M.; Sano, K.; Sugawara, Y.; Takayama, T.; Makuuchi, M. Prognostic impact of anatomic resection for hepatocellular carcinoma. *Ann. Surg.* **2005**, *242*, 252–259. [CrossRef]
3. Shindoh, J.; Makuuchi, M.; Matsuyama, Y.; Mise, Y.; Arita, J.; Sakamoto, Y.; Hasegawa, K.; Kokudo, N. Complete removal of the tumor-bearing portal territory decreases local tumor recurrence and improves disease-specific survival of patients with hepatocellular carcinoma. *J. Hepatol.* **2016**, *64*, 594–600. [CrossRef] [PubMed]
4. Morimoto, M.; Tomassini, F.; Berardi, G.; Mori, Y.; Shirata, C.; Abu Hilal, M.; Asbun, H.; Cherqui, D.; Gotohda, N.; Han, H.S.; et al. Glissonean approach for hepatic inflow control in minimally invasive anatomic liver resection: A systematic review. *J. Hepatobiliary Pancreat. Sci.* **2022**, *29*, 51–65. [CrossRef] [PubMed]
5. Berardi, G.; Igarashi, K.; Li, C.J.; Ozaki, T.; Mishima, K.; Nakajima, K.; Honda, M.; Wakabayashi, G. Parenchymal sparing anatomical liver resections with full laparoscopic approach: Description of technique and short-term results. *Ann. Surg.* **2021**, *273*, 785–791. [CrossRef]
6. Kato, Y.; Sugioka, A.; Kojima, M.; Kiguchi, G.; Tanahashi, Y.; Uchida, Y.; Yoshikawa, J.; Yasuda, A.; Nakajima, S.; Takahara, T.; et al. Laparoscopic isolated liver segmentectomy 8 for malignant tumors: Techniques and comparison of surgical results with the open approach using a propensity score-matched study. *Langenbecks Arch. Surg.* **2022**, *407*, 2881–2892. [CrossRef] [PubMed]
7. Ibrahim, D.; Lainas, P.; Carloni, A.; Caillard, C.; Champault, A.; Smadja, C.; Franco, D. Laparoscopic liver resection for hepatocellular carcinoma. *Surg. Endosc.* **2008**, *22*, 372–378.
8. Lee, J.H.; Han, D.H.; Jang, D.S.; Choi, G.H.; Choi, J.S. Robotic extrahepatic Glissonean pedicle approach for anaomic liver resection in the right liver: Techniques and perioperative outcomes. *Surg. Endosc.* **2016**, *30*, 3882–3888. [CrossRef]
9. Liao, K.; Yang, K.; Cao, L.; Lu, Y.; Zheng, B.; Li, X.; Wang, X.; Li, J.; Chen, J.; Zhenf, S. Laparoscopic anatomical versus non-anatomical hepatectomy in the treatment of hepatocellular carcinoma: A randomized controlled trial. *Int. J. Surg.* **2022**, *102*, 106652. [CrossRef]
10. Strasberg, S.M.; Belghiti, J.; Clavien, P.A.; Gadzijev, E.; Garden, J.O.; Lau, W.Y.; Makuuchi, M.; Strong, R.W. The Brisbane 2000 Terminology of Liver Anatomy and Resections. *HPB* **2000**, *2*, 333–339. [CrossRef]
11. Couinaud, C. *Le Foie: Etudes Anatomiques et Chirurgicales*; Masson: Paris, France, 1957; pp. 9–12.
12. Wakabayashi, G.; Cherqui, D.; Geller, D.A.; Abu Hilal, M.; Berardi, G.; Ciria, R.; Abe, Y.; Aoki, T.; Asbun, H.J.; Chan, A.C.Y.; et al. The Tokyo 2020 terminology of liver anatomy and resections: Updates of the Brisbane 2000 system. *J. Hepatobiliary Pancreat. Sci.* **2022**, *29*, 6–15. [CrossRef] [PubMed]

13. Kato, Y.; Sugioka, A.; Tanahashi, Y.; Kojima, M.; Nakajima, S.; Yasuda, A.; Yoshikawa, J.; Uyama, I. Standardization of isolated caudate lobectomy by extrahepatic Glissonean pedicle isolation and HV root-at first one-way resection based on Laennec's capsule: Open and laparoscopic approaches. *Surg. Gastroenterol. Oncol.* **2020**, *25*, 89–92. [CrossRef]
14. Makuuchi, M.; Kosuge, T.; Takayama, T.; Yamazaki, S.; Kakazu, T.; Miyagawa, S.; Kawasaki, S. Surgery for small liver cancers. *Semin. Surg. Oncol.* **1993**, *9*, 298–304. [CrossRef]
15. Ban, D.; Tanabe, M.; Ito, H.; Otsuka, Y.; Nitta, H.; Abe, Y.; Hasegawa, Y.; Katagiri, T.; Takagi, C.; Itano, O.; et al. A novel difficulty scoring system for laparoscopic liver resection. *J. Hepatobiliary Pancreat. Sci.* **2014**, *21*, 745–753. [CrossRef] [PubMed]
16. Liver Cancer Study Group of Japan. *General Rules for the Clinical and Pathological Study of Primary Liver Cancer*, 6th ed.; Kokudo, N., Ed.; Kanehara: Tokyo, Japan, 2015; p. 26.
17. Berardi, G.; Wakabayashi, G.; Igarashi, K.; Ozaki, T.; Toyota, N.; Tsuchiya, A.; Nishikawa, K. Full laparoscopic anatomical segment 8 resection for hepatocellular carcinoma using the Glissonian approach with indocyanine green dye fluorescence. *Ann. Surg. Oncol.* **2019**, *26*, 2577–2578. [CrossRef] [PubMed]
18. Sugioka, A.; Kato, Y.; Tanahashi, Y. Systematic extrahepatic Glissonean pedicle isolation for anatomical liver resection based on Laennec's capsule: Proposal of a novel comprehensive surgical anatomy of the liver. *J. Hepatobiliary Pancreat. Sci.* **2017**, *24*, 17–23. [CrossRef]
19. Sugioka, A.; Kato, Y.; Tanahashi, Y.; Yoshikawa, J.; Kiguchi, G.; Kojima, M.; Yasuda, A.; Nakajima, S.; Uyama, I. Standardization of anatomic liver resection based on Laennec's capsule. *Surg. Gastroenterol. Oncol.* **2020**, *25*, 57–66. [CrossRef]
20. Dindo, D.; Demartines, N.; Clavien, P.A. Classification of surgical complications: A new proposal with evaluation in a cohort of 6336 patients and results of a survey. *Ann. Surg.* **2004**, *240*, 205–213. [CrossRef] [PubMed]
21. Yin, Z.; Huang, X.; Ma, T.; Jin, H.; Lin, Y.; Yu, M.; Jian, Z. Postoperative complications affect long-term survival outcomes following hepatic resection for colorectal liver metastasis. *World J. Surg.* **2015**, *39*, 1818–1827. [CrossRef] [PubMed]
22. Fernandez-Moreno, M.C.; Dorcaratto, D.; Garces-Albir, M.; Munoz, E.; Arvizu, R.; Ortega, J.; Sabater, L. Impact of type and severity of postoperative complications on long-term outcomes after colorectal liver metastases resection. *J. Surg. Oncol.* **2020**, *122*, 212–225. [CrossRef]
23. Kato, Y.; Sugioka, A.; Kojima, M.; Kiguchi, G.; Mii, S.; Uchida, Y.; Takahara, T.; Uyama, I. Initial experience with robotic liver resection: Audit of 120 consecutive cases at a single center and comparison with open and laparoscopic approaches. *J. Hepatobiliary Pancreat. Sci.* **2023**, *30*, 72–90. [CrossRef] [PubMed]
24. Hu, J.X.; Dai, W.D.; Miao, X.Y.; Zhong, D.W.; Huang, S.F.; Wen, Y.; Xiong, S.Z. Anatomic resection of segment VIII of liver for hepatocellular carcinoma in cirrhotic patients based on an intrahepatic Glissonian approach. *Surgery* **2009**, *146*, 854–860. [CrossRef] [PubMed]
25. Conrad, C.; Ogiso, S.; Inoue, Y.; Shivathirthan, N.; Gayet, B. Laparoscopic parenchymal-sparing liver resections in the central segments: Feasible, safe, and effective. *Surg. Endosc.* **2015**, *29*, 2410–2417. [CrossRef] [PubMed]
26. Takahara, T.; Wakabayashi, G.; Beppu, T.; Aihara, A.; Hasegawa, K.; Gotohda, N.; Hatano, E.; Tanahashi, Y.; Mizuguchi, T.; Kamiyama, T.; et al. Long-term and perioperative outcomes of laparoscopic versus open liver resection for hepatocellular carcinoma with propensity score matching: A multi-institutional Japanese study. *J. Hepatobiliary Pancreat. Sci.* **2015**, *22*, 721–727. [CrossRef]
27. Tozzi, F.; Berardi, G.; Vierstraete, M.; Kasai, M.; de Carvalho, L.A.; Vivarelli, M.; Montalti, R.; Troisi, R.I. Laparoscopic versus open approach for formal right and reft hepatectomy: A propensity score matching analysis. *World J. Surg.* **2018**, *42*, 2627–2634. [CrossRef]
28. Untereiner, X.; Cagniet, A.; Memeo, R.; Cherkaoui, Z.; Piardi, T.; Severac, F.; Mutter, D.; Kianmanesh, R.; Wakabayashi, T.; Sommacale, D.; et al. Laparoscopic hepatectomy versus open hepatectomy for the management of hepatocellular carcinoma: A comparative study using a propensity score matching. *World J. Surg.* **2019**, *43*, 615–625. [CrossRef]
29. Cheung, T.T.; Dai, W.C.; Tsang, S.H.; Chan, A.C.; Chok, K.S.; Chan, S.C.; Lo, C.M. Pure laparoscopic hepatectomy versus openhepatectomy for hepatocellular carcinoma in 110 patients with liver cirrhosis: A propensity analysis at a single center. *Ann. Surg.* **2016**, *264*, 612–620. [CrossRef]
30. Lim, C.; Salloum, C.; Tudisco, A.; Ricci, C.; Osseis, M.; Napoli, N.; Lahat, E.; Boggi, U.; Azoulay, D. Short- and Long-term Outcomes after Robotic and Laparoscopic Liver Resection for Malignancies: A Propensity Score-Matched Study. *World J. Surg.* **2019**, *43*, 1594–1603. [CrossRef]
31. Chong, C.C.; Fuks, D.; Lee, K.F.; Zhao, J.J.; Choi, G.H.; Sucandy, I.; Chiow, A.K.H.; Marino, M.V.; Gastaca, M.; Wang, X.; et al. Propensity score-matched analysis comparing robotic and laparoscopic right and extended right hepatectomy. *JAMA Surg.* **2022**, *157*, 436–444. [CrossRef]
32. Yang, H.Y.; Choi, G.H.; Chin, K.H.; Choi, S.H.; Syn, N.L.; Cheung, T.T.; Chiow, A.K.H.; Sucandy, I.; Marino, M.V.; Prieto, M.; et al. Robotic and laparoscopic right anterior sectionectomy and central hepatectomy: Multicentre propensity score-matched analysis. *Br. J. Surg.* **2022**, *109*, 311–314. [CrossRef]
33. Sucandy, I.; Rayman, S.; Lai, E.C.; Tang, C.N.; Chong, Y.; Efanov, M.; Fuks, D.; Choi, G.H.; Chong, C.C.; Chiow, A.K.H.; et al. Robotic versus laparoscopic left and extended left hepatectomy: An international multicenter study propensity score-matched analysis. *Ann. Surg. Oncol.* **2022**, *29*, 8398–8406. [CrossRef] [PubMed]

34. Nakauchi, M.; Suda, K.; Shibasaki, S.; Nakamura, K.; Kadoya, S.; Kikuchi, K.; Inaba, K.; Uyama, I. Prognostic factors of minimally invasive surgery for gastric cancer: Does robotic gastrectomy bring oncological benefit? *World J. Gastroenterol.* **2021**, *27*, 6659–6672. [CrossRef] [PubMed]
35. Nakayama, H.; Okamura, Y.; Higaki, T.; Moriguchi, M.; Takayama, T. Effect of blood product transfusion on the prognosis on patients undergoing hepatectomy for hepatocellular carcinoma: A propensity score matching analysis. *J. Gastroenterol.* **2023**, *58*, 171–181. [CrossRef] [PubMed]

Disclaimer/Publisher's Note: The statements, opinions and data contained in all publications are solely those of the individual author(s) and contributor(s) and not of MDPI and/or the editor(s). MDPI and/or the editor(s) disclaim responsibility for any injury to people or property resulting from any ideas, methods, instructions or products referred to in the content.

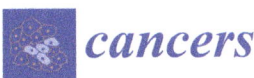

Review

Minimally Invasive ALPPS Procedure: A Review of Feasibility and Short-Term Outcomes

Luigi Cioffi [1,*], Giulio Belli [2], Francesco Izzo [3], Corrado Fantini [4], Alberto D'Agostino [5], Gianluca Russo [4,6], Renato Patrone [3], Vincenza Granata [7] and Andrea Belli [3]

1 Department of General Surgery, Ospedale del Mare, 80147 Naples, Italy
2 Department of General and HPB Surgery, Loreto Nuovo Hospital, 80127 Naples, Italy
3 Division of Epatobiliary Surgical Oncology, Istituto Nazionale Tumori IRCCS Fondazione Pascale-IRCCS di Napoli, 80131 Naples, Italy
4 Department of General Surgery, Pellegrini Hospital, 80134 Naples, Italy; gianlu_russo@hotmail.com (G.R.)
5 Department of General Surgery, San Paolo Hospital, 80125 Naples, Italy
6 Department of General Surgery, University of Campania Luigi Vanvitelli, 80131 Naples, Italy
7 Division of Radiology, Istituto Nazionale Tumori IRCCS Fondazione Pascale-IRCCS di Napoli, 80131 Naples, Italy
* Correspondence: drluicioffi@gmail.com; Tel.: +39-81-18775110

Simple Summary: Associated liver partition with portal vein ligation for staged hepatectomy (ALPPS) represents a recent and promising strategy to perform extensive hepatic resection and limit the risk of post-operative liver failure. Significant morbidity and mortality rates in its pioneering stage has limited acceptance of this treatment. The aim of this review is to evaluate the feasibility, safety, and clinical outcomes of this strategy following application of laparoscopic approach and technical modifications. An evaluation of the data has highlighted that a mini-invasive approach, a less invasive technique in first stage and a better selection of patients could account for potentially better results after ALPPS procedure in terms of blood loss, morbidity, and mortality rate in comparison with outcomes of open series.

Abstract: Background: Associated liver partition with portal vein ligation for staged hepatectomy (ALPPS) represents a recent strategy to improve resectability of extensive hepatic malignancies. Recent surgical advances, such as the application of technical variants and use of a mini-invasive approach (MI-ALPPS), have been proposed to improve clinical outcomes in terms of morbidity and mortality. Methods: A total of 119 MI-ALPPS cases from 6 series were identified and discussed to evaluate the feasibility of the procedure and short-term clinical outcomes. Results: Hepatocellular carcinoma were widely the most common indication for MI-ALPPS. The median estimated blood loss was 260 mL during Stage 1 and 1625 mL in Stage 2. The median length of the procedures was 230 min in Stage 1 and 184 in Stage 2. The median increase ratio of future liver remnant volume was 87.8%. The median major morbidity was 8.14% in Stage 1 and 23.39 in Stage 2. The mortality rate was 0.6%. Conclusions: MI-ALPPS appears to be a feasible and safe procedure, with potentially better short-term outcomes in terms of blood loss, morbidity, and mortality rate if compared with those of open series.

Keywords: ALPPS; laparoscopic ALPPS; RALPPS

Citation: Cioffi, L.; Belli, G.; Izzo, F.; Fantini, C.; D'Agostino, A.; Russo, G.; Patrone, R.; Granata, V.; Belli, A. Minimally Invasive ALPPS Procedure: A Review of Feasibility and Short-Term Outcomes. *Cancers* **2023**, *15*, 1700. https://doi.org/10.3390/cancers15061700

Academic Editor: Hiromitsu Hayashi

Received: 27 December 2022
Revised: 27 February 2023
Accepted: 5 March 2023
Published: 10 March 2023

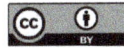

Copyright: © 2023 by the authors. Licensee MDPI, Basel, Switzerland. This article is an open access article distributed under the terms and conditions of the Creative Commons Attribution (CC BY) license (https://creativecommons.org/licenses/by/4.0/).

1. Introduction

Associated liver partition with portal vein ligation for staged hepatectomy (ALPPS) represents a recent and promising strategy to perform extensive hepatic resection in order to obtain a negative resection margin (R0) and to limit the risk of post-operative liver failure (PHLF).

At present, the standard strategy in the case of extensive hepatic resection with bilobar distribution and presumed insufficient future liver remnant volume (FLRV) is a two-stage hepatectomy with or without preoperative induction of a parenchymal hypertrophy using portal vein embolization (PVE), or, if technically feasible, a one-stage parenchymal sparing hepatectomy. The two-stage hepatectomy has been widely applied with good results in recent decades, allowing an increase of FLRV of 11.9–38% average after 4–8 weeks [1,2]. Nevertheless, patient drop-out, either for insufficient liver hypertrophy or for disease progression between the two stages, still represents the major drawback of such approach.

Therefore, the surgical community has accepted the introduction of ALPPS as an alternative strategy for R0 resection in a condition of estimated insufficient liver remnant with great expectations. The original ALPPS technique provided two operative times:

- Stage 1: portal vein ligation without dissection of the remaining structures of the pedicle combined with in situ splitting of the liver;
- Stage 2: completion of resection of the de-portalized liver via a right or extended right hepatectomy after an accelerated hypertrophy of portalized liver [3].

Nevertheless, after the pioneering phase described in several series [4–6], validity and full approval of ALPPS has been strongly debated due to the higher morbidity rate when compared to PVE (33–58 vs. 16%). In fact, poor outcomes in terms of morbidity/mortality data jeopardized potential benefits regarding magnitude and quickness of hypertrophy.

Over time, in order to preserve the potential benefits of a promising strategy, a more accurate patient selection was pursued and several efforts were made to improve short- and long-term outcomes by promoting different technical variants of "in situ splitting" with the aim of reducing the invasiveness of the first stage:

- partial ALPPS: limiting the depth and extent of parenchymal transection, allowing a FLR hypertrophy that is comparable to complete transection with a significantly lower morbidity (38.1% vs. 88.9%; $p = 0.049$) and near-zero mortality [7,8] (Figure 1);
- radiofrequency (RF)- or microwave (MW)-assisted ALPPS (RALPPS or MW-ALPPS) (Figure 2): obtaining a functional liver partition by a "necrotic groove" using RF o MW ablation and allowing a rate of hypertrophy that is comparable to resection associated with a lower morbidity [9,10];
- tourniquet ALPPS (ALTPS): providing application of a tourniquet around a parenchymal groove of 1 cm in the future transection line [11];
- mini-ALPPS: combining a partial ALPPS and intraoperative PVE, avoiding dissection of *porta hepatis* [12];
- hybrid ALPPS: consisting of three steps: in situ splitting, radiological PVE, and completion of hepatectomy [13,14].

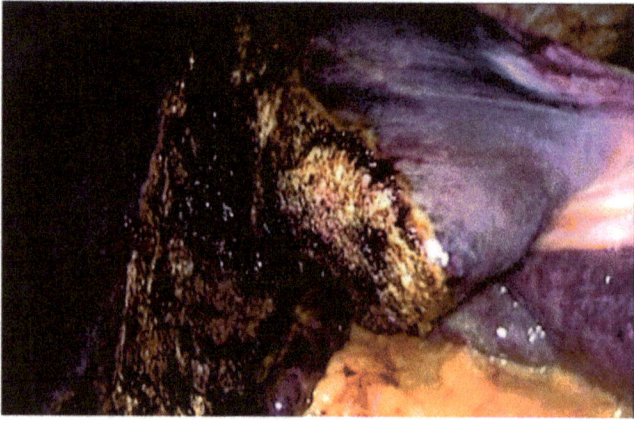

Figure 1. Intraoperative view of Split in situ during laparoscopic partial ALPPS.

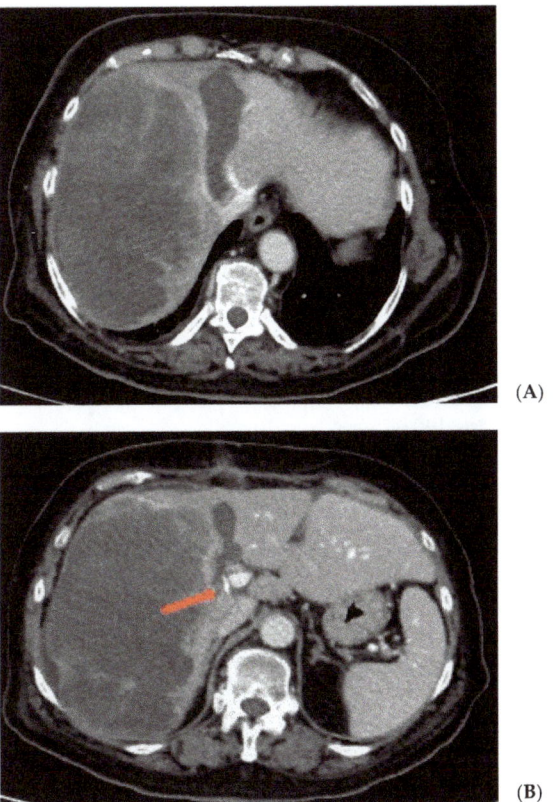

Figure 2. (**A**) CT scan after Stage 1 of RALPPS procedure showing the ablated future transection line. (**B**) CT scan after Stage 1 of RALPPS procedure showing the sectioned right portal vein (red arrow).

Minimally invasive laparoscopic and robotic approaches (MI-ALPPS) have also been advocated in order to assign the well-known benefits of a minimally invasive approach with the aim of reducing the morbidity/mortality rate of this promising surgical strategy.

The aim of this review is to evaluate the currently available data about the feasibility and safety of MI-ALPPS. Analysis of short-term clinical outcomes of MI-ALPPS in terms of FLVR hypertrophy, length of surgery, blood loss, hospital stay, morbidity, and mortality of the procedure and comparison with the outcomes of open standard ALPPS procedures are the secondary end-points.

2. Materials and Methods

2.1. Search Strategy

A review of the literature, based on predetermined criteria, was independently performed by two authors (L.C. and A.B.) in 3 databases (PubMed, Scopus, and Cochrane databases) in order to maximize articles capturing data. Boolean search terms 'ALPPS' OR 'Associating liver partition for portal vein ligation for staged hepatectomy' AND 'laparoscopic' OR 'minimally invasive' OR 'robotic' were used, with no restriction on publishing date. The last search was conducted on October 2022. The identified abstracts were reviewed independently by the two aforementioned authors (L.C. and A.B.) and discrepancies in data collection, synthesis, and analysis were solved by consensus of all authors.

2.2. Inclusion Criteria

The inclusion criteria were: (1) English language studies, (2) patients that were operated for an ALPPS procedure with a minimally invasive approach in at least one of the two stages, and (3) studies reporting at least one intra-operative and post-operative outcome as defined below.

2.3. Exclusion Criteria

The exclusion criteria included: (1) animal studies; (2) non-English studies; (3) conference abstracts, expert opinions, case reports, editorials, meta-analysis, reviews, and letter to the editors; (4) studies reporting inadequate clinical data; and (5) studies reporting less than 4 patients that were operated on with a minimally invasive approach in at least one of the two stages of an ALPPS procedure. (Figure 3).

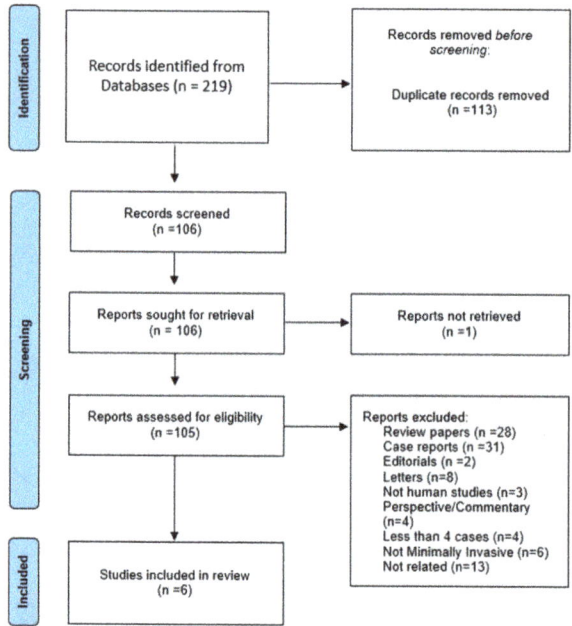

Figure 3. Search strategy and reason for exclusion of studies.

2.4. Data Extraction and Outcomes

Data extraction was conducted separately by two authors (L.C. and A.B.). Patient characteristics included age, tumor type, and percent ratio sFLVR/weight body (sFLVR/WB%) before Stage 1. Perioperative data included surgical techniques in both stages, length of surgery, estimated blood loss, interval between two stages, and % FLR hypertrophy. Post-operative data included the length of hospital stay, major morbidity rate for two stages, defined as Grade $\geq$ 3a according to Clavien–Dindo classification [15], and 90-day mortality.

3. Results

The outcomes from 119 patients undergoing laparoscopic ALPPS and its variants, extrapolated from six papers that met the inclusion criteria were described in this study.

The patient's background features are summarized in Table 1.

Table 1. Patients features.

References	Age (Mean)	n	Type of Tumor (n)				FLRV/Body Weight Ratio Prior Stage 1
			CRLM	HCC	CCA	other	
Gall et al. [16]	62	5	5	0	0	0	0.5
Truant et al. [17]	60.8	4	4	0	0	0	0.4
Jiao et al. [18]	62.4	26	20	1	0	5	0.23
Machado et al. [19]	58	10	9	0	0	1	0.19
Serenari et al. [20]	64	14	0	14	0	0	0.51
Jie et al. [21]	46.8	60	13	44	3	0	0.78
Overall	59	119	52 (43.5%)	59 (49.5%)	3 (2%)	6 (5%)	0.43

CRLM, Colorectal liver metastasis; HCC, Hepatocellular carcinoma; CCA, Cholangiocarcinoma; FLRV, Future liver remnant volume.

Hepatocellular carcinoma (HCC) represented the primary indication for surgery for a total 59 patients (49.6%) undergoing MI-ALPPS, included in three [18,20,21] of the selected studies, although 44 of them were part of a single center study from China [21]. Instead, colorectal liver metastasis (CRLM) represented the most common surgical indication for MI-ALPPS in four of the selected studies [16–19], for a total of 38 out of 45 patients (84.44%). The intra- and peri-operative data are summarized in Table 2.

Table 2. Perioperative data MI-ALPPS.

References	ALPPS, n		Length of Surgery, Median in Min (Range)		Estimated Blood Loss, Median in Mls (Range)		Interstage Time, Median in Days, (Range)	FLVR Hypertrophy, Median in ±% (Range)
	Stage 1	Stage 2	Stage 1	Stage 2	Stage 1	Stage 2		
Gall et al. [16]	Laparoscopic RALPPS n = 4	Right Hepatectomy n = 4 open	140 (105–140)	-	-	-	23 (12–34)	+62 (53.1–95.4)
Truant et al. [17]	Laparoscopic partial ALPPS n = 5	Right extended hepatectomy n = 5 open	270 (190–400)	188 (150–280)	250 (100–500)	550 (100–1400)	7.6 (6–13)	+60 (18.6–108.1)
Jiao et al. [18]	Laparoscopic RALPPS n = 24 Robotic RALPPS n = 2	Right hepatectomy n = 19: • 14 open • 4 laparoscopic • 1 robotic Right extended hepatectomy n = 5: • 4 open • 1 laparoscopic Not completed n = 2	90 (60–125)	180 (110–390)	310 (20–480)	300 (50–3200)	20 (14–36)	+80.7 (67–103.4)
Machado et al. [19]	Laparoscopic ALPPS n = 10	Right Hepatectomy n = 3 laparoscopic Right extended hepatectomy n = 7 laparoscopic	300 (208–340)	180 (140–300)	200 (110–330)	320 (150–800)	21 (9–30)	+118 (42–157)
Serenari et al. [20]	Laparoscopic ALPPS n = 7 Laparoscopic mini-ALPPS n = 6 Robotic ALPPS n = 1 (Laparoscopic partial ALPPS in 11/14)	Right hepatectomy n = 2 laparoscopic Right extended hepatectomy n = 5 laparoscopic (Converted = 2) Not completed n = 7	205 (187–257)	305 (280–360)	-	-	20 (12–27)	+62 (37–91)

Table 2. Cont.

References	ALPPS, n		Length of Surgery, Median in Min (Range)		Estimated Blood Loss, Median in Mls (Range)		Interstage Time, Median in Days, (Range)	FLVR Hypertrophy, Median in ±% (Range)
	Stage 1	Stage 2	Stage 1	Stage 2	Stage 1	Stage 2		
Jie et al. [21]	Laparoscopic RALPPS n = 60	Right hepatectomy n = 32 open Right extended hepatectomy n = 28 open	156.8 (102–227)	305.3 (218–407)	165 (80–280)	628 (350–960)	16.4	+45.7
Overall Median (range)	n = 119	n = 110	230 (60–400)	258.5 (110–407)	260 (20–500)	1625 (50–3200)	21 (6–36)	87.8 (18.6–157)

FLRV, Future liver remnant volume; RALPPS, Radiofrequency-assisted ALPPS.

In Stage 1, a classic split in situ technique was performed in 10.92% of patients, while modified procedures were performed in 89.07%. The laparoscopic RALPPS technique was performed in 88 patients, robotic RALPPS in 2 patients, laparoscopic classic ALPPS in 13 patients, and laparoscopic partial ALPPS in 16 patients (1 of them robotic and 6 mini-ALPPS, with intraoperative PVE, avoiding hilar dissection). Mini-invasive RALPPS (laparoscopic + robotic) was performed in 90 patients (75.63%) and represented the most common minimally invasive strategy that was applied at the first stage. Partial transection was performed in 16 laparoscopic ALPPS (27%).

Stage 2 was performed using an open approach in 87 patients, laparoscopic approach in 21 patients, and robotic in in 1 patient. Specifically, 11 right extended hepatectomy and 9 right hepatectomy were completed using laparoscopic approach, and 1 right hepatectomy by robotic approach (Table 3).

Table 3. Indications and technical features.

	MI-ALPPS
Type of tumors, n (%)	
CRLM	52 (43.69%)
HCC	59 (49.57%)
CCA	3 (2.52%)
Other	6 (5.04%)
Split in situ variant Stage 1, n (%)	
Classic	13 (10.92%)
Modified	106 (89.07%)
Type of hepatectomy Stage 2, n (%)	
Right hepatectomy	60 (54.54%)
Right extended hepatectomy	50 (45.45%)
Left extended hepatectomy	0

CRLM, Colorectal liver metastasis; HCC, Hepatocellular carcinoma; CCA, Cholangiocarcinoma.

A total of nine patients did not complete the second stage of ALPPS because of insufficient liver hypertrophy, progression of disease, or intra-operative complications that occurred during completion of hepatectomy.

The post-operative data are summarized in Table 4.

Table 4. Post-operative data MI-ALPPS.

References	Length of Hospital Stay (Median, Range in Days)			CD Classification Grade ≥ 3a (%)		90 Days Mortality (%)
	Stage 1	Stage 2	Stage 1 + 2	Stage 1	Stage 2	
Gall et al. [16]	-	-	-	20 - Pulmonary thromboembolism;	-	0
Truant et al. [17]	7 (5–9)	12 (6–18)	19 (11–27)	0	40 - Biliary fistula - Intra-abdominal collection	0
Jiao et al. [18]	9.5 (2–17)	8 (4–32)	27.5 (6–49)	3.85 - Limb compartment syndrome	15.38 - Intra-abdominal collection - Pleural effusion - Post-operative ileus - Small bowel ischemia	3.8
Machado et al. [19]			14 (8–20)	0		0
Serenari et al. [20]	6.5 (4–9)	12 (11–17)	20.5 (15–26)	14.2	8.3	0
Jie et al. [21]	-	23.24	-	13.3	53.3	0
Overall Median (range)	9.5 (2–17)	18 (4–32)	27.5 (6–49)	8.14 (0–20)	23.39 (0–53.3)	0.6 (0–3.8)

CD Classification, Clavien–Dindo Classification.

The estimated blood loss during two ALPPS stages was reported for 101 patients from four papers [17–19,21]. A total of three of them exclusively investigated a technical variant. In classic ALPPS [21], the range was 110–330 mL and 150–800 mL, in laparoscopic RALPPS [18,21] 20–480 mL and 80–280 mL, and 50–3200 mL and 350–960 mL, respectively, for Stage 1 and 2. The overall median that was observed was 260 mL in Stage 1 and 1625 mL in Stage 2. Details of the perioperative data are summarized in Table 5.

Table 5. Details of perioperative data MI-ALPPS.

	MI-ALPPS
Interstage time, median in days ± IQR	21 (6–36)
FLVR hypertrophy, median in % ± IQR	87.8 (18.6–157)
Length of surgery, Stage 1, median in min ± IQR	230 (60–400)
Length of surgery, Stage 2, median in min ± IQR	250 (110–407)
Estimated blood loss, Stage 1, median in mls ± IQR	260 (20–500)
Estimated blood loss, Stage 2, median in mls ± IQR (Stage 1 and 2)	1625 (50–3200)
CD classification Grade > 3a, Stage 1. median in % ± IQR	8.14 (0–24)
CD classification Grade > 3a, Stage 2, median in % ± IQR	23.39 (0–53.3)
Total length of hospital stay, median in days ± IQR	27.5 (6–49)
90 days mortality, median in % ± IQR	0.8 (0–3.8)

IQR, Inter-quantile ratio; FLRV, Future liver remnant volume; CD Classification, Clavien–Dindo Classification.

The median length of procedures was 230 min in Stage 1 and 250 in Stage 2.

The median increase ratio of FLVR was +87.8% in MI-ALPPS; a median value of +118% was reported in a series of patients that were undergoing laparoscopic classic ALPPS [20].

The time between the two stages ranged from 6 days in a single patient undergoing mini-ALPSS to 36 days in a single patient who underwent a laparoscopic RALPPS. The overall median value was 21 days.

The hospital stay ranged from 2 to 17 days in Stage 1 and 4 to 17 in Stage 2, with minimum values in Stage 1 for patients that were undergoing the RALPPS technique. The median hospital stay value was 22.5 days.

The overall major morbidity was 8.14% in Stage 1, with 6 cases of biliary fistula requiring percutaneous drainage (Clavien–Dindo Grade IIIa) in the series by Jie et al. [21]. The 90-day mortality was reported in one case after Stage 2 (0.8%) following severe peritonitis after mechanical ischemic obstruction of the small bowel.

4. Discussion

PHLF due to insufficient future liver remnant volume (FLRV) represents a key limiting factor for extensive hepatectomy in oncological liver surgery. It is generally agreed that FLRV should be at least 25–30% of the total volume, up to 40% if liver function is compromised because of neoadjuvant chemotherapy or underlying diseases [9]. At the time, the standard strategy to limit PHLF in extensive hepatic resection is a two-stage hepatectomy (with surgical clearance of the FLR in case of bilobar disease) with or without pre-operative induction of parenchymal hypertrophy using PVE or ligation. This approach allows an increase of the estimated FLRV of 11.9–38% after 4–8 weeks. The major morbidity of PVE was seen in 2.2%, while mortality was negligible [1].

Nevertheless, patient drop-out for insufficient liver hypertrophy or for disease progression between the two stages still represents the major drawback of such a strategy. Since its advent, ALPPS appeared as a possible and promising strategy in order to limit both the risk of PHLF in case of extensive liver resection and dropout rate because of progression of disease associated with two-stage hepatectomy.

After its pioneering stage, in which unacceptable morbidity and mortality rates have limited the acceptance of this strategy, a better selection of patients, a refinement in timing of Stage 2, and promotion of several technical variants of the original technique limiting invasiveness of first stage have been proposed in order to take advantage of potential benefits of ALPPS [7–14]. In this direction, minimally invasive approaches, such as laparoscopic and robotic, have been suggested to assign to ALPPS the well-known advantages of laparoscopy, which include reduced blood loss and induction of adhesions between the two stages, minor abdominal wall trauma, faster recovery and shorter hospital stay, and a lower incidence of ascites and liver failure in cirrhotic patients [22–25]. On the other hand, ALPPS is a technically challenging procedure where a laparoscopic or robotic approach can require both additional expertise in the hands of hepatic surgeon and prolonged operative times. Therefore, the diffusion of minimally invasive ALPPS has been greatly limited because of the related technical difficulties means that only six studies, mainly descriptive case series, including more than four patients that underwent MI-ALPPS, are currently available in the literature.

The analyzed studies showed several discrepancies, dissimilar design, and different levels of accuracy, as MI-ALPPS approach has been associated with different technical variants in Stage 1. Considering the aforementioned limits, some observations can be proposed.

The current ALPPS strategy has been profoundly subverted compared to the past as it provides, for the lightening of Stage 1, less invasive techniques such as laparoscopy and a reduced or "virtual" liver split in situ to postpone a more aggressive intervention in Stage 2. Indeed, the well-known benefits of laparoscopy could play in synergy with a limited hilar and pericaval dissection, an incomplete liver mobilization, and a reduced parenchymal partition in improving safety of first stage of MI-ALPPS.

Effectively, modified procedures of Stage 1 were performed in 89.07% of patients in the MI-ALPPS series with a prevalence of the mini-invasive RALPPS technique (75.6%) versus 10.16% which was reported for open series in a systematic review by Kawka et al. [26]. Only 23 out of 110 patients (20.9%) that underwent a mini-invasive approach in Stage 1 were submitted to the laparoscopic approach also in Stage 2. These data highlight how the technical difficulties that are connected with Stage 2, which is associated with higher blood loss and a higher incidence of post-operative major complications, currently limit a widespread use of the minimally invasive approach.

Considering the whole MI-ALPPS series, major morbidity rate for Stage 1 was 8.14%, apparently lower than 11% that was reported for open ALPPS series [24], and 23.39% for Stage 2, surprisingly higher than 14.4% that was reported for open series [24]. This higher morbidity rate in MI-ALPPS cases could be related to the influence of series reported by Jie et al. [21] which included HCC as the most frequent indication for surgery (44 patients which 8 Child–Pugh B) taking into account that, on the other side, the majority of the cases in open ALPPS series had been performed for CRLM.

Indeed, a better selection of patients, associated with the lightening of surgical techniques, may have affected the better outcomes in MI-ALPPS cases in four [16–19] out of the analyzed series in which colorectal liver metastasis (CRLM) represented the main indication for ALPPS procedures, reporting a median major morbidity of 5.96% after Stage 1 and of 15.92% after Stage 2. The mortality rate was 0.6% versus 8.45 for open series.

This positive trend does appear in accordance with the "paradigm" that was proposed by De Santibanes et al. for which improving short-term outcomes depends mainly on a minor aggressiveness of Stage 1 and full recovery of patients before the second stage, regardless of how the completion surgery was approached [12].

Perihilar and intra-hepatic cholangiocarcinoma (CCA) represented 2% (3/119) of indications in the MI-ALPPS groups. To our knowledge, only three other cases of CCA treatments [27–29] have been described for the MI-ALPPS technique, not allowing us to define the role of procedure in the treatment of a tumor where cholestatic features of liver could contribute to the poor outcomes that were reported.

Blood loss reached the lowest value (20 mL) in Stage 1 and the highest value (3200 mL) in Stage 2. These aspects can corroborate that the most challenging surgical step in MI-ALPPS procedures has been postponed in the second stage of the procedure and a full MI-ALPPS in both stages is still rarely performed due to the related technical difficulties.

Interstage time seemed to be shorter and the FLVR ratio higher in open series [16] than in MI-ALPPS series. Nevertheless, 110 out of 119 patients have completed the second stage of ALPPS, highlighting efficiency of a mini-invasive approach in avoiding PHLF, despite the reduced performance in terms of quickness and magnitude of hypertrophy.

Only two studies have reported on the oncologic outcomes for MI-ALPPS [20,21]. In the series of Serenari et al., the median overall survival (OS) did not significantly differ between MI-ALPPS and open-ALPPS (22.6 months versus 17.9 months, $p = 0.278$), while in the study by Jie et al. [21], the median OS of the series was reported to be 22.4 months (3.2–31.4) not allowing us to extrapolate outcomes for different indications.

In addition, the paucity of a homogeneous series in terms of employed surgical techniques and indications for surgery, makes it difficult to assess the specific impact of technical variations of ALPPS on post-operative clinical outcomes. In fact, among the published series focusing on open standard and modified ALPPS, a direct comparison between classic versus partial ALPPS is reported in only two studies. In detail, Chan et al. [30], compared 12 complete versus 13 partial ALPPS for the treatment of HCC, highlighting a more rapid FLR hypertrophy after classic procedures and a non-statistically significant different incidence of post-operative major complications between the two groups in patients with chronic liver disease. On the other hand, Linecker et al. [31] demonstrated that a partial parenchymal partition of at least 50% of the transection line at Stage 1 results in a FLR hypertrophy that is comparable to that reported after complete ALPPS but with a lower rate of minor complications and liver failure (0% vs. 27%; $p = 0.001$) which is similar to those that were reported for MI-ALPPS.

Nevertheless, the lack of comparative data between the open modified ALPPS and modified MI-ALPPS hinder the evaluation of the specific impact of a minimally invasive approach in this setting. In fact, among the studies that focused on MI-ALPPS, merely the early experience of Truant et al. [17] reported a homogeneous series consisting of only five patients undergoing partial ALPPS, which are potentially comparable with the aforementioned open series of Linecker et al. in terms of surgical techniques that were used and indications to surgery. However, the limited sample size that was available in both the modified open and MI-ALPPS precludes any meaningful statistical analysis.

5. Conclusions

Over the past few years, a new strategy consisting in a mini-invasive approach, a less invasiveness version of employed techniques in first stage, and a better selection of patients could account for potentially better short-term outcomes after ALPPS procedure in terms of blood loss, morbidity, and mortality rate. Taking into account the actual lack of MI-ALLPS series reported in the literature, the real impact of the minimally invasive approach in the setting of the ALPPS procedures is still to be determined. More comparative data between open ALPPS and MI-ALLPS are needed to determinate the specific impact of the minimally invasive approach.

Author Contributions: Conceptualization: L.C. and A.B.; writing—review and editing: L.C., A.B., C.F., F.I., R.P., V.G., A.D.A., G.R. and G.B.; supervision: G.B. All authors have read and agreed to the published version of the manuscript.

Funding: This research received no external funding.

Conflicts of Interest: The authors declare no conflict of interest.

References

1. Abulkhir, A.; Limongelli, P.; Healey, A.J.; Damrah, O.; Tait, P.; Jackson, J.; Habib, N.; Jiao, L.R. Preoperative portal vein embolization for major liver resection: A meta-analysis. *Ann. Surg.* **2008**, *247*, 49–57. [CrossRef]
2. van Lienden, K.P.; van den Esschert, J.W.; de Graaf, W.; Bipat, S.; Lameris, J.S.; van Gulik, T.M.; Van Delden, O.M. Portal vein embolization before liver resection: A systematic review. *CardioVascular Interv. Radiol.* **2013**, *36*, 25–34. [CrossRef]
3. Schnitzbauer, A.A.; Lang, S.A.; Goessmann, H.; Nadalin, S.; Baumgart, J.; Farkas, S.A.; Fichtner-Feigl, S.; Lorf, T.; Goralcyk, A.; Hörbelt, R.; et al. Right portal vein ligation combined with in situ splitting induces rapid left lateral liver lobe hypertrophy enabling 2-staged extended right hepatic resection in small-forsize settings. *Ann. Surg.* **2012**, *255*, 405–414. [CrossRef] [PubMed]
4. Schlegel, A.; Lesurtel, M.; Melloul, E.; Limani, P.; Tschuor, C.; Graf, R.; Humar, B.; Clavien, P.A. ALPPS: From human to mice highlighting accelerated and novel mechanisms of liver regeneration. *Ann. Surg.* **2014**, *260*, 83–87. [CrossRef] [PubMed]
5. Schadde, E.; Ardiles, V.; Robles-Campos, R.; Malago, M.; Machado, M.; Hernandez-Alejandro, R.; Soubrane, O.; Schnitzbauer, A.A.; Raptis, D.; Tschuor, C.; et al. Early survival and safety of ALPPS: First report of the international ALPPS registry. *Ann. Surg.* **2014**, *260*, 82–88. [CrossRef] [PubMed]
6. Sandstrom, P.; Rosok, B.I.; Sparrelid, E.; Larsen, P.N.; Larsson, A.L.; Lindell, G.; Schultz, N.A.; Bjørnbeth, B.A.; Isaksson, B.; Rizell, M.; et al. ALPPS improves resectability compared with conventional two-stage hepatectomy in patients with advanced colorectal liver metastasis: Results from a Scandinavian multicenter randomized controlled trial (LIGRO trial). *Ann. Surg.* **2018**, *267*, 833–840. [CrossRef]
7. Alvarez, F.A.; Ardiles, V.; de Santibanes, M.; Pekolj, J.; de Santibanes, E. Associating liver partition and portal vein ligation for staged hepatectomy offers high oncological feasibility with adequate patient safety: A prospective study at a single center. *Ann. Surg.* **2015**, *261*, 723–732. [CrossRef] [PubMed]
8. Petrowsky, H.; Györi, G.; de Oliveira, M.; Lesurtel, M.; Clavien, P.A. Is partial-ALPPS safer than ALPPS? A single-center experience. *Ann. Surg.* **2015**, *261*, e90–e92. [CrossRef]
9. Qiang, W.; Jun, Y.; Xiabin, F.; Geng, C.; Feng, X.; Xiaowu, L.; Kuansheng, M.; Ping, B. Safety and efficacy of radiofrequency-assisted ALPPS (RALPPS) in patients with cirrhosis-related hepatocellular carcinoma. *Int. J. Hyperth.* **2017**, *33*, 846–852. [CrossRef]
10. Cillo, U.; Gringeri, E.; Feltracco, P.; Bassi, D.; D'Amico, F.E.; Polacco, M.; Boetto, R. Totally laparoscopic microwave ablation and portal vein ligation for staged hepatectomy: A new minimally invasive two-stage hepatectomy. *Ann. Surg. Oncol.* **2015**, *22*, 2787–2788. [CrossRef]
11. Robles, R.; Parrilla, P.; López-Conesa, A.; Brusain, R.; de la Peña, J.; Fuster, M.; Garcia-López, J.A.; Hernandez, E. Tourniquet modification of the associating liver partition and portal ligation for staged hepatectomy procedure. *BJS* **2014**, *101*, 1129–1134. [CrossRef] [PubMed]
12. de Santibañes, E.; Alvarez, F.A.; Ardiles, V.; Pekolj, J.; de Santibañes, M. Inverting the ALPPS paradigm by minimizing first stage impact: The Mini-ALPPS technique. *Langenbecks Arch. Surg.* **2016**, *401*, 557–563. [CrossRef] [PubMed]
13. Baili, E.; Tsilimigras, D.I.; Moris, D.; Sahara, K.; Pawlik, T.M. Technical modifications and outcomes after Associating Liver Partition and Portal Vein Ligation for Staged Hepatectomy (ALPPS) for primary liver malignancies: A systematic review. *Surg. Oncol.* **2020**, *33*, 70–80. [CrossRef] [PubMed]
14. Lai, Q.; Melandro, F.; Rossi, M. Hybrid partial ALPPS: A feasible approach in case of right trisegmentectomy and microvascular invasion. *Ann. Surg.* **2018**, *267*, e80–e82. [CrossRef] [PubMed]

15. Dindo, D.; Demartines, N.; Clavien, P.A. Classification of surgical complications: A new proposal with evaluation in a cohort of 6336 patients and results of a survey. *Ann. Surg.* 2004, *240*, 205–213. [CrossRef] [PubMed]
16. Gall, T.M.; Sodergren, M.H.; Frampton, A.E.; Fan, R.; Spalding, D.R.; Habib, N.A.; Pai, M.M.; Jackson, J.E.F.; Tait, P.F.; Jiao, L.R.M. Radio-frequency-assisted liver partition with portal vein ligation (RALPP) for liver regeneration. *Ann. Surg.* 2015, *261*, 45. [CrossRef]
17. Truant, S.; El Amrani, M.; Baillet, C.; Ploquin, A.; Lecolle, K.; Ernst, O.; Hebbar, M.; Huglo, D.; Pruvot, F.-R. Laparoscopic partial ALPPS: Much Better than ALPPS! *Ann. Hepatol.* 2018, *18*, 269–273. [CrossRef]
18. Jiao, L.R.; Fajardo Puerta, A.B.; Gall, T.M.H.; Sodergren, M.H.; Frampton, A.E.; Pencavel, T.; Nagendran, M.; Habib, N.A.; Darzi, A.; Pai, M.; et al. Rapid induction of liver regeneration for major hepatectomy (REBIRTH): A randomized controlled trial of portal vein embolization versus ALPPS assisted2 with radiofrequency. *Cancers* 2019, *11*, 302. [CrossRef]
19. Machado, M.A.; Makdissi, F.F.; Surjan, R.C.; Basseres, T.; Schadde, E. Transition from open to laparoscopic ALPPS for patients with very small FLR: The initial experience. *HPB* 2017, *19*, 9–66. [CrossRef]
20. Serenari, M.; Ratti, F.; Zanello, M.; Guglielmo, N.; Mocchegiani, F.; Di Benedetto, F.; Nardo, B.; Mazzaferro, V.; Cillo, U.; Massani, M.; et al. Minimally Invasive Stage 1 to Protect Against the Risk of Liver Failure: Results from the Hepatocellular Carcinoma Series of the Associating Liver Partition and Portal Vein Ligation for Staged Hepatectomy Italian Registry. *J. Laparoendosc. Adv. Surg. Tech. A.* 2020, *30*, 1082–1089. [CrossRef]
21. Jie, L.; Guang-Sheng, Y.; Ke-Jian, S.; Yan, M.; Xiao-Wang, B.; Xu, H. Clinical evaluation of modified ALPPS procedures based on risk-reduced strategy for staged hepatectomy. *Ann. Hepatol.* 2021, *20*, 100245. [CrossRef]
22. Dagher, I.; Lainas, P.; Carloni, A.; Caillard, C.; Champault, A.; Smadja, C.; Franco, D. Laparoscopic liver resection for hepatocellular carcinoma. *Surg. Endosc.* 2008, *22*, 372–378. [CrossRef] [PubMed]
23. Belli, G.; Fantini, C.; D'Agostino, A.; Cioffi, L.; Langella, S.; Russolillo, N.; Belli, A. Laparoscopic versus open liver resection for hepatocellular carcinoma in patients with histologically proven cirrhosis: Short- and middle-term results. *Surg. Endosc.* 2007, *21*, 2004–2011. [CrossRef] [PubMed]
24. Belli, A.; Fantini, C.; Cioffi, L.; D'Agostino, A.; Belli, G. MILS for HCC: The state of art. *Updates Surg.* 2015, *67*, 105–109. [CrossRef]
25. Belli, G.; Limongelli, P.; Fantini, C.; D'Agostino, A.; Cioffi, L.; Belli, A.; Russo, G. Laparoscopic and open treatment of hepatocellular carcinoma in patients with cirrhosis. *Br. J. Surg.* 2009, *96*, 1041–1048. [CrossRef]
26. Kawka, M.; Mak, S.; Gall, T.; Jiao, L. A better route to ALPPS: Minimally invasive vs open. *Surg. End.* 2020, *34*, 2379–2389. [CrossRef]
27. Balci, D.; Kirimker, O.E.; Üstüner, E.; Yilmaz, A.A.; Azap, A. Stage I-laparoscopy partial ALPPS procedure for perihilar cholangiocarcinoma. *J. Surg. Oncol.* 2020, *121*, 1022–1026. [CrossRef]
28. Di Benedetto, F.; Magistri, P.; Guerrini, G.P.; Di Sandro, S. Robotic liver partition and portal vein embolization for staged hepatectomy for perihilar cholangiocarcinoma. *Updates Surg.* 2022, *74*, 773–777. [CrossRef]
29. Boggi, U.; Napoli, N.; Kauffmann, E.F.; Presti, G.L.; Moglia, A. Laparoscopic microwave liver ablation and portal vein ligation: An alternative approach to the conventional ALPPS procedure in hilar cholangiocarcinoma. *Ann. Surg. Oncol.* 2016, *23*, 884. [CrossRef]
30. Chan, A.C.Y.; Chok, K.; Dai, J.W.C.; Lo, C.M. Impact of split completeness on future liver remnant hypertrophy in associating liver partition and portal vein ligation for staged hepatectomy (ALPPS) in hepatocellular carcinoma: Complete-ALPPS versus partial-ALPPS. *Surgery* 2017, *161*, 357–364. [CrossRef]
31. Linecker, M.; Kambakamba, P.; Reiner, C.S.; Linh Nguyen-Kim, T.D.; Stavrou, G.A.; Jenner, R.M.; Oldhafer, K.J.; Björnsson, B.; Schlegel, A.; Györi, G.; et al. How much liver needs to be transected in ALPPS? A translational study investigating the concept of less invasiveness. *Surgery* 2017, *16*, 453–464. [CrossRef] [PubMed]

Disclaimer/Publisher's Note: The statements, opinions and data contained in all publications are solely those of the individual author(s) and contributor(s) and not of MDPI and/or the editor(s). MDPI and/or the editor(s) disclaim responsibility for any injury to people or property resulting from any ideas, methods, instructions or products referred to in the content.

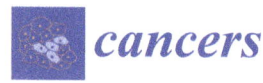

Article

Laparoscopic Right Hemihepatectomy after Future Liver Remnant Modulation: A Single Surgeon's Experience

Tijs J. Hoogteijling [1,2,3], Jasper P. Sijberden [1,2,3], John N. Primrose [4], Victoria Morrison-Jones [4], Sachin Modi [5], Giuseppe Zimmitti [1], Marco Garatti [1], Claudio Sallemi [6], Mario Morone [6] and Mohammad Abu Hilal [1,4,*]

[1] Department of Surgery, Poliambulanza Foundation Hospital, 25124 Brescia, Italy
[2] Amsterdam UMC Location University of Amsterdam, Department of Surgery, Meibergdreef 9, 1105 AZ Amsterdam, The Netherlands
[3] Cancer Center Amsterdam, Cancer Treatment and Quality of Life, 1081 HV Amsterdam, The Netherlands
[4] Department of Surgery, University Hospital Southampton NHS Foundation Trust, Southampton SO16 6YD, UK
[5] Department of Interventional Radiology, University Hospital Southampton NHS Foundation Trust, Southampton SO16 6YD, UK
[6] Department of Interventional Radiology, Poliambulanza Foundation Hospital, 25124 Brescia, Italy
* Correspondence: abuhilal9@gmail.com

Simple Summary: Laparoscopic right hemihepatectomy (L-RHH) after future liver remnant modulation (FLRM) is considered a technically challenging procedure. This study included consecutive L-RHHs performed by a single surgeon, both with and without prior FLRM. The analysis included 59 patients who underwent L-RHH between October 2007 and March 2023, of which 33 patients received FLRM. L-RHH after FLRM was more technically challenging, as it required longer operative time and Pringle duration. However, there were no significant differences in intraoperative blood loss, conversion rates, or postoperative outcomes such as hospital stay, morbidity rates, and textbook outcome. When performed by experienced laparoscopic hepatobiliary surgeons, L-RHH after FLRM is a safe and feasible procedure.

Abstract: Background: Laparoscopic right hemihepatectomy (L-RHH) is still considered a technically complex procedure, which should only be performed by experienced surgeons in specialized centers. Future liver remnant modulation (FLRM) strategies, including portal vein embolization (PVE), and associating liver partition and portal vein ligation for staged hepatectomy (ALPPS), might increase the surgical difficulty of L-RHH, due to the distortion of hepatic anatomy, periportal inflammation, and fibrosis. Therefore, this study aims to evaluate the safety and feasibility of L-RHH after FLRM, when compared with ex novo L-RHH. Methods: All consecutive right hemihepatectomies performed by a single surgeon in the period between October 2007 and March 2023 were retrospectively analyzed. The patient characteristics and perioperative outcomes of L-RHH after FLRM and ex novo L-RHH were compared. Results: A total of 59 patients were included in the analysis, of whom 33 underwent FLRM. Patients undergoing FLRM prior to L-RHH were most often male (93.9% vs. 42.3%, $p < 0.001$), had an ASA-score > 2 (45.5% vs. 9.5%, $p = 0.006$), and underwent a two-stage hepatectomy (45.5% vs. 3.8% $p < 0.001$). L-RHH after FLRM was associated with longer operative time (median 360 vs. 300 min, $p = 0.008$) and Pringle duration (31 vs. 24 min, $p = 0.011$). Intraoperative blood loss, unfavorable intraoperative incidents, and conversion rates were similar in both groups. There were no significant differences in length of hospital stay and 30-day overall and severe morbidity rates. Radical resection margin (R0) and textbook outcome rates were equal. One patient who underwent an extended RHH in the FLRM group deceased within 90 days of surgery, due to post-hepatectomy liver failure. Conclusion: L-RHH after FLRM is more technically complex than L-RHH ex novo, as objectified by longer operative time and Pringle duration. Nevertheless, this procedure appears safe and feasible in experienced hands.

Citation: Hoogteijling, T.J.; Sijberden, J.P.; Primrose, J.N.; Morrison-Jones, V.; Modi, S.; Zimmitti, G.; Garatti, M.; Sallemi, C.; Morone, M.; Abu Hilal, M. Laparoscopic Right Hemihepatectomy after Future Liver Remnant Modulation: A Single Surgeon's Experience. *Cancers* **2023**, *15*, 2851. https://doi.org/10.3390/cancers15102851

Academic Editor: David Wong

Received: 13 April 2023
Revised: 11 May 2023
Accepted: 19 May 2023
Published: 21 May 2023

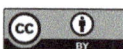

Copyright: © 2023 by the authors. Licensee MDPI, Basel, Switzerland. This article is an open access article distributed under the terms and conditions of the Creative Commons Attribution (CC BY) license (https://creativecommons.org/licenses/by/4.0/).

Keywords: liver neoplasms; right hemihepatectomy; laparoscopic liver resection; future liver remnant modulation; treatment outcome

1. Introduction

Right hemihepatectomy (RHH) is a complex liver resection that is classified as a major surgical procedure, requiring a high level of technical skill [1,2]. The safety of this procedure has been proven with both the open and the minimally invasive approach, but careful attention should be paid to its specific potential complications [3,4]. Resecting the right hemi liver (segments V–VIII) or, in case of an extended right hemihepatectomy, segments IV (or part of IV) –VIII, is associated to an increased risk of post-hepatectomy liver failure (PHLF), which is the main cause of postoperative mortality after major liver resections [5,6]. Such increased risk is related to the potentially insufficient volume of the future liver remnant (FLR), which, on average, corresponds to 35% and 16% of the total liver volume, following RHH and extended right hepatectomy, respectively [7]. For such reasons, in order to reduce the risk of PHLF, FLR volume should always be determined before a major liver resection is performed, as this is strongly associated with the liver's functional capacity [8–10]. Most experts agree that an FLR volume of 20–25% in noncirrhotic, >30–40% in steatotic and cholestatic livers, and >50% in cirrhotic livers should be pursued [11]. In addition, it is advised to perform a functional assessment through hepatobiliary scintigraphy (HBS) with ^{99m}Tc-mebrofenin, indocyanine green retention test at 15 min (ICGR15), or newer imaging techniques, such as dynamic hepatocyte-specific contrast-enhanced MRI (DHCE-MRI) with gadolinium ethoxybenzyl diethylenetriaminepentaacetic acid (Gd-EOB-DTPA) [9,12–16].

When the preoperatively determined FLR volume is insufficient, various strategies of future liver remnant modulation (FLRM) have been developed. They include portal vein embolization (PVE) and associating liver partition and portal vein ligation for staged hepatectomy (ALPPS), which stimulate compensatory hypertrophy of the contralateral liver parenchyma, thereby increasing FLR volume and function [9,17–19]. Both PVE (in the setting of single- or two-stage hepatectomy) and ALPPS have increased the pool of patients that are eligible for a liver resection [20,21]. However, due to the FLR hypertrophy, the overall liver anatomy can be distorted, making it harder to recognize anatomical landmarks during RHH. In addition, PVE and ALPPS are associated with periportal inflammation and fibrosis, leading to increased difficulty in hilar dissection [22].

Another technical breakthrough of the last decades has been the development of laparoscopic liver surgery (LLS). The implementation of LLS was initially slow, but the first consensus statement in Louisville generated enormous enthusiasm for this novel technique [23]. Now, LLS is considered the standard of care in minor liver resections, and is being increasingly used for technically and anatomically major liver resections [1]. In addition, the indications for LLS kept widening, which enabled surgeons in specialized centers to adopt laparoscopy for increasingly difficult resections [24–27]. Since then, there have been several studies showing favorable outcomes of laparoscopic right hemihepatectomy (L-RHH), and, finally, the Southampton guidelines stated that L-RHH should be expanded further in specialized centers [28–32]. However, studies investigating the results of L-RHH after FLRM are scarce. In this study, we aim to assess the safety and feasibility of L-RHH after FLRM, when compared with L-RHH not preceded by FLRM (ex novo).

2. Methods

This is a retrospective analysis of the prospectively maintained databases of two tertiary referral hepatobiliary centers. All consecutive laparoscopic right or extended right hemihepatectomies performed by a single surgeon (MAH) in the period between October 2007 and March 2023 were included. Patients were stratified in two study groups: those who did and those who did not undergo preoperative FLRM. Baseline characteristics and perioperative outcomes of patients in the two study groups were compared.

2.1. Definitions and Outcomes

The term 'future liver remnant modulation' (FLRM) was used to describe either a PVE or a first stage of ALPPS prior to RHH. Resections that were not preceded by FLRM were labeled as 'ex novo'. Data were collected from electronic health records. Baseline characteristics included patient demographics, body mass index (BMI), American Society of Anesthesiologists (ASA) score, presence of, and, if present, grade (Child-Pugh) of cirrhosis, history of hepatic surgery, neoadjuvant chemotherapy, disease characteristics (pathology, number, and size of lesions), and operative information (type of hemihepatectomy and multiple resections). The Brisbane 2000 terminology was used to define the type and extent of RHH, defining RHH as resection of the right hemi liver (segment 5, 6, 7, 8) and extended right hemihepatectomy (ERHH) as resection of the right hemi liver plus left medial section (segment 4, 5, 6, 7, 8) [33]. Perioperative outcomes consisted of resection margin status, application of Pringle maneuver and Pringle-duration, operative time, intraoperative blood loss, intraoperative transfusion, intraoperative incidents, conversion to an open procedure, length of hospital stay, 30-day morbidity, post hepatectomy liver failure, 30-day readmission, 30-day reintervention, and 90-day or in-hospital mortality. Intraoperative incidents and postoperative morbidity were respectively graded according to the Oslo and the Clavien-Dindo classifications [34,35]. In addition, the rate of textbook outcome in liver surgery (TOLS) was evaluated. TOLS was defined as: the absence of intraoperative incidents of grade 2 or higher, postoperative bile leak grade B or C, severe postoperative complications, readmission within 30 days after discharge, in-hospital mortality, and the presence of an R0 resection margin (in case of malignancy) [36].

2.2. Technique

A number of publications by our group have detailed the radiological and surgical techniques employed in L-RHH ex novo and following FLRM [3,4,22]. Concisely summarized, the techniques are as follows.

2.2.1. Patient Selection

Patients requiring a liver resection for any indication are discussed in a multidisciplinary team (MDT) meeting with (hepatobiliary) surgeons, pathologists, oncologists, hepatologists, and (interventional) radiologists. In our center, we maintain the following cut-off values for FLR volume: more than 30% in normal background livers, 35% following neoadjuvant chemotherapy, and 40% in the case of underlying chronic liver disease or portal hypertension. HBS is not implemented in our practice, however, in selected cases, ICGR15 tests are performed to assess the functional status of the FLR. All patients needing FLRM first received PVE, and, only if a sufficient FLR hypertrophy was not obtained, a salvage ALPPS was considered.

2.2.2. PVE

PVE is performed via a trans-hepatic percutaneous ipsilateral approach. Patients are typically treated under sedation and local anesthesia. Under ultrasound guidance, a peripheral vein from the right portal branch is punctured and a vascular sheath is introduced. Portal venography is performed prior to the actual selective embolization. FLR hypertrophy is evaluated by a CT scan 4 weeks after PVE.

2.2.3. Laparoscopic Right Hemihepatectomy Surgical Technique

Port placement for L-RHH is shown in Figure 1: in order to be in line with the transection plane, which is moved more right due to the left liver hypertrophy, in the group of FLRM, all the ports are usually placed 2 cm right, compared to the ex novo L-RHH group. After accessing the abdominal cavity, a thorough intraoperative ultrasound (IOUS) is performed. The liver is mobilized by first dissecting the round and falciform ligament back to the hepatocaval confluence. Thereafter, the right triangular and coronary ligaments are divided. As the right liver is lifted up and rotated to the left, the inferior retrohepatic vena cava is exposed, and eventual accessory hepatic veins can be identified, dissected, clipped, and divided. The Makuuchi ligament is dissected, slinged, and stapled using a powered vascular stapler (PVS) (ECHELON FLEX™, Ethicon, Johnson & Johnson, New Brunswick, NJ, USA) and the right hepatic vein is isolated and encircled with an elastic tape. After the right liver has been mobilized, the hepatic pedicle is encircled with a cotton tape for Pringle maneuver and the hepatic hilum is dissected, in order to identify the right portal vein (RPV) and the right hepatic artery (RHA), which are dissected and slinged. It should be noted that, after FLRM, this step can be more challenging, due to distorted anatomy and periportal fibrosis [22,37,38]. Typically, the Pringle maneuver is performed by placing a nylon tape around the porta hepatis from the most laterally placed trocar. To facilitate this maneuver, the liver is retracted to the left, thereby putting tension on the hepatoduodenal ligament and exposing the foramen of Winslow. Alternatively, when passing the foramen of Winslow is not possible, due to the earlier mentioned fibrosis, the Pringle maneuver can be applied from the left side of the porta hepatis. To facilitate this more difficult approach, the Goldfinger (Blunt Dissector and Suture Retrieval System, Ethicon Endo Surgery, Johnson & Johnson, New Brunswick, NJ, USA) can be used.

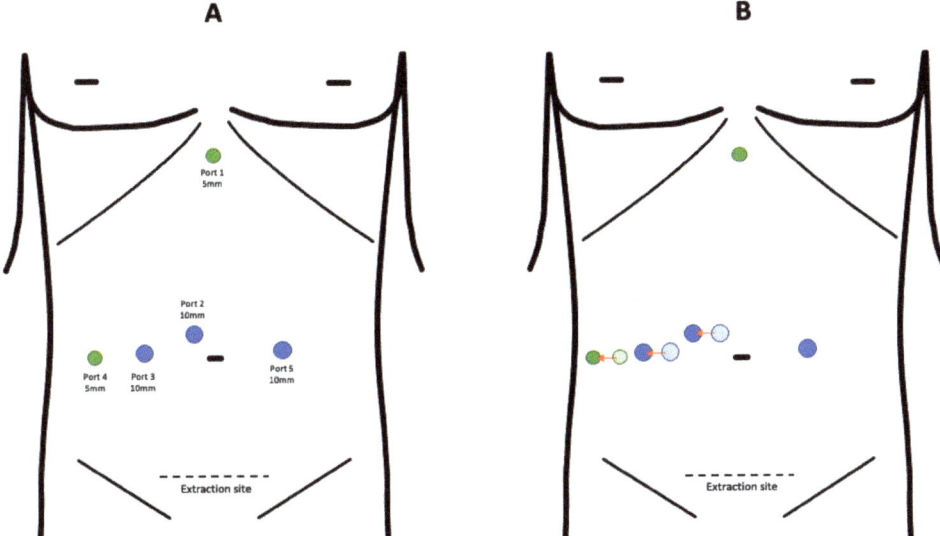

Figure 1. Port placement in L-RHH (**A**) and in L-RHH after FLRM (**B**).

Accurate preoperative CT imaging must be performed in order to better understand the vascular anatomy. By placing a bulldog on the RHA and RPV, the ischemia line on the liver surface between the right and left liver can be identified. In addition, with IOUS and color Doppler, we check the presence of venous and arterial flow in the left, and absence of venous and arterial flow in the right, lobe. Moreover, in the last five years, indocyanine green (ICG) is administered at a dose of 0.3 mg/kg to confirm the negative staining in the right lobe and to ensure the rightness of the ischemic Glissonean line. The RHA is then transected between Hem-o-Lock clips (Weck Closure Systems, Research Triangle Park, NC, USA). The RPV can be divided in a similar fashion, or using a PVS. After FLRM, RPV transection is not necessary, as it has already been embolized or ligated.

After reassessing the intraparenchymal anatomy with IOUS, the parenchymal transection phase starts. In our center, we use an ultrasonic dissector to transect the Glissonean sheath and the superficial part of the liver parenchyma, and the Cavitron Ultrasonic Surgical Aspirator (CUSA) (Integra Lifesciences, Princeton, NJ, USA) for the deep parenchyma dissection. Titanium or Hem-o-Lock clips are used to control small-medium Glissonean and venous branches. Major vessels, such as the RHD, RPV, and right hepatic vein (RHV), are dissected intraparenchymally and usually transected with a stapler. During the parenchymal transection phase, a good vision of the transection plane is paramount. We use a 30° camera and assert traction on the two sides of the parenchyma to open the liver and maintain a field of vision that is in line with the transection plane. It should be noted that parenchymal dissection can be challenging, due to the presence of embolic material and related inflammation; hence, special attention should be paid to possible stapler failure.

2.2.4. Salvage ALPPS Surgical Technique

Ports are positioned as in L-RHH and intra operative ultrasound is regularly performed. No liver mobilization is performed.

The first step is the identification of the right hepatic artery (RHA), which is slinged and controlled with a bulldog clamp. At this stage, due to the previously performed right portal vein embolization, a clear ischemia line is identified. The right liver ischemia and the adequate arterial and portal flow in the FLR are further confirmed, using intraoperative ultrasound with color Doppler and ICG test, as described previously. The transection line is marked, except in the case of lesion extension in segment IV, in which case the line is deviated further to the left. Thereafter, parenchymal transection is performed with a similar technique to the one described above. The parenchymal transection is extended deep enough to ensure that all major communicating outflow and venous structures are divided (mini ALPPS). After careful assessment of the resection margin, a drain between the resection planes is placed and a PDS-1 10 cm loop is left around the RHA.

2.3. Statistical Analysis

Categorical variables, reported as counts and percentages, were compared between the treatment groups (FLRM and ex novo) using Chi-squared or Fisher's exact tests, when appropriate. Normally distributed continuous variables were reported as the mean with its standard deviation and compared between treatment groups using an unpaired T-test. Not normally distributed continuous variables were reported as the median with its range and compared between treatment groups using the Mann-Whitney U test. Normality was assessed by visually inspecting histograms and Q-Q plots. A two-sided p-value < 0.05 was considered statistically significant. As exploratory analysis, due to the small sample size, unadjusted (univariate) and adjusted (multivariate) regression analyses were performed for the endpoints TOLS, Pringle duration, and operative time. Logistic and linear regression was performed for binary and continuous outcomes, respectively. Besides the exposure (FLRM), potential confounding factors were added as covariates in the adjusted regression analyses when they were significantly (Cut-off: $p \leq 0.20$) associated with the outcome of interest in the unadjusted analyses. Data were analyzed using R for Mac OS X version 4.2.1 (R Foundation for Statistical Computing, Vienna, Austria).

3. Results

Overall, 59 patients that underwent a laparoscopic right or extended right hemihepatectomy were included. As shown in Figure 2, 33 patients underwent L-RHH after FLRM, and 26 patients underwent an ex novo L-RHH. Among the included patients, 45 were operated on in the University Hospital of Southampton, United Kingdom, between October 2007 and October 2019. In November 2019, the operating surgeon (MAH) moved to Fondazione Poliambulanza Hospital in Brescia, Italy, where the remaining 14 patients were treated. In the FLRM group, 28 patients received PVE and five underwent first-stage ALPPS prior to L-RHH.

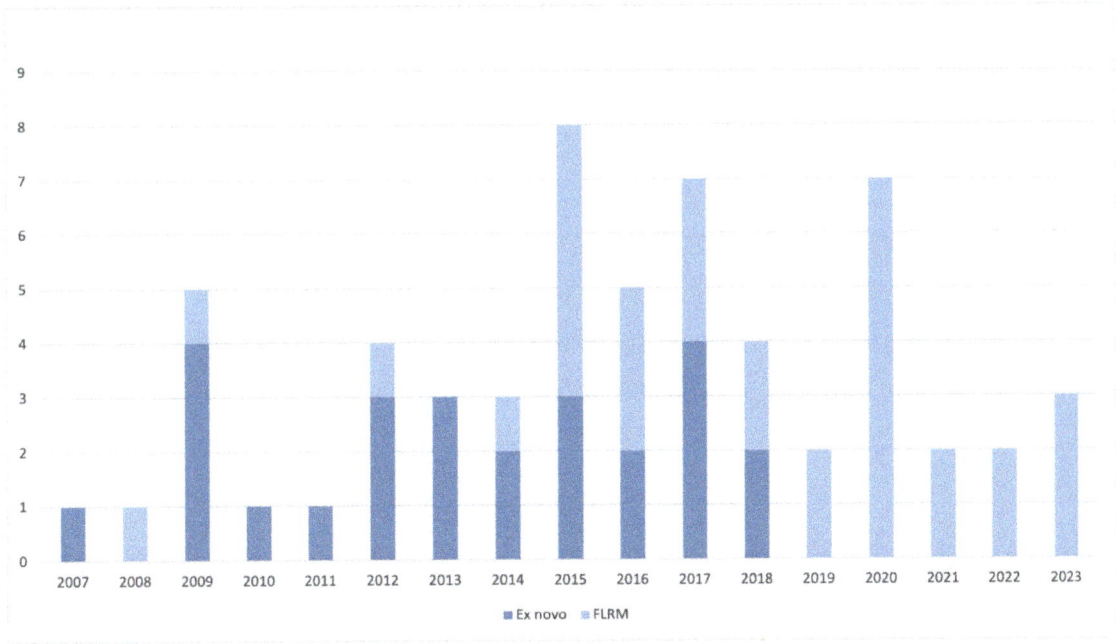

Figure 2. Proportion of L-RHH after FLRM and ex novo per year.

3.1. Baseline, Procedural, and Disease Characteristics

The baseline, procedural, and disease characteristics are shown in Table 1. Both groups were well balanced, in terms of median age, median BMI, and median tumor size. The proportion of male patients and patients with higher ASA scores was significantly higher in the FLRM group than in the ex novo group (93.9% vs. 42.3%, $p < 0.001$, and 45.5% vs. 9.5%, $p = 0.006$, respectively). Significantly more patients in the FLRM group underwent surgery in the setting of a two-stage hepatectomy (45.5% vs. 3.8% $p < 0.001$). The majority of patients ($n = 32$) were treated for colorectal liver metastases (CRLM), whilst 16 were treated for hepatocellular carcinoma (HCC), one was treated for intrahepatic cholangiocarcinoma (CCA), three were treated for non-colorectal liver metastases (NCRLM), and six were treated for benign lesions. The proportion of malignancy was well balanced between the two groups. In the FLRM group, two patients underwent extended right hemihepatectomy.

Table 1. Baseline Characteristics.

	FLRM ($n = 33$)	Ex Novo ($n = 26$)	p
AgeatOp (median [IQR])	64.00 [58.00, 70.00]	60.63 [48.22, 75.42]	0.306
BMI (median [IQR])	28.40 [25.00, 29.70]	27.07 [24.95, 31.00]	0.942
Male Gender (%)	31 (93.9)	11 (42.3)	<0.001
ASA > 2 (%)	15 (45.5)	2 (9.5)	0.006
Cirrhosis (%)			0.036
No	25 (83.3)	24 (100.0)	
Yes *	5 (16.7)	0 (0.0)	
Neoadjuvant Chemotherapy (%)	21 (63.6)	12 (46.2)	0.179
Previous Liver Surgery (%)	15 (46.9)	2 (7.7)	0.001

Table 1. Cont.

	FLRM (n = 33)	Ex Novo (n = 26)	p
Pathology (%)			0.040
CRLM	20 (60.6)	12 (48.0)	
HCC	11 (33.3)	5 (20.0)	
CCA	1 (3.0)	0 (0.0)	
Benign	1 (3.0)	5 (20.0)	
NCRLM	0 (0.0)	3 (12.0)	
Malignancy (%)	32 (97.0)	22 (84.6)	0.091
Size Largest Lesion, mm (median [IQR])	40.00 [15.00, 70.00]	44.50 [31.50, 68.50]	0.571
Number of Lesions (median [IQR])	2.00 [1.00, 4.00]	1.00 [1.00, 2.00]	0.124
Type of FLRM (%)			
None	0 (0.0)	26 (100.0)	<0.001
PVE	28 (84.8)	0 (0.0)	
ALPPS	5 (15.2)	0 (0.0)	
Time Interval PVE to Surgery (median [IQR])	43.00 [39.00, 61.00]	-	-
Two-stage Hepatectomy (%)	15 (45.5)	1 (3.8)	<0.001
Extended Right Hemihepatectomy (%)	2 (6.1)	0 (0.0)	0.202
Multiple Resections (%)	4 (12.1)	3 (11.5)	0.945

Abbreviations: FLRM = Future Liver Remnant Modulation; IQR = Inter Quartile Range; BMI = Body Mass Index; ASA = American Society of Anesthesiologists; CRLM = Colorectal Liver Metastasis; HCC = Hepatocellular Carcinoma; CCA = Cholangiocarcinoma; NCRLM = Non-colorectal Liver Metastasis; PVE = Portal Vein Embolization; ALPPS = Associating Liver Partition and Portal vein ligation for Staged hepatectomy. * All patients had Child-Pugh A cirrhosis.

3.2. Intra- and Postoperative Outcomes

Intra- and postoperative outcomes are shown in Table 2. FLRM was associated with longer operative times (Median 360 [IQR 300–427.50] vs. 300 min [IQR 240–360], $p = 0.008$) and a longer Pringle duration (Median 31 [IQR 25–43] vs. 24 min [IQR 20–30], $p = 0.011$). The rate of unfavorable intraoperative incidents, conversion to open surgery, and amount of intraoperative blood loss were similar in both groups. The R0 rates did not significantly differ between the FLRM and ex novo groups (90.3% vs. 90%, $p = 0.970$). Postoperatively, the median length of stay, 30-day morbidity, 30-day readmission, and 30-day reintervention rates were comparable and did not statistically differ. The TOLS rates were comparable in the FLRM and ex novo groups (74.2% vs. 70.6%, $p = 0.788$). One patient who underwent an extended L-RHH after FLRM deceased as a result of ISGLS grade B PHLF.

Table 2. Perioperative Outcomes.

	FLRM (n = 33)	Ex Novo (n = 26)	p
Pringle Maneuver (%)	30 (93.8)	20 (76.9)	0.065
Pringle Duration (median [IQR]) †	31.00 [25.00, 43.00]	24.00 [20.00, 30.00]	0.011
Operating Time, minutes (median [IQR])	360.00 [300.00, 427.50]	300.00 [240.00, 360.00]	0.008
Intraoperative Blood Loss, mL (median [IQR])	700.00 [400.00, 1200.00]	500.00 [312.50, 737.50]	0.162
Intraoperative Blood Transfusion (%)	9 (28.1)	3 (13.0)	0.182
Intraoperative Incidents, OSLO-classification (%)			0.678
0	26 (83.9)	18 (75.0)	
1	2 (6.5)	3 (12.5)	
2	3 (9.7)	3 (12.5)	
Conversion (%)	2 (6.1)	3 (11.5)	0.453
Length of Hospital Stay, days (median [IQR])	6.00 [5.00, 8.25]	6.00 [5.00, 8.00]	0.537
30-day Complication (%)	8 (24.2)	11 (47.8)	0.067
Severe Postoperative Complications (%)	5 (15.2)	1 (4.2)	0.182
Post-hepatectomy Liver Failure (%)	2 (6.5) ‡	0 (0.0)	0.331
30-day Readmission (%)	6 (18.8)	2 (7.7)	0.225

Table 2. Cont.

	FLRM (n = 33)	Ex Novo (n = 26)	p
30-day Reintervention (%)	3 (9.4)	1 (5.0)	0.565
90-day Mortality (%)	1 (3.0)	0 (0.0)	0.371
R0 Resection Margin(%)	28 (90.3)	18 (90.0)	0.970
TOLS (%)	23 (74.2)	12 (70.6)	0.788

Abbreviations: FLRM = Future Liver Remnant Modulation; IQR = Inter Quartile Range; OSLO = Oslo classification of intraoperative incidents; ISGLS = International Study Group on Liver Surgery; PHLF = Post Hepatectomy Liver Failure; TOLS = Textbook Outcome in Liver Surgery. Missing data: counts may not add up, due to missing data. Missing values for continuous data: BMI 26; Size of largest lesion 3; Pringle duration 4; Operative time 2; intraoperative blood loss 2; length of stay 2. † Analysis of Pringle duration, only when Pringle maneuver was applied. ‡ One patient had ISGLS grade A, and one had grade B PHLF.

The additional, exploratory, adjusted analyses (Supplementary Table S1) confirmed these findings, although the observed difference in operative time no longer reached statistical significance.

4. Discussion

The present study reports on the 17-year experience of a single surgeon in performing L-RHH, ex novo and after FLRM [39]. It shows that the added difficulty of anatomical and structural changes after FLRM in L-RHH resulted in a significantly longer operative time and pringle duration. However, importantly, there were no significant differences in intraoperative blood loss, unfavorable incidents, conversion rate and resection margin status between L-RHH after FLRM and ex novo. Importantly, these resections were performed in tertiary referral centers specialized in LLS, and by a surgeon with extensive experience in both laparoscopic and open liver surgery.

L-RHH after FLRM remains a technical challenge. The Southampton guidelines, which stated that the implementation of LLS should be realized in a stepwise manner, owing to the extensive learning curve associated with the more difficult resections, considers L-RHH among the most challenging resections and recommends exploring the technique only in highly specialized centers [30]. FLRM further increases the technical difficulty of L-RHH. FLRM is usually performed in patients with extensive uni- or bilobar disease, who have a high disease burden, and is often used in the context of staged hepatectomy: in this case, the FLR is cleared of lesions during the first stage, followed by PVE and by RHH or extended right hepatectomy during the second stage. Alternatively, during the first stage of ALPPS, the liver parenchyma is (partially) transected before ligation or embolization of the portal vein. A history of previous liver surgery is a well-known factor of increased surgical difficulty [2,40,41]. More importantly, FLR modulation with PVE or ALPPS leads to an important anatomical distortion and periportal fibrosis, which significantly increase the technical difficulty of L-RHH [9]. As a result, evidence regarding the safety and feasibility of these procedures is limited [42].

In this single surgeon experience study, we included all consecutive L-RHH, including two-stage hepatectomies and second-stage ALPPS procedures. Patients in the FLRM group, predictably, were associated with more extensive disease. In addition, FLRM is often performed in the setting of staged hepatectomy, which can be seen from the higher portion of staged hepatectomies in the FLRM group. It is fair to assume that these factors have resulted in the longer operative time and Pringle duration in the FLRM group, even if they did not result in significantly worse intra- and postoperative outcomes. In the current experience, blood loss, transfusion, and conversion rates are largely consistent with previously published series. A study by Fuks et al. (2015), of 26 patients undergoing second-stage L-RHH for CRLM, reported a median blood loss of 250 mL, transfusion rate of 15%, a conversion rate of 15%, a major morbidity rate of 27%, and 9 days length of hospital stay [37]. Another study by Okumura et al. (2019), of 38 patients undergoing second-stage L-RHH for CRLM, reported a median blood loss of 225 mL, 13% transfusion rate, 11% conversion rate, 18% major morbidity rate, and 9 days length of stay [43]. It should be noted that, in the latter analysis, 13 of the 38 patients did not undergo FLRM prior to the second-stage hepatectomy. The most recent analysis was published by Taillieu et al. (2022), reporting the outcomes of seven patients who underwent L-RHH after FLRM. This analysis showed a median intraoperative blood loss of 240 mL, 0% transfusion rate, 1 (14%) conversion, 18% major morbidity, and 4 days hospital stay [44]. In addition, the increased surgical difficulty did not negatively impact oncological efficiency, with an R0 rate approaching 90%, which is comparable to both the ex novo group, and to the reports by Fuks et al., Okumara et al., and Taillieu et al. [37,43,44].

Recently, textbook outcome has been introduced in different surgical disciplines [45]. Based on an all-or-nothing principle, these composite outcome measures incorporate multiple clinical and pathological outcomes to give a more comprehensive picture of patient-level hospital performance [36]. Textbook outcome in liver surgery (TOLS) was defined by Gorgec et al. through a survey among the members of the European African Hepato-Pancreato-Biliary Association (E-AHPBA) and the International Hepato-Pancreato-Biliary Association (I-HPBA), and was subsequently validated in a large retrospective database [36]. As patients undergoing FLRM were excluded from the analyses by Gorgec et al., TOLS is not validated for the patients in the present study. Interestingly, however, when we did apply TOLS to our analysis, the rates in both groups were around 70%, which is consistent with the results reported by Gorgec et al. in the general population of patients undergoing liver surgery [36].

This study has several limitations. First, the small sample size and retrospective nature of the analysis produce an inevitable risk of bias. The baseline characteristics between the two groups differ significantly in terms of gender, history of previous liver surgery, and number of patients with multiple lesions. However, this is one of the largest series reported to date, and we do believe that some baseline differences are inevitable when comparing these two clinically different groups; hence, we chose not to address this by means of statistical techniques such as propensity-score matching. The exploratory, adjusted analyses confirmed that FLRM is associated with a longer Pringle duration, but non-inferior TOLS rates. In these analyses, the FLRM group also tended to have longer operative times, although this finding no longer reached statistical significance. However, the results of these analyses need to be interpreted with extreme caution, due to the very small sample size, making regression analyses notoriously unreliable.

Another issue is the relatively large proportion (56%) of patients who underwent FLRM prior to L-RHH, which is higher than other series [28]. In our center, an effort is made to be as parenchyma-sparing as possible. RHH is typically reserved for patients who have extensive disease, characterized by a large number of lesions or lesions located deep in the parenchyma and in close proximity to major Glissonean or venous vessels. In such scenarios, performing FLRM is often necessary.

Another limitation is that the current results refer to a single surgeon with a wide experience in open and minimally invasive liver surgery, who gradually expanded the indications during the years, whilst accumulating more experience in MILS, thus these results should not be seen as a green light for the liberal adoption of the minimally invasive approach for such complex cases, unless experience is developed and a learning curve has been completed. However, a large single-surgeon series reduces potential confounding factors, thus permitting a more reliable analysis.

5. Conclusions

The results of this analysis suggest that, despite the increased technical difficulty, L-RHH after FLRM is feasible and safe for carefully selected patients, assuming that such complex procedures are performed by surgeons highly experienced in LLS.

Supplementary Materials: The following supporting information can be downloaded at: https://www.mdpi.com/article/10.3390/cancers15102851/s1, Table S1: Univariable and Multivariable Regression Analysis.

Author Contributions: Study conception and design: T.J.H., J.P.S. and M.A.H.; Acquisition of data: All authors; Analysis and interpretation of data: T.J.H., J.P.S. and M.A.H.; Drafting of manuscript: T.J.H., J.P.S. and M.A.H.; Critical revision: All authors. All authors have read and agreed to the published version of the manuscript.

Funding: This research received no external funding.

Institutional Review Board Statement: Ethical approval was obtained in accordance with UK and Italian (NP. 5403) legislature.

Informed Consent Statement: The medical ethical committee of Brescia approved this study and waived the need to obtain informed consent, due to its retrospective nature and the use of pseudonymized data. (Judgement's reference number: NP 5403).

Data Availability Statement: The data that support the findings of this study are available from the corresponding author, Mohammed Abu Hilal, upon reasonable request. The data are not publicly available, since this could compromise the privacy of research participants.

Conflicts of Interest: The authors declare no conflict of interest.

References

1. Buell, J.F.; Cherqui, D.; Geller, D.A.; O'Rourke, N.; Iannitti, D.; Dagher, I.; Koffron, A.J.; Thomas, M.; Gayet, B.; Han, H.S.; et al. The international position on laparoscopic liver surgery: The Louisville Statement, 2008. *Ann. Surg.* **2009**, *250*, 825–830. [CrossRef]
2. Halls, M.C.; Berardi, G.; Cipriani, F.; Barkhatov, L.; Lainas, P.; Harris, S.; D'Hondt, M.; Rotellar, F.; Dagher, I.; Aldrighetti, L.; et al. Development and validation of a difficulty score to predict intraoperative complications during laparoscopic liver resection. *Br. J. Surg.* **2018**, *105*, 1182–1191. [CrossRef]
3. Pearce, N.W.; Di Fabio, F.; Teng, M.J.; Syed, S.; Primrose, J.N.; Abu Hilal, M. Laparoscopic right hepatectomy: A challenging, but feasible, safe and efficient procedure. *Am. J. Surg.* **2011**, *202*, e52–e58. [CrossRef] [PubMed]
4. Abu Hilal, M.; Di Fabio, F.; Teng, M.J.; Lykoudis, P.; Primrose, J.N.; Pearce, N.W. Single-Centre Comparative Study of Laparoscopic Versus Open Right Hepatectomy. *J. Gastrointest. Surg.* **2011**, *15*, 818–823. [CrossRef] [PubMed]
5. Pulitano, C.; Crawford, M.; Joseph, D.; Aldrighetti, L.; Sandroussi, C. Preoperative assessment of postoperative liver function: The importance of residual liver volume. *J. Surg. Oncol.* **2014**, *110*, 445–450. [CrossRef]
6. Mullen, J.T.; Ribero, D.; Reddy, S.K.; Donadon, M.; Zorzi, D.; Gautam, S.; Abdalla, E.K.; Curley, S.A.; Capussotti, L.; Clary, B.M.; et al. Hepatic insufficiency and mortality in 1059 noncirrhotic patients undergoing major hepatectomy. *J. Am. Coll. Surg.* **2007**, *204*, 854–862, discussion 862–854. [CrossRef]
7. Abdalla, E.K.; Denys, A.; Chevalier, P.; Nemr, R.A.; Vauthey, J.N. Total and segmental liver volume variations: Implications for liver surgery. *Surgery* **2004**, *135*, 404–410. [CrossRef]
8. van den Broek, M.A.; Olde Damink, S.W.; Dejong, C.H.; Lang, H.; Malagó, M.; Jalan, R.; Saner, F.H. Liver failure after partial hepatic resection: Definition, pathophysiology, risk factors and treatment. *Liver Int.* **2008**, *28*, 767–780. [CrossRef] [PubMed]
9. Memeo, R.; Conticchio, M.; Deshayes, E.; Nadalin, S.; Herrero, A.; Guiu, B.; Panaro, F. Optimization of the future remnant liver: Review of the current strategies in Europe. *Hepatobiliary Surg. Nutr.* **2021**, *10*, 350–363. [CrossRef] [PubMed]
10. Truant, S.; Oberlin, O.; Sergent, G.; Lebuffe, G.; Gambiez, L.; Ernst, O.; Pruvot, F.R. Remnant liver volume to body weight ratio > or =0.5%: A new cut-off to estimate postoperative risks after extended resection in noncirrhotic liver. *J. Am. Coll. Surg.* **2007**, *204*, 22–33. [CrossRef]
11. Gruttadauria, S.; Vasta, F.; Minervini, M.I.; Piazza, T.; Arcadipane, A.; Marcos, A.; Gridelli, B. Significance of the Effective Remnant Liver Volume in Major Hepatectomies. *Am. Surg.* **2005**, *71*, 235–240. [CrossRef] [PubMed]
12. de Graaf, W.; van Lienden, K.P.; Dinant, S.; Roelofs, J.J.; Busch, O.R.; Gouma, D.J.; Bennink, R.J.; van Gulik, T.M. Assessment of future remnant liver function using hepatobiliary scintigraphy in patients undergoing major liver resection. *J. Gastrointest. Surg.* **2010**, *14*, 369–378. [CrossRef]
13. Bennink, R.J.; Tulchinsky, M.; de Graaf, W.; Kadry, Z.; van Gulik, T.M. Liver function testing with nuclear medicine techniques is coming of age. *Semin. Nucl. Med.* **2012**, *42*, 124–137. [CrossRef] [PubMed]
14. Rassam, F.; Zhang, T.; Cieslak, K.P.; Lavini, C.; Stoker, J.; Bennink, R.J.; van Gulik, T.M.; van Vliet, L.J.; Runge, J.H.; Vos, F.M. Comparison between dynamic gadoxetate-enhanced MRI and ^{99m}Tc-mebrofenin hepatobiliary scintigraphy with SPECT for quantitative assessment of liver function. *Eur. Radiol.* **2019**, *29*, 5063–5072. [CrossRef] [PubMed]
15. Sunagawa, Y.; Yamada, S.; Kato, Y.; Sonohara, F.; Takami, H.; Inokawa, Y.; Hayashi, M.; Nakayama, G.; Koike, M.; Kodera, Y. Perioperative assessment of indocyanine green elimination rate accurately predicts postoperative liver failure in patients undergoing hepatectomy. *J. Hepatobiliary Pancreat. Sci.* **2021**, *28*, 86–94. [CrossRef]
16. Le Roy, B.; Grégoire, E.; Cossé, C.; Serji, B.; Golse, N.; Adam, R.; Cherqui, D.; Mabrut, J.Y.; Le Treut, Y.P.; Vibert, E. Indocyanine Green Retention Rates at 15 min Predicted Hepatic Decompensation in a Western Population. *World J. Surg.* **2018**, *42*, 2570–2578. [CrossRef]

17. Schnitzbauer, A.A.; Lang, S.A.; Goessmann, H.; Nadalin, S.; Baumgart, J.; Farkas, S.A.; Fichtner-Feigl, S.; Lorf, T.; Goralcyk, A.; Hörbelt, R.; et al. Right portal vein ligation combined with in situ splitting induces rapid left lateral liver lobe hypertrophy enabling 2-staged extended right hepatic resection in small-for-size settings. *Ann. Surg.* **2012**, *255*, 405–414. [CrossRef]
18. van Lienden, K.P.; van den Esschert, J.W.; de Graaf, W.; Bipat, S.; Lameris, J.S.; van Gulik, T.M.; van Delden, O.M. Portal vein embolization before liver resection: A systematic review. *Cardiovasc. Interv. Radiol.* **2013**, *36*, 25–34. [CrossRef]
19. Del Basso, C.; Gaillard, M.; Lainas, P.; Zervaki, S.; Perlemuter, G.; Chagué, P.; Rocher, L.; Voican, C.S.; Dagher, I.; Tranchart, H. Current strategies to induce liver remnant hypertrophy before major liver resection. *World J. Hepatol.* **2021**, *13*, 1629–1641. [CrossRef]
20. Sandström, P.; Røsok, B.I.; Sparrelid, E.; Larsen, P.N.; Larsson, A.L.; Lindell, G.; Schultz, N.A.; Bjørnbeth, B.A.; Isaksson, B.; Rizell, M.; et al. ALPPS Improves Resectability Compared with Conventional Two-stage Hepatectomy in Patients with Advanced Colorectal Liver Metastasis: Results From a Scandinavian Multicenter Randomized Controlled Trial (LIGRO Trial). *Ann. Surg.* **2018**, *267*, 833–840. [CrossRef]
21. Azoulay, D.; Castaing, D.; Smail, A.; Adam, R.; Cailliez, V.; Laurent, A.; Lemoine, A.; Bismuth, H. Resection of nonresectable liver metastases from colorectal cancer after percutaneous portal vein embolization. *Ann. Surg.* **2000**, *231*, 480–486. [CrossRef]
22. Görgec, B.; Suhool, A.; Al-Jarrah, R.; Fontana, M.; Tehami, N.A.; Modi, S.; Abu Hilal, M. Surgical technique and clinical results of one- or two-stage laparoscopic right hemihepatectomy after portal vein embolization in patients with initially unresectable colorectal liver metastases: A case series. *Int. J. Surg.* **2020**, *77*, 69–75. [CrossRef] [PubMed]
23. Abu Hilal, M. Why do we need guidelines in laparoscopic liver surgery? *HPB* **2017**, *19*, 287–288. [CrossRef]
24. Wakabayashi, G.; Cherqui, D.; Geller, D.A.; Buell, J.F.; Kaneko, H.; Han, H.S.; Asbun, H.; O'Rourke, N.; Tanabe, M.; Koffron, A.J.; et al. Recommendations for laparoscopic liver resection: A report from the second international consensus conference held in Morioka. *Ann. Surg.* **2015**, *261*, 619–629.
25. Abu Hilal, M.; Tschuor, C.; Kuemmerli, C.; López-Ben, S.; Lesurtel, M.; Rotellar, F. Laparoscopic posterior segmental resections: How I do it: Tips and pitfalls. *Int. J. Surg.* **2020**, *82*, 178–186. [CrossRef]
26. Coles, S.R.; Besselink, M.G.; Serin, K.R.; Alsaati, H.; Di Gioia, P.; Samim, M.; Pearce, N.W.; Abu Hilal, M. Total laparoscopic management of lesions involving liver segment 7. *Surg. Endosc.* **2015**, *29*, 3190–3195. [CrossRef] [PubMed]
27. Cipriani, F.; Shelat, V.G.; Rawashdeh, M.; Francone, E.; Aldrighetti, L.; Takhar, A.; Armstrong, T.; Pearce, N.W.; Abu Hilal, M. Laparoscopic Parenchymal-Sparing Resections for Nonperipheral Liver Lesions, the Diamond Technique: Technical Aspects, Clinical Outcomes, and Oncologic Efficiency. *J. Am. Coll. Surg.* **2015**, *221*, 265–272. [CrossRef]
28. Cipriani, F.; Alzoubi, M.; Fuks, D.; Ratti, F.; Kawai, T.; Berardi, G.; Barkhatov, L.; Lainas, P.; Van der Poel, M.; Faoury, M.; et al. Pure laparoscopic versus open hemihepatectomy: A critical assessment and realistic expectations—A propensity score-based analysis of right and left hemihepatectomies from nine European tertiary referral centers. *J. Hepatobiliary Pancreat. Sci.* **2020**, *27*, 3–15. [CrossRef]
29. Pietrasz, D.; Fuks, D.; Subar, D.; Donatelli, G.; Ferretti, C.; Lamer, C.; Portigliotti, L.; Ward, M.; Cowan, J.; Nomi, T.; et al. Laparoscopic extended liver resection: Are postoperative outcomes different? *Surg. Endosc.* **2018**, *32*, 4833–4840. [CrossRef] [PubMed]
30. Abu Hilal, M.; Aldrighetti, L.; Dagher, I.; Edwin, B.; Troisi, R.I.; Alikhanov, R.; Aroori, S.; Belli, G.; Besselink, M.; Briceno, J.; et al. The Southampton Consensus Guidelines for Laparoscopic Liver Surgery: From Indication to Implementation. *Ann. Surg.* **2018**, *268*, 11–18. [CrossRef]
31. Wang, Z.Y.; Chen, Q.L.; Sun, L.L.; He, S.P.; Luo, X.F.; Huang, L.S.; Huang, J.H.; Xiong, C.M.; Zhong, C. Laparoscopic versus open major liver resection for hepatocellular carcinoma: Systematic review and meta-analysis of comparative cohort studies. *BMC Cancer* **2019**, *19*, 1047. [CrossRef]
32. Ciria, R.; Cherqui, D.; Geller, D.A.; Briceno, J.; Wakabayashi, G. Comparative Short-term Benefits of Laparoscopic Liver Resection: 9000 Cases and Climbing. *Ann. Surg.* **2016**, *263*, 761–777. [CrossRef]
33. Strasberg, S.M.; Belghiti, J.; Clavien, P.A.; Gadzijev, E.; Garden, J.O.; Lau, W.Y.; Makuuchi, M.; Strong, R.W. The Brisbane 2000 Terminology of Liver Anatomy and Resections. *HPB* **2000**, *2*, 333–339. [CrossRef]
34. Kazaryan, A.M.; Røsok, B.I.; Edwin, B. Morbidity Assessment in Surgery: Refinement Proposal Based on a Concept of Perioperative Adverse Events. *ISRN Surg.* **2013**, *2013*, 625093. [CrossRef]
35. Dindo, D.; Demartines, N.; Clavien, P.A. Classification of surgical complications: A new proposal with evaluation in a cohort of 6336 patients and results of a survey. *Ann. Surg.* **2004**, *240*, 205–213. [CrossRef] [PubMed]
36. Görgec, B.; Benedetti Cacciaguerra, A.; Lanari, J.; Russolillo, N.; Cipriani, F.; Aghayan, D.; Zimmitti, G.; Efanov, M.; Alseidi, A.; Mocchegiani, F.; et al. Assessment of Textbook Outcome in Laparoscopic and Open Liver Surgery. *JAMA Surg.* **2021**, *156*, e212064. [CrossRef]
37. Fuks, D.; Nomi, T.; Ogiso, S.; Gelli, M.; Velayutham, V.; Conrad, C.; Louvet, C.; Gayet, B. Laparoscopic two-stage hepatectomy for bilobar colorectal liver metastases. *Br. J. Surg.* **2015**, *102*, 1684–1690. [CrossRef]
38. Rotellar, F.; Pardo, F.; Benito, A.; Martí-Cruchaga, P.; Zozaya, G.; Bellver, M. Laparoscopic right hepatectomy extended to middle hepatic vein after right portal vein embolization. *Ann. Surg. Oncol.* **2014**, *21*, 165–166. [CrossRef]
39. Jain, G.; Parmar, J.; Mohammed, M.M.; Bryant, T.; Kitteringham, L.; Pearce, N.; Abu Hilal, M. "Stretching the limits of laparoscopic surgery": Two-stage laparoscopic liver resection. *J. Laparoendosc. Adv. Surg. Tech. A* **2010**, *20*, 51–54. [CrossRef] [PubMed]

40. Kawaguchi, Y.; Fuks, D.; Kokudo, N.; Gayet, B. Difficulty of Laparoscopic Liver Resection: Proposal for a New Classification. *Ann. Surg.* **2018**, *267*, 13–17. [CrossRef] [PubMed]
41. Ban, D.; Tanabe, M.; Ito, H.; Otsuka, Y.; Nitta, H.; Abe, Y.; Hasegawa, Y.; Katagiri, T.; Takagi, C.; Itano, O.; et al. A novel difficulty scoring system for laparoscopic liver resection. *J. Hepatobiliary Pancreat. Sci.* **2014**, *21*, 745–753. [CrossRef] [PubMed]
42. Bozkurt, E.; Sijberden, J.P.; Abu Hilal, M. Safety and Feasibility of Laparoscopic Right or Extended Right Hemi Hepatectomy Following Modulation of the Future Liver Remnant in Patients with Colorectal Liver Metastases: A Systematic Review. *J. Laparoendosc. Adv. Surg. Tech. A* **2023**. [CrossRef]
43. Okumura, S.; Goumard, C.; Gayet, B.; Fuks, D.; Scatton, O. Laparoscopic versus open two-stage hepatectomy for bilobar colorectal liver metastases: A bi-institutional, propensity score-matched study. *Surgery* **2019**, *166*, 959–966. [CrossRef] [PubMed]
44. Taillieu, E.; De Meyere, C.; D'Hondt, M. The role of the laparoscopic approach in two-stage hepatectomy for colorectal liver metastases: A single-center experience. *Surg. Endosc.* **2022**, *36*, 559–568. [CrossRef] [PubMed]
45. Pretzsch, E.; Koliogiannis, D.; D'Haese, J.G.; Ilmer, M.; Guba, M.O.; Angele, M.K.; Werner, J.; Niess, H. Textbook outcome in hepato-pancreato-biliary surgery: Systematic review. *BJS Open* **2022**, *6*, zrac149. [CrossRef]

Disclaimer/Publisher's Note: The statements, opinions and data contained in all publications are solely those of the individual author(s) and contributor(s) and not of MDPI and/or the editor(s). MDPI and/or the editor(s) disclaim responsibility for any injury to people or property resulting from any ideas, methods, instructions or products referred to in the content.

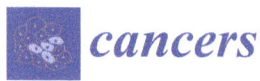

Review

Multiple Laparoscopic Liver Resection for Colorectal Liver Metastases

Alexandra Nassar [1,*], Stylianos Tzedakis [1], Alix Dhote [1], Marie Strigalev [1], Romain Coriat [2], Mehdi Karoui [3], Anthony Dohan [4], Martin Gaillard [1], Ugo Marchese [1] and David Fuks [1]

1. Department of Hepato-Pancreatic-Biliary and Endocrine Surgery, Cochin Hospital, Assistance Publique-Hôpitaux de Paris Centre, Université Paris Cité, 75014 Paris, France
2. Department of Gastroenterology and Digestive Oncology, Cochin Hospital, Assistance Publique-Hôpitaux de Paris Centre, Université Paris Cité, 75014 Paris, France
3. Department of General Digestive Surgery and Cancerology, Hopital Européen Georges Pompidou, Université Paris Cité, 75015 Paris, France
4. Department of Radiology, Cochin Hospital, Assistance Publique-Hôpitaux de Paris Centre, Université Paris Cité, 75014 Paris, France
* Correspondence: alexandra.nassar@free.fr; Tel.: +33-1-58-41-17-24

Simple Summary: Colorectal liver metastases are multiple in 80% of cases, and surgical resection is still the best treatment known in terms of survival. Laparoscopic multiple liver resections are yet not recommended, and no dedicated comparative study has been published. This literature review aimed to assess feasibility of laparoscopic liver resection for multiple colorectal liver metastases, whether by parenchymal-sparing multiple resections or two-stage resections. The purpose of this review is to guide the implementation of this minimal invasive technique for multiple colorectal liver metastases.

Abstract: Over the past decades, liver cancer's minimally invasive approach has primarily become as a new standard of oncological care. Colorectal liver metastases (CRLM) are one of the most developed indications of laparoscopic liver resection (LLR). CRLM resection is still the best treatment known in terms of survival. As multiple CRLM are found in up to 80% of cases at diagnosis (Manfredi S. and al, Annals of Surgery 2006), a lot of possible technical management approaches are described. With the development of the parenchymal-sparing strategy, multiple concomitant laparoscopic liver resections (LLR) are gaining acceptance. However, no recommendation is available regarding its indications and feasibility. Also, laparoscopic two-stage hepatectomy is developing for bilobar CRLM, and this also does not have established recommendation. The purpose of this paper was to highlight novelty and updates in the field of multiple minimally invasive liver resections. A review of the international literature was performed. The feasibility of laparoscopic concomitant multiple LLR and two-stage hepatectomy for CRLM as well as their outcomes were discussed. These clarifications could further guide the implementation of minimal resection in multiple colorectal liver metastases therapies.

Keywords: laparoscopic liver resections; colorectal liver metastases; multiple laparoscopic resections

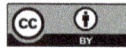

Citation: Nassar, A.; Tzedakis, S.; Dhote, A.; Strigalev, M.; Coriat, R.; Karoui, M.; Dohan, A.; Gaillard, M.; Marchese, U.; Fuks, D. Multiple Laparoscopic Liver Resection for Colorectal Liver Metastases. *Cancers* **2023**, *15*, 435. https://doi.org/10.3390/cancers15020435

Academic Editors: Zenichi Morise and Tomoharu Yoshizumi

Received: 24 November 2022
Revised: 29 December 2022
Accepted: 7 January 2023
Published: 10 January 2023

Copyright: © 2023 by the authors. Licensee MDPI, Basel, Switzerland. This article is an open access article distributed under the terms and conditions of the Creative Commons Attribution (CC BY) license (https://creativecommons.org/licenses/by/4.0/).

1. Introduction

During the past decades, the laparoscopic approach in liver surgery has gained popularity, due to its various advantages compared to open surgery, which has led to its acceptance as a future new standard of care [1]. Yet, laparoscopic liver resection (LLR) has been one of the latest indications of laparoscopy, due to its prolonged learning curve and technicality [2].

Knowing that liver resection is the is the only treatment that currently offers a chance of long-term survival for colorectal liver metastases (CRLM) [3], the laparoscopic approach has been widely developed for CRLM, and LLR has shown its benefits compared to the open approach in this indication [4–6]. Paradoxically, despite two decades of the diffusion of laparoscopy, many surgeons do not perform more than 4–5 concomitant LLR for CRLM, and experts are still reluctant to recommend it [7,8]. This statement is due to the theoretical difficulty of performing multiple LLR and the lack of evidence in the literature, as many studies have a median number of one or two lesions resected at once [9].

However, the one-stage parenchymal-sparing strategy has shown its benefits compared to major hepatectomy [10,11] and to two-stage hepatectomy [12] in the open approach. Parenchymal-sparing hepatectomy in the laparoscopic approach has also shown its benefits [13–15]. Moreover, the better understanding of liver anatomy with the development of intraoperative ultrasonography in laparoscopy [16–18] should allow multiple concomitant LLR in CRLM.

The purpose of this article was to highlight updates in the field of multiple concomitant LLR for colorectal liver metastases in order to clarify its indications and help further its implementation. The international literature was reviewed and compared to our team's experience to discuss several topics: feasibility of multiple concomitant LLR for CRLM; available guidance techniques in laparoscopy for liver surgery; Short-term and long-term outcomes after multiple LLR for CRLM; feasibility and results of laparoscopic two-stage hepatectomy.

2. Feasibility of Multiple Concomitant LLR

In the study from Russolillo et al. [19], the authors aimed to assess the best outcomes in LLR based on surgical difficulty by using benchmarking. In this trial, 819 patients who underwent multiple LLR (i.e. more than one resection during the same intervention) were described, including 438 who experienced CRLM. Unfortunately, no details about the exact number of resections performed was mentioned. In the meta-analysis conducted by J Kalil et al. [14], which aimed to assess feasibility and the limitation of laparoscopic parenchymal-sparing hepatectomy, included 10 studies, from which 92 patients reported having undergone multiple LLR. In this trial, the highest number of resections reported was seven. Those two studies did not only include CRLM, which represented 58% of patients in the J Kalil et al. study. Other indications were hepatocellular carcinoma, metastatic neuroendocrine tumors, liver adenoma, and intrahepatic cholangiocarcinoma.

Only three studies specifically compared multiple and single laparoscopic resections for CRLM [20–22], and one study specifically described multiple LLR for CRLM [23]. Overall, 271 patients underwent multiple concomitant LLR for CRLM in these studies, including 69 (25.5%) patients with three to five, and 24 (8.9%) patients with more than five resections. Lesions were bilobar in 153 (56.5%) patients [20,21,23]. No difference was found regarding the maximal tumor size between multiple and single LLR [21,22].

The type of hepatectomy [20–22] is described in Table 1. Most of the patients underwent multiple atypical LLR (126 patients). For patients who underwent resections in the right lobe of the liver, 3 patients underwent multiple anterior LLR, and 11 underwent posterior LLR. The majority of the studies [20,22,23] included only limited multiple resections. No difference was found in terms of grade of difficulty according to the IMM classification [24] according to the number of LLR in Nassar et al. [22]. However, multiple LLR were significantly less associated with grade III than with single resections in the Russolillo et al. trial [19].

Compared to single resections, multiple LLR did not impact blood loss [20,22], except in the series reported by D'Hondt et al. [21]. Significantly higher blood loss for bilobar CRLM (250 mL vs. 100 mL) was described in this study. However, this result was also associated with a significantly higher rate of major resections in the bilobar LLR group (32 out of 36 patients), while other studies only reported minor hepatectomies in both multiple and single resection groups.

The conversion rate was not influenced by the number of LLR [20–22], with only 11 (4.1%) patients who required a conversion to open. As expected, operative time was significantly longer for multiple LLR than for single LLR in all studies. Operative time also significantly increased with the number of LLR, as described in Nassar et al [22] (175.3 min vs. 200.4 min vs. 234.1 min for <3, 3–5, >5 resections respectively, $p = 0.039$). Table 2 summarizes the per-operative outcomes for multiple LLR.

Table 1. Number and type of resections described in concomitant multiple LLR for CRLM.

Variable	Number of Patients Reported [20–23]	Kazaryan et al. [20] (n = 104)	D'Hondt et al. [21] (n = 36)	Nassar et al. [22] (n = 39)	Aghayan et al. [23] (n = 92)
Number of LLR					
2	178 (65.7%)				
3–4	69 (25.5%)				
≥5	24 (8.9%)				
Variable	Number of Patients Reported	Kazaryan et al. [20] (n = 104)	D'Hondt et al. [21] (n = 36)	Nassar et al. [22] (n = 39)	Aghayan et al. [23] (n = 92)
Type of LLR					Not described
Left lateral sectionectomy with right atypical	29	20	9		
Left hemihepatectomy with right atypical	1	1			
Multiple atypical resections	126	83	23	20	
Left	13/126 (10.3%)	6		7	
Right	36/126 (28.6%)	22		14	
Bilateral	77/126 (61.1%)	54	23		
Right bi-segmentectomy or hemihepatectomy with left atypical	5	1	4		

Table 2. Per-operative outcomes for patients who underwent multiple laparoscopic liver resections.

Article	Tumor Maximum Size (mm)	p (vs. Single)	Mean Blood Loss (mL Range)	p (vs. Single)	Mean Operative Time (min (Range)	p (vs. Single)	Conversion Rate	p (vs. Single)
Karazyan et al. [20] (n = 104)	22	0.12	300 (50–5000)	0.75	186 (75–390)	0.26	2.9%	0.41
D'Hondt et al. [21] (n = 36)	Not described		250 (150–450)	<0.001, higher for multiple	200 (170–230)	<0.001, longer for multiple	8.3%	0.07
Nassar et al. [22] (n = 39)	23.9	0.69	188.9 (0–1000)	0.39	217.3 (90–369)	0.039, longer for multiple	0%	0.88

In our experience, 20% of patients considered for multiple LLR needed more than three concomitant resections. Patients who underwent multiple LLR had a mean number of 2.8 lesions. In 50% of cases, multiple LLR involved only multiple atypical resections. Conversion occurred in less than 10% of patients. Operative time steeply increased with the number of LLR performed.

Overall, multiple concomitant LLR for CRLM seem to be feasible and safe. The tumor location, maximal size, or number should not be an indication to perform a single larger resection in place of multiple small resections. Parenchymal-sparing strategy seems feasible by laparoscopy for multiple CRLM. However, operative time seems to increase with the number of resections performed, but without impacting the conversion rate or blood loss.

3. Ultrasonography and Other Operative Guidance in Multiple LLR for CRLM

Intraoperative ultrasound (IOUS) is nowadays well established in liver surgery to help identify anatomic landmarks and guide liver resection. Laparoscopic IOUS is particularly interesting in LLR and used to compensate for the lack of palpation [18]. Figure 1. shows an example of laparoscopic IOUS performed by our team for multiple colorectal liver metastases localization and their relation to anatomical structure. Due to its technicality and positioning difficulties, laparoscopic IOUS can appear to be more challenging than in an open approach, especially in multiple CRLM cases. However, its performance for staging liver tumors in laparoscopy is similar compared to an open approach [25], and it should be integrated into the surgeons' habits and formation [26]. Some expert teams, in particular in Italy, proposed specific masterclasses on IOUS during liver surgery.

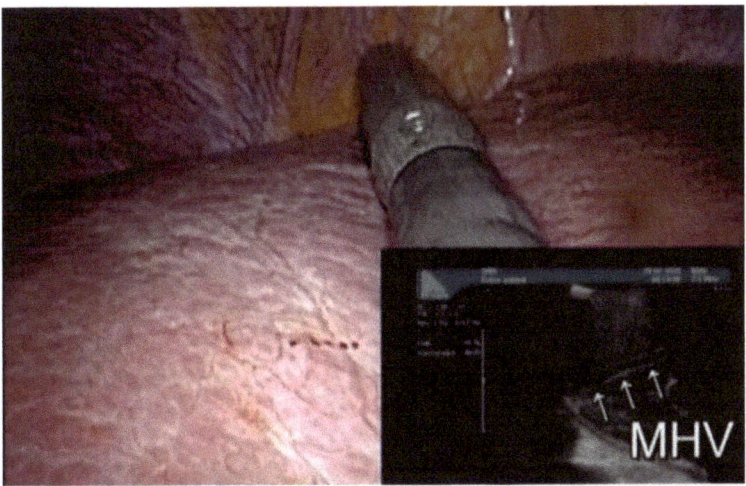
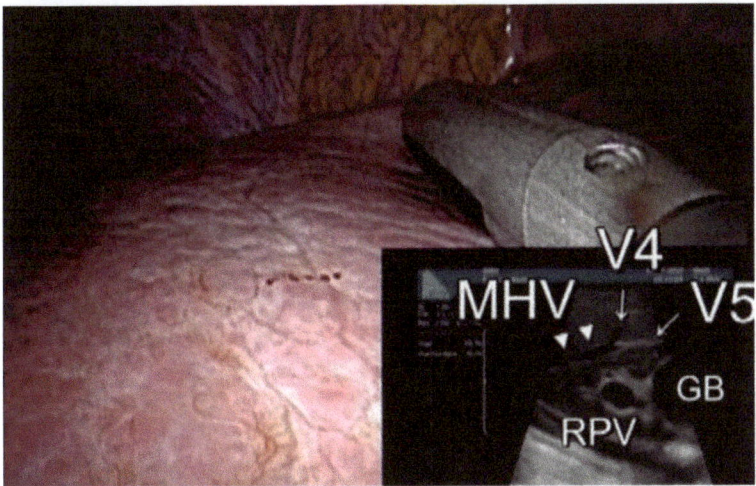

Figure 1. Laparoscopic intraoperative ultrasonography guidance. (MHV: median hepatic vein; RPV: right portal vein; GB: gall bladder; V4 and V5: hepatic veins of segment 4 and 5).

IOUS has demonstrated its accuracy in bilobar multiple one-stage resections for CRLM in the open approach [17]. No study has specifically been conducted to determine the accuracy of IOUS in multiple LLR for CRLM. However, IOUS was always described in different studies investigating multiple LLR [20–22] to guide parenchymal transection. Also, the IOUS map technique has been described recently in laparoscopy [27] and was performed in 25 patients who underwent multiple concomitant LLR. This study confirms the technical feasibility of IOUS for multiple LLR, and also suggests its effectiveness to prevent bleeding, with no major bleeding (>1000 mL) reported.

Indocyanine green (ICG) has also gained popularity as an intraoperative aid to delineating segmental boundaries and CRLM locations in LLR [28]. Showing margins of the tumors, ICG also improve complete R0 resection. Unfortunately, no study has been conducted to investigate its efficiency for multiple LLR for CRLM, and most studies published do not include multiple resections. Lu et al. [29] described ICG navigation in LLR, which included eight patients with bilobar involvement, and showed its efficiency in this indication. Figure 2 shows an example of the use of ICG for bilobar CRLM in a laparoscopic approach performed by our team.

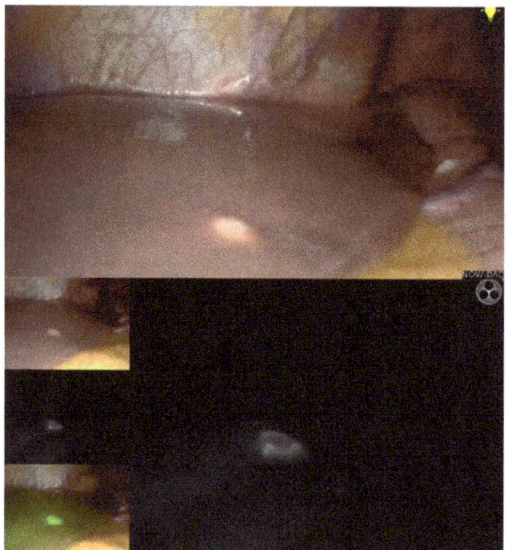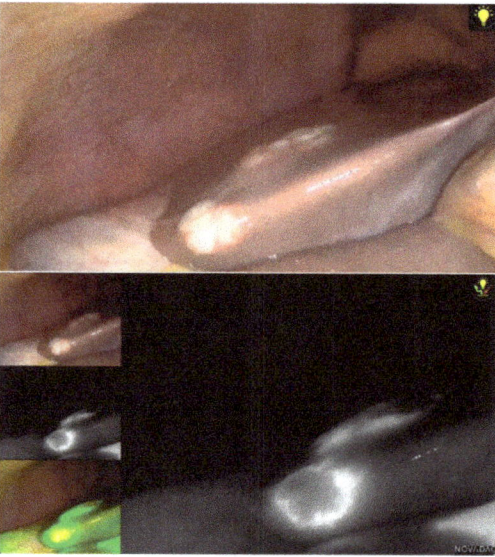

Figure 2. Laparoscopic use of ICG for multiple colorectal liver metastases. This figure is a case of multiple bilobar CRLM (upper images), and shows the effectiveness of laparoscopic ICG to determine CRLM location and margins, to ensure complete resection.

However, ICG has some limitations, mostly due to its inefficiency to identify deep lesions in the liver parenchyma [30]. However, some green staining during the parenchymal transection can guide the surgeon intraoperatively. If IOUS still offers the best assistance to locate deep lesions [30], ICG has demonstrated its capacity to have a real-time visualization of tumor margins when they are peripherical. Both IOUS and ICG are capable of detecting lesions that are not visible on preoperative CT-scans [30]. As a consequence, both IOUS and ICG could modified the operative strategy and improve complete resection.

Intraoperative real-time navigation by 3D models based on preoperative CT-scan models has demonstrated its help in an open approach for parenchymal-sparing hepatectomy in multiple CRLM [31] by estimating future liver remnants. Three-dimensional modelling has not yet been validated for the laparoscopic approach, but it could help to plan complex LLR, such as multiple resections [32]. However, 3D models could be unreliable if lesions are not detected by the preoperative CT-scan, and they should always be combined with IOUS.

The description of advantages and disadvantages of these guidance techniques are presented in Table 3.

To sum up, IOUS should remain as an aid to determine a tumor's location and burdens, but further studies should be conducted to validate indocyanine green and/or 3D modeling for multiple LLR.

Table 3. Description of available laparoscopic guidance techniques for CRLM resections.

Technique	Location of Tumors Detected	Tumor Margins	Detection of Missing Tumors from Preoperative CT Scan	Availability in OR	Disadvantages
Intraoperative ultrasound	Superficial or deep	Location relative to veins	Yes	Available	Technicality
Indocyanine green fluorescence	Only superficial	Real-time visualization	Yes, if superficial	Available	No deep lesion visualization
3D models	Superficial and deep	Location relative to anatomical structures	No	Not available	Location of tumor detected only if by preoperative CT-scan

4. Postoperative Short-Term Outcomes after Multiple LLR

No dedicated study has been made to compare the laparoscopic and open approach for multiple CRLM. However, a OSLO-COMET randomized trial [4], which compared open and laparoscopic parenchyma-sparing resections on short-term outcomes for CRLM, included multiple resections and did not reveal it as a factor of worse outcomes in the laparoscopic group.

When compared to single resections, multiple LLR were not associated with higher postoperative overall morbidity [20–22] or 90-day mortality [21,22]. Multiple LLR were even associated with significantly less liver failure in Kazaryan et al. [20] (0% vs. 8.3% for single resections), but the single LLR group in this study included 27.8% of major hepatectomy outcomes and only one in the multiple LLR group. The number of LLR did not impact the length of hospital stay [22]. The number of LLR also did not influence the achievement of the textbook outcomes [22,33]. Table 4 summarizes the postoperative outcomes for multiple LLR.

However, Russolillo et al. [19] described multiple concomitant LLR as an independent risk factor for morbidity in multivariate analysis, along with difficulty in the IMM grade of resection, bowel resection and cirrhosis, whereas it was not associated with major morbidity (i.e. Clavien III–V) [34]. Also, in this trial, patients who underwent multiple LLR had significantly higher risks of pulmonary infection (3.1%) and bowel complications (2.6%) compared to those who had single LLR. However, 11.3% of patients who had multiple LLR also had bowel resection, and the proportion of minor or major resection in the multiple LLR subgroup was unknown.

All in all, results concerning postoperative pulmonary complications are conflicting. A higher risk of pulmonary infection could be due to longer operative time [35]. However, multiple LLR for CRLM does not seems to increase major complications or postoperative mortality.

Table 4. Postoperative short- and long-term outcomes for patients who underwent multiple laparoscopic liver resection.

Article	90-Days Morbidity Rate	p (vs. Single)	Major Complication (Clavien III-IV)	p (vs. Single)	90-Days Mortality Rate (n)	p (vs. Single)	Length of Stay (Days)	p (vs. Single)	5-Year OS	p (vs. Single)	5-Year RFS	p (vs. Single)
Karazyan et al. [20] (n = 104)	20 (19.2%)	0.17	14 (13.4%)	Not described	1 (0.96%)		3 (1–26)	0.62	42%	0.62	16%	0.14
D'Hondt et al. [21] (n = 36)	2 (5.6%)	1.0	1 (2.8%)	1.0	0 (0%)	1.0	5 (4–7)	0.015, longer for multiple	66%	0.49	28%	0.62
Nassar et al. [22] (n = 39)	14 (27.5%)	0.82	1 (1.9%)	0.45	0 (0%)	0.94	5.5	0.59	Not described		Not described	

5. Oncological Outcomes after Multiple LLR for CRLM

As CRLM are numerous at the diagnosis in 80% of patients [36], and liver resection is still the best-known treatment for survival [3], many studies have investigated the impacts of multiple liver resection on long-term outcomes for CRLM.

Montalti et al. [15] described that multiple liver tumors were significantly associated with the risk of R1 margins (<1 mm), but the number of LLR performed was not specifically studied. In the three papers specifically studying multiple concomitant LLR for CRLM, the rate of R0 surgical margins was not significantly different between single and multiple LLR [20–22]. Lu et al. [29] described ICG in multiple LLR, but failed to show the difference regarding R0 margins compared to the non-ICG group.

No dedicated study has been made to compare the outcomes of a laparoscopic or an open approach for multiple CRLM. However, a recent randomized trial from Aghayan et al. [37] compared long-term outcomes between laparoscopic and open parenchymal-sparing resections for CRLM, and their findings suggested that multiple (>1) and bilobar CRLM resections did not impact overall (OS) or recurrence-free survival (RFS) in this cohort.

A trial by Bolton et al. [38] described that complex metastatic disease (defined by at least four unilobar CRLM or at least two bilobar CRLM) had a 5-year survival rate of 37% after the open approach resection. A recent multicentric study [39] described long-term outcomes in 142 patients who underwent LLR for CRLM, with a 37.1% 5-year overall survival (OS) and a median survival of 39 months. Aghayan et al. [23] described a 5-year OS of 44% in 80 patients in a multiple LLR subgroup (defined by more than two concomitant resections) who had no extrahepatic metastases.

When compared to single resections, only two studies described long-term outcomes [20,21] of multiple concomitant LLR in 140 patients with CRLM. Multiple concomitant LLR did not seem to impact OS nor RFS when compared to single resections in those studies.

Five-year OSs and RFSs are described in Table 4.

Recurrence was a liver recurrence in 74 (52.9%) patients, and liver only occurred in 43 (30.7%) patients in these two studies. Kazaryan et al. [20] described the possibility of repeat surgical procedures to treat liver recurrence for 35% of patients, without significant difference compared to single resections (25%).

In short, multiple concomitant resections do not seem to impact R0 margins rate or oncological outcomes compared to single resections. Parenchymal-sparing multiple LLR could allow for the simplest repeat hepatectomy for recurrence [23].

6. Two-Stage Laparoscopic Hepatectomy

For patients with initially unresectable bilobar extensive CRLM (i.e. multiple lesions which cannot be resected in upfront single stage surgery with R0 margins), the realization of one-stage hepatectomy is limited, due to the risk of liver failure. For those patients, two-stage hepatectomy (TSH) improved their resectability [40] and demonstrated its advantages in an open approach [41,42].

Seven studies described the role of the laparoscopic approach in TSH for CRLM [43–49]. Descriptions of the patients included in these studies are detailed in Table 5.

Overall, 131 patients were described in those studies for a median number of lesions of 5.3 CRLM [43–45,47], with 119 patients who underwent laparoscopic first-stage hepatectomy, and 87 who underwent laparoscopic second-stage hepatectomy. Between the two stages, 63 patients had portal vein embolization, and 7 patients had right portal vein ligation during the first stage. The second stage was performed after a mean interval of 3.0 months [43–45,47]. However, 18 patients dropped out between the two stages, due to tumor progression (16 patients) or insufficient future liver remnant volume (2 patients). A total of 4 patients (3.4%) in the first stage and 11 patients (12.6%) in the second stage required conversion to an open approach. The first-stage hepatectomies consisted mostly in atypical left resections (107 patients, 89.9%), and the second-stage hepatectomies consisted mostly in right hepatectomy (71 patients, 81.6%) or right-extended hepatectomy (10 patients, 11.5%).

Table 5. Data for laparoscopic two-stage hepatectomy.

Article	1st Stage Laparoscopy	2nd Stage Laparoscopy	Interval Time (Months)	Mean Number of CRLM	Conversion Rate 1st/2nd	90-Day Morbidity Rate 1st/2nd
Fuks et al. [42]	34	26	3		2/4	
Okumura et al. [43]	38	38	2.8	6	1/4	16%/26%
Kilburn et al. [44]	7	1	3.4	5.2	0/1	0%/0%
Taillieu et al. [45]	23	7	1.9	Not described	1/1	0%/14%
Di Fabio et al. [46]	8	3	2.9	4	0/1	0%/Not described
Görgec et al. [47]	Not described	12	Not described	3.6	-/2	Not described/17%
Levi Sandri et al. [48]	5	0	2.2	6.6	0/-	Not described

Compared to open TSH [44,46], laparoscopic TSH had significantly less blood loss, significantly shorter length of hospital stay, and less overall postoperative complications for both the first and second stage when realized in laparoscopy.

In our experience, all patients with totally laparoscopic TSH had right hepatectomy or right extended hepatectomy as the second stage. More than 90% of patients underwent PVE before the second hepatectomy. The 90-day morbidity rate after the first stage was less than 5%, with no major complications (Clavien III–IV). After the second stage, the 90-day morbidity was around 30%. Postoperative 90-day mortality was nil after both the first and second stage.

In terms of long-term outcomes, the OS and RFS was not different from the open TSH [43,44], with a significantly higher possibility to perform repeat hepatectomy for liver recurrences [44] (58.8% of liver recurrence was treated by repeat hepatectomy in laparoscopic TSH vs. 11.8% in the open approach). Overall survival was significantly better for the patients who completed the two stages than for the patients who did not complete the second stage.

Overall, for bilobar extended CRLM that have been initially considered unresectable, laparoscopic TSH is feasible and safe, with similar oncological outcomes to the open approach. Also, as for multiple concomitant resections, laparoscopic approach seems to simplify repeat hepatectomy for hepatic recurrence.

7. Conclusions

CRLM are one of the most developed indications of LLR. Still, surgeons tend to perform multiple liver resections in the open approach. Most of the large studies comparing the laparoscopic to the open approach for CRLM do not include multiple resections. Indeed, most surgeons favor performing LLR unilobar metastases and a limited number of nodules in the context of nonrandomized trials [50]. This review suggests that multiple concomitant LLR for CRLM seems to be feasible and safe, without impacting major short-term or long-term outcomes. The feasibility of laparoscopic liver resection does not seem to be affected by the number of lesions. However, the operative time increases with the number of resections, and could impact the postoperative pulmonary complication rate. Thus, from our point of view, for patients requiring more than five concomitant resections, laparoscopy should be considered for those selected patients and managed in expert centers. In our experience, patients with multiple CRLM have been selected to undergo multiple resections or TSH in laparoscopy when they have no history of upper abdominal surgery performed in an open approach or anesthetic contraindication to laparoscopy, as well as when no difficult resection is needed (venous reconstruction / bile duct resection). Laparoscopic TSH is also a safe alternative for initially unresectable bilobar CRLM. Moreover, laparoscopic approach for multiple CRLM, resected in one or two-stages, could improve the feasibility of repeat hepatectomy for liver recurrence of CRLM. Further dedicated studies, and more prospective comparative studies, are needed to confirm those findings. Meta-analysis on this matter should also be performed when enough material is available.

Author Contributions: Conceptualization, A.N., D.F.; Methodology, A.N., D.F.; Validation, S.T., U.M., M.G., A.D. (Alix Dhote), M.K., R.C.; Formal Analysis, A.N.; Investigation, A.N.; Resources, A.N., A.D. (Alix Dhote), M.S.; Data Curation, A.N., A.D. (Alix Dhote), M.S., Writing—Original Draft Preparation, A.N.; Writing—Review and Editing, S.T., A.D. (Alix Dhote), M.S., R.C., M.K., A.D. (Anthony Dohan), U.M., M.G., D.F.; Visualization, A.N., D.F.; Supervision, D.F.; Project Administration, D.F. All authors have read and agreed to the published version of the manuscript.

Funding: This research received no external funding.

Conflicts of Interest: The authors declare no conflict of interest.

References

1. Abu Hilal, M.; Aldrighetti, L.; Dagher, I.; Edwin, B.; Troisi, R.I.; Alikhanov, R.; Aroori, S.; Belli, G.; Besselink, M.; Briceno, J.; et al. The Southampton Consensus Guidelines for Laparoscopic Liver Surgery: From Indication to Implementation. *Ann. Surg.* **2018**, *268*, 11–18. [CrossRef] [PubMed]
2. Halls, M.C.; Alseidi, A.; Berardi, G.; Cipriani, F.; Van der Poel, M.; Davila, D.; Ciria, R.; Besselink, M.; D'Hondt, M.; Dagher, I.; et al. A Comparison of the Learning Curves of Laparoscopic Liver Surgeons in Differing Stages of the IDEAL Paradigm of Surgical Innovation: Standing on the Shoulders of Pioneers. *Ann. Surg.* **2019**, *269*, 221–228. [CrossRef]
3. Phelip, J.M.; Tougeron, D.; Léonard, D.; Benhaim, L.; Desolneux, G.; Dupré, A.; Michel, P.; Penna, C.; Tournigand, C.; Louvet, C.; et al. Metastatic Colorectal Cancer (MCRC): French Intergroup Clinical Practice Guidelines for Diagnosis, Treatments and Follow-up (SNFGE, FFCD, GERCOR, UNICANCER, SFCD, SFED, SFRO, SFR). *Dig. Liver Dis.* **2019**, *51*, 1357–1363. [CrossRef] [PubMed]
4. Fretland, Å.A.; Dagenborg, V.J.; Bjørnelv, G.M.W.; Kazaryan, A.M.; Kristiansen, R.; Fagerland, M.W.; Hausken, J.; Tønnessen, T.I.; Abildgaard, A.; Barkhatov, L.; et al. Laparoscopic Versus Open Resection for Colorectal Liver Metastases: The OSLO-COMET Randomized Controlled Trial. *Ann. Surg.* **2018**, *267*, 199–207. [CrossRef]
5. Robles-Campos, R.; Lopez-Lopez, V.; Brusadin, R.; Lopez-Conesa, A.; Gil-Vazquez, P.J.; Navarro-Barrios, Á.; Parrilla, P. Open versus Minimally Invasive Liver Surgery for Colorectal Liver Metastases (LapOpHuva): A Prospective Randomized Controlled Trial. *Surg. Endosc.* **2019**, *33*, 3926–3936. [CrossRef] [PubMed]
6. Zhang, X.-L.; Liu, R.-F.; Zhang, D.; Zhang, Y.-S.; Wang, T. Laparoscopic versus Open Liver Resection for Colorectal Liver Metastases: A Systematic Review and Meta-Analysis of Studies with Propensity Score-Based Analysis. *Int. J. Surg.* **2017**, *44*, 191–203. [CrossRef]
7. Buell, J.F.; Cherqui, D.; Geller, D.A.; O'Rourke, N.; Iannitti, D.; Dagher, I.; Koffron, A.J.; Thomas, M.; Gayet, B.; Han, H.S.; et al. The International Position on Laparoscopic Liver Surgery: The Louisville Statement, 2008. *Ann. Surg.* **2009**, *250*, 825–830. [CrossRef]
8. Wakabayashi, G.; Cherqui, D.; Geller, D.A.; Buell, J.F.; Kaneko, H.; Han, H.S.; Asbun, H.; O'Rourke, N.; Tanabe, M.; Koffron, A.J.; et al. Recommendations for Laparoscopic Liver Resection: A Report from the Second International Consensus Conference Held in Morioka. *Ann. Surg.* **2015**, *261*, 619–629. [CrossRef]
9. van der Werf, L.R.; Kok, N.F.M.; Buis, C.I.; Grünhagen, D.J.; Hoogwater, F.J.H.; Swijnenburg, R.J.; den Dulk, M.; Dejong, K.C.H.C.; Klaase, J.M. Dutch Hepato Biliary Audit Group Implementation and First Results of a Mandatory, Nationwide Audit on Liver Surgery. *HPB* **2019**, *21*, 1400–1410. [CrossRef]
10. Alvarez, F.A.; Sanchez Claria, R.; Oggero, S.; de Santibañes, E. Parenchymal-Sparing Liver Surgery in Patients with Colorectal Carcinoma Liver Metastases. *World J. Gastrointest. Surg.* **2016**, *8*, 407–423. [CrossRef]
11. Gold, J.S.; Are, C.; Kornprat, P.; Jarnagin, W.R.; Gönen, M.; Fong, Y.; DeMatteo, R.P.; Blumgart, L.H.; D'Angelica, M. Increased Use of Parenchymal-Sparing Surgery for Bilateral Liver Metastases from Colorectal Cancer Is Associated with Improved Mortality without Change in Oncologic Outcome: Trends in Treatment over Time in 440 Patients. *Ann. Surg.* **2008**, *247*, 109–117. [CrossRef]
12. Torzilli, G.; Viganò, L.; Cimino, M.; Imai, K.; Vibert, E.; Donadon, M.; Mansour, D.; Castaing, D.; Adam, R. Is Enhanced One-Stage Hepatectomy a Safe and Feasible Alternative to the Two-Stage Hepatectomy in the Setting of Multiple Bilobar Colorectal Liver Metastases? A Comparative Analysis between Two Pioneering Centers. *Dig. Surg.* **2018**, *35*, 323–332. [CrossRef] [PubMed]
13. Okumura, S.; Tabchouri, N.; Leung, U.; Tinguely, P.; Louvet, C.; Beaussier, M.; Gayet, B.; Fuks, D. Laparoscopic Parenchymal-Sparing Hepatectomy for Multiple Colorectal Liver Metastases Improves Outcomes and Salvageability: A Propensity Score-Matched Analysis. *Ann. Surg. Oncol.* **2019**, *26*, 4576–4586. [CrossRef] [PubMed]
14. Kalil, J.A.; Poirier, J.; Becker, B.; Van Dam, R.; Keutgen, X.; Schadde, E. Laparoscopic Parenchymal-Sparing Hepatectomy: The New Maximally Minimal Invasive Surgery of the Liver-a Systematic Review and Meta-Analysis. *J. Gastrointest. Surg.* **2019**, *23*, 860–869. [CrossRef] [PubMed]

15. Montalti, R.; Tomassini, F.; Laurent, S.; Smeets, P.; De Man, M.; Geboes, K.; Libbrecht, L.J.; Troisi, R.I. Impact of Surgical Margins on Overall and Recurrence-Free Survival in Parenchymal-Sparing Laparoscopic Liver Resections of Colorectal Metastases. *Surg. Endosc.* **2015**, *29*, 2736–2747. [CrossRef]
16. Ferrero, A.; Lo Tesoriere, R.; Russolillo, N.; Viganò, L.; Forchino, F.; Capussotti, L. Ultrasound-Guided Laparoscopic Liver Resections. *Surg. Endosc.* **2015**, *29*, 1002–1005. [CrossRef]
17. Torzilli, G.; Procopio, F.; Botea, F.; Marconi, M.; Del Fabbro, D.; Donadon, M.; Palmisano, A.; Spinelli, A.; Montorsi, M. One-Stage Ultrasonographically Guided Hepatectomy for Multiple Bilobar Colorectal Metastases: A Feasible and Effective Alternative to the 2-Stage Approach. *Surgery* **2009**, *146*, 60–71. [CrossRef]
18. Langella, S.; Russolillo, N.; D'Eletto, M.; Forchino, F.; Lo Tesoriere, R.; Ferrero, A. Oncological Safety of Ultrasound-Guided Laparoscopic Liver Resection for Colorectal Metastases: A Case-Control Study. *Updates Surg.* **2015**, *67*, 147–155. [CrossRef]
19. Russolillo, N.; Aldrighetti, L.; Cillo, U.; Guglielmi, A.; Ettorre, G.M.; Giuliante, F.; Mazzaferro, V.; Dalla Valle, R.; De Carlis, L.; Jovine, E.; et al. Risk-Adjusted Benchmarks in Laparoscopic Liver Surgery in a National Cohort. *Br. J. Surg.* **2020**, *107*, 845–853. [CrossRef]
20. Kazaryan, A.M.; Aghayan, D.L.; Barkhatov, L.I.; Fretland, Å.A.; Edwin, B. Laparoscopic Multiple Parenchyma-Sparing Concomitant Liver Resections for Colorectal Liver Metastases. *Surg. Laparosc. Endosc. Percutan. Tech.* **2019**, *29*, 187–193. [CrossRef]
21. D'Hondt, M.; Pironet, Z.; Parmentier, I.; De Meyere, C.; Besselink, M.; Pottel, H.; Vansteenkiste, F.; Verslype, C. One-Stage Laparoscopic Parenchymal Sparing Liver Resection for Bilobar Colorectal Liver Metastases: Safety, Recurrence Patterns and Oncologic Outcomes. *Surg. Endosc.* **2022**, *36*, 1018–1026. [CrossRef] [PubMed]
22. Nassar, A.; Tribillon, E.; Marchese, U.; Faermark, N.; Bonnet, S.; Beaussier, M.; Gayet, B.; Fuks, D. Feasibility and Outcomes of Multiple Simultaneous Laparoscopic Liver Resections. *Surg. Endosc.* **2022**, *36*, 2466–2472. [CrossRef]
23. Aghayan, D.L.; Pelanis, E.; Avdem Fretland, Å.; Kazaryan, A.M.; Sahakyan, M.A.; Røsok, B.I.; Barkhatov, L.; Bjørnbeth, B.A.; Jakob Elle, O.; Edwin, B. Laparoscopic Parenchyma-Sparing Liver Resection for Colorectal Metastases. *Radiol. Oncol.* **2018**, *52*, 36–41. [CrossRef]
24. Kawaguchi, Y.; Fuks, D.; Kokudo, N.; Gayet, B. Difficulty of Laparoscopic Liver Resection: Proposal for a New Classification. *Ann. Surg.* **2018**, *267*, 13–17. [CrossRef]
25. Viganò, L.; Ferrero, A.; Amisano, M.; Russolillo, N.; Capussotti, L. Comparison of laparoscopic and open intraoperative ultrasonography for staging liver tumours. *Br. J. Surg.* **2013**, *100*, 535–542. [CrossRef] [PubMed]
26. Kamiyama, T.; Kakisaka, T.; Orimo, T. Current role of intraoperative ultrasonography in hepatectomy. *Surg. Today* **2021**, *51*, 1887–1896. [CrossRef] [PubMed]
27. Ferrero, A.; Lo Tesoriere, R.; Russolillo, N. Ultrasound Liver Map Technique for Laparoscopic Liver Resections. *World J. Surg.* **2019**, *43*, 2607–2611. [CrossRef]
28. Wang, X.; Teh, C.S.C.; Ishizawa, T.; Aoki, T.; Cavallucci, D.; Lee, S.-Y.; Panganiban, K.M.; Perini, M.V.; Shah, S.R.; Wang, H.; et al. Consensus Guidelines for the Use of Fluorescence Imaging in Hepatobiliary Surgery. *Ann. Surg.* **2021**, *274*, 97–106. [CrossRef]
29. Lu, H.; Gu, J.; Qian, X.-F.; Dai, X.-Z. Indocyanine Green Fluorescence Navigation in Laparoscopic Hepatectomy: A Retrospective Single-Center Study of 120 Cases. *Surg. Today* **2021**, *51*, 695–702. [CrossRef]
30. Takahashi, H.; Zaidi, N.; Berber, E. An initial report on the intraoperative use of indocyanine green fluorescence imaging in the surgical management of liver tumorss. *J. Surg. Oncol.* **2016**, *114*, 625–629. [CrossRef]
31. Procopio, F.; Cimino, M.; Viganò, L.; Colombo, A.E.; Franchi, E.; Costa, G.; Donadon, M.; Del Fabbro, D.; Torzilli, G. Prediction of Remnant Liver Volume Using 3D Simulation Software in Patients Undergoing R1vasc Parenchyma-Sparing Hepatectomy for Multiple Bilobar Colorectal Liver Metastases: Reliability, Clinical Impact, and Learning Curve. *HPB* **2021**, *23*, 1084–1094. [CrossRef] [PubMed]
32. Witowski, J.; Budzyński, A.; Grochowska, A.; Ballard, D.H.; Major, P.; Rubinkiewicz, M.; Złahoda-Huzior, A.; Popiela, T.J.; Wierdak, M.; Pędziwiatr, M. Decision-making based on 3D printed models in laparoscopic liver resections with intraoperative ultrasound: A prospective observational study. *Eur. Radiol.* **2020**, *30*, 1306–1312. [CrossRef] [PubMed]
33. Tsilimigras, D.I.; Sahara, K.; Moris, D.; Mehta, R.; Paredes, A.Z.; Ratti, F.; Marques, H.P.; Soubrane, O.; Lam, V.; Poultsides, G.A.; et al. Assessing Textbook Outcomes Following Liver Surgery for Primary Liver Cancer Over a 12-Year Time Period at Major Hepatobiliary Centers. *Ann. Surg. Oncol.* **2020**, *27*, 3318–3327. [CrossRef] [PubMed]
34. Dindo, D.; Demartines, N.; Clavien, P.-A. Classification of Surgical Complications: A New Proposal with Evaluation in a Cohort of 6336 Patients and Results of a Survey. *Ann. Surg.* **2004**, *240*, 205–213. [CrossRef] [PubMed]
35. Nobili, C.; Marzano, E.; Oussoultzoglou, E.; Rosso, E.; Addeo, P.; Bachellier, P.; Jaeck, D.; Pessaux, P. Multivariate Analysis of Risk Factors for Pulmonary Complications after Hepatic Resection. *Ann. Surg.* **2012**, *255*, 540–550. [CrossRef]
36. Manfredi, S.; Lepage, C.; Hatem, C.; Coatmeur, O.; Faivre, J.; Bouvier, A.-M. Epidemiology and Management of Liver Metastases from Colorectal Cancer. *Ann. Surg.* **2006**, *244*, 254–259. [CrossRef]
37. Aghayan, D.L.; Kazaryan, A.M.; Dagenborg, V.J.; Røsok, B.I.; Fagerland, M.W.; Waaler Bjørnelv, G.M.; Kristiansen, R.; Flatmark, K.; Fretland, Å.A.; Edwin, B.; et al. Long-Term Oncologic Outcomes After Laparoscopic Versus Open Resection for Colorectal Liver Metastases: A Randomized Trial. *Ann. Intern. Med.* **2021**, *174*, 175–182. [CrossRef]
38. Bolton, J.S.; Fuhrman, G.M. Survival after Resection of Multiple Bilobar Hepatic Metastases from Colorectal Carcinoma. *Ann. Surg.* **2000**, *231*, 743–751. [CrossRef]

39. Gumbs, A.A.; Croner, R.; Lorenz, E.; Cacciaguerra, A.B.; Tsai, T.-J.; Starker, L.; Flanagan, J.; Yu, N.J.; Chouillard, E.; Abu Hilal, M. Survival Study: International Multicentric Minimally Invasive Liver Resection for Colorectal Liver Metastases (SIMMILR-2). *Cancers* **2022**, *14*, 4190. [CrossRef]
40. Adam, R.; Laurent, A.; Azoulay, D.; Castaing, D.; Bismuth, H. Two-Stage Hepatectomy: A Planned Strategy to Treat Irresectable Liver Tumors. *Ann. Surg.* **2000**, *232*, 777–785. [CrossRef]
41. Jaeck, D.; Oussoultzoglou, E.; Rosso, E.; Greget, M.; Weber, J.-C.; Bachellier, P. A Two-Stage Hepatectomy Procedure Combined with Portal Vein Embolization to Achieve Curative Resection for Initially Unresectable Multiple and Bilobar Colorectal Liver Metastases. *Ann. Surg.* **2004**, *240*, 1037–1049; discussion 1049–1051. [CrossRef]
42. Wicherts, D.A.; Miller, R.; de Haas, R.J.; Bitsakou, G.; Vibert, E.; Veilhan, L.-A.; Azoulay, D.; Bismuth, H.; Castaing, D.; Adam, R. Long-Term Results of Two-Stage Hepatectomy for Irresectable Colorectal Cancer Liver Metastases. *Ann. Surg.* **2008**, *248*, 994–1005. [CrossRef]
43. Fuks, D.; Nomi, T.; Ogiso, S.; Gelli, M.; Velayutham, V.; Conrad, C.; Louvet, C.; Gayet, B. Laparoscopic Two-Stage Hepatectomy for Bilobar Colorectal Liver Metastases. *Br. J. Surg.* **2015**, *102*, 1684–1690. [CrossRef]
44. Okumura, S.; Goumard, C.; Gayet, B.; Fuks, D.; Scatton, O. Laparoscopic versus Open Two-Stage Hepatectomy for Bilobar Colorectal Liver Metastases: A Bi-Institutional, Propensity Score-Matched Study. *Surgery* **2019**, *166*, 959–966. [CrossRef]
45. Kilburn, D.J.; Chiow, A.K.H.; Lewin, J.; Kienzle, N.; Cavallucci, D.J.; Bryant, R.; O'Rourke, N. Laparoscopic Approach to a Planned Two-Stage Hepatectomy for Bilobar Colorectal Liver Metastases. *ANZ J. Surg.* **2016**, *86*, 811–815. [CrossRef]
46. Taillieu, E.; De Meyere, C.; D'Hondt, M. The Role of the Laparoscopic Approach in Two-Stage Hepatectomy for Colorectal Liver Metastases: A Single-Center Experience. *Surg. Endosc.* **2022**, *36*, 559–568. [CrossRef] [PubMed]
47. Di Fabio, F.; Whistance, R.; Rahman, S.; Primrose, J.N.; Pearce, N.W.; Abu Hilal, M. Exploring the Role of Laparoscopic Surgery in Two-Stage Hepatectomy for Bilobar Colorectal Liver Metastases. *J. Laparoendosc. Adv. Surg. Tech. A* **2012**, *22*, 647–650. [CrossRef] [PubMed]
48. Görgec, B.; Suhool, A.; Al-Jarrah, R.; Fontana, M.; Tehami, N.A.; Modi, S.; Abu Hilal, M. Surgical Technique and Clinical Results of One- or Two-Stage Laparoscopic Right Hemihepatectomy after Portal Vein Embolization in Patients with Initially Unresectable Colorectal Liver Metastases: A Case Series. *Int. J. Surg.* **2020**, *77*, 69–75. [CrossRef]
49. Levi Sandri, G.B.; Santoro, R.; Vennarecci, G.; Lepiane, P.; Colasanti, M.; Ettorre, G.M. Two-Stage Hepatectomy, a 10 Years Experience. *Updates Surg.* **2015**, *67*, 401–405. [CrossRef] [PubMed]
50. Cheng, Y.; Zhang, L.; Li, H.; Wang, L.; Huang, Y.; Wu, L.; Zhang, Y. Laparoscopic versus open liver resection for colorectal liver metastases: A systematic review. *J. Surg. Res.* **2017**, *220*, 234–246. [CrossRef]

Disclaimer/Publisher's Note: The statements, opinions and data contained in all publications are solely those of the individual author(s) and contributor(s) and not of MDPI and/or the editor(s). MDPI and/or the editor(s) disclaim responsibility for any injury to people or property resulting from any ideas, methods, instructions or products referred to in the content.

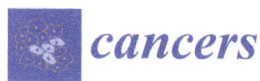

Article

Surgical and Oncological Outcomes of Salvage Hepatectomy for Locally Recurrent Hepatocellular Carcinoma after Locoregional Therapy: A Single-Institution Experience

Takuya Minagawa [1], Osamu Itano [1,*], Minoru Kitago [2], Yuta Abe [2], Hiroshi Yagi [2], Taizo Hibi [3], Masahiro Shinoda [1], Hidenori Ojima [4], Michiie Sakamoto [4] and Yuko Kitagawa [2]

[1] Department of Hepato-Biliary-Pancreatic and Gastrointestinal Surgery, School of Medicine, International University of Health and Welfare, Chiba 286-0124, Japan; tminagawa@iuhw.ac.jp (T.M.); masa02114@yahoo.co.jp (M.S.)
[2] Departments of Surgery, Keio University School of Medicine, Tokyo 160-8582, Japan; dragonpegasus427@gmail.com (M.K.); abey3666@gmail.com (Y.A.); hy0624@gmail.com (H.Y.); kitagawa.a3@keio.jp (Y.K.)
[3] Department of Pediatric Surgery and Transplantation, Kumamoto University Graduate School of Medical Sciences, Kumamoto 860-8556, Japan; taizohibi@gmail.com
[4] Departments of Pathology, Keio University School of Medicine, Tokyo 160-8582, Japan; hojima@a3.keio.jp (H.O.); msakamot@z5.keio.jp (M.S.)
* Correspondence: itano@iuhw.ac.jp; Tel.: +81-476-35-5600

Simple Summary: For 35 patients with recurrent HCC after primary hepatectomy and 67 patients with recurrent HCC after locoregional therapies, surgical and oncological outcomes were examined. Pathologic review revealed 30 patients with locally recurrent HCC after locoregional therapy (LR-HCC). Background liver function was significantly worse in patients with recurrent HCC after locoregional therapy. Serum levels of AFP and AFP-L3 were significantly higher in patients with LR-HCC. Perioperative morbidities were observed in significantly more patients with recurrent HCC after locoregional therapies. Long-term outcomes of recurrent HCC after locoregional therapies were worse than those after hepatectomy, though there was no prognostic difference according to the recurrence patterns after locoregional therapies. Multivariate analyses showed that prognostic factors for resected recurrent HCC were previous locoregional therapy, multiple HCCs, and portal venous invasion, whereas LR-HCC was not a prognostic factor. In conclusion, salvage hepatectomy for LR-HCC showed worse surgical outcomes but a favorable prognosis.

Abstract: Surgical and oncological outcomes of hepatectomy for recurrent hepatocellular carcinoma (HCC) after locoregional therapy, including locally recurrent HCC (LR-HCC), were examined. Among 273 consecutive patients who underwent hepatectomy for HCC, 102 with recurrent HCC were included and retrospectively reviewed. There were 35 patients with recurrent HCC after primary hepatectomy and 67 with recurrent HCC after locoregional therapies. Pathologic review revealed 30 patients with LR-HCC. Background liver function was significantly worse in patients with recurrent HCC after locoregional therapy ($p = 0.002$). AFP ($p = 0.031$) and AFP-L3 ($p = 0.033$) serum levels were significantly higher in patients with LR-HCC. Perioperative morbidities were significantly more frequently observed with recurrent HCC after locoregional therapies ($p = 0.048$). Long-term outcomes of recurrent HCC after locoregional therapies were worse than those after hepatectomy, though there was no prognostic difference according to the recurrence patterns after locoregional therapies. Multivariate analyses showed that prognostic factors for resected recurrent HCC were previous locoregional therapy (hazard ratio [HR] 2.0; $p = 0.005$), multiple HCCs (HR 2.8; $p < 0.001$), and portal venous invasion (HR 2.3; $p = 0.001$). LR-HCC was not a prognostic factor. In conclusion, salvage hepatectomy for LR-HCC showed worse surgical outcomes but a favorable prognosis.

Citation: Minagawa, T.; Itano, O.; Kitago, M.; Abe, Y.; Yagi, H.; Hibi, T.; Shinoda, M.; Ojima, H.; Sakamoto, M.; Kitagawa, Y. Surgical and Oncological Outcomes of Salvage Hepatectomy for Locally Recurrent Hepatocellular Carcinoma after Locoregional Therapy: A Single-Institution Experience. *Cancers* **2023**, *15*, 2320. https://doi.org/10.3390/cancers15082320

Academic Editor: Alessandro Vitale

Received: 17 February 2023
Revised: 8 April 2023
Accepted: 12 April 2023
Published: 16 April 2023

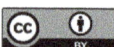

Copyright: © 2023 by the authors. Licensee MDPI, Basel, Switzerland. This article is an open access article distributed under the terms and conditions of the Creative Commons Attribution (CC BY) license (https://creativecommons.org/licenses/by/4.0/).

Keywords: hepatocellular carcinoma; salvage hepatectomy; locoregional therapy; radiofrequency ablation; transarterial chemoembolization; local recurrence

1. Introduction

Hepatocellular carcinoma (HCC) is the fifth most fatal disease in the world, and it is especially prevalent in Eastern Asia [1]. The recurrence rate remains high even after curative treatment is performed. The incidence of intrahepatic recurrence within 2 years after primary resection for primary HCC is almost 70% [2]. It is important to develop an optimal strategy for improving the prognosis. The treatment strategy for HCC is proposed depending on the tumor status and the patient's liver function. Although several guidelines indicate the staging and recommend optimal treatment for primary HCC [3–6], there has not been any suggested treatment for recurrent HCC after locoregional therapy such as radiofrequency ablation (RFA) or transarterial chemoembolization (TACE). It has been noted in the Japanese guidelines for HCC that a curative treatment strategy that takes hepatic functional reserve into account should be designed for recurrent HCC after RFA [4]. However, the guidelines fall short on the specifics. In clinical practice, because of impaired liver function or declined performance status of the patient, sequential local therapy tends to be selected even after local recurrence.

In addition, no definitive strategy has been clarified in any guidelines according to patterns of recurrence: multicentric recurrence, intrahepatic metastasis, and local recurrence. Locally recurrent HCC after RFA has been thought to be more invasive and needs extensive liver resection [7–11]. Although 5-year recurrence-free survival (RFS) after salvage surgery for recurrent HCC was reported as 0–33%, 5-year overall survival (OS) was revealed to be 43–67% [9–11]. On the other hand, the prognosis of the remaining viable HCC after repeated TACE is not fully understood. It is also still unclear whether salvage surgery for locally recurrent HCC after TACE is beneficial.

In this study, we retrospectively evaluated the clinical characteristics of recurrent HCC after locoregional therapy, in particular, locally recurrent HCC after locoregional therapy (LR-HCC). We also studied the perioperative and oncological outcomes of salvage surgery for LR-HCC.

2. Materials and Methods

2.1. Study Population

A retrospective review of an HCC database was performed. Consecutive patients who had undergone hepatectomy with curative intent between January 2004 and April 2015 were analyzed. This study only included patients who had undergone curative hepatectomy as the first treatment for recurrent HCC. Patients who had undergone re-hepatectomy for recurrent HCC were analyzed, whereas those who had undergone a second or more hepatectomy for recurrent HCC were excluded because they were at risk of double counting as participants in this study. All patients had a confirmed pathologic diagnosis of HCC. The study was approved by the institutional review board of Keio University School of Medicine (unique number: 20122080) and met the standards of the Declaration of Helsinki and the Ethical Guidelines for Clinical Studies of the Ministry of Health, Labour, and Welfare of Japan. This study was registered with the University Hospital Medical Information Network Center (UMIN000014691).

2.2. Diagnostic Criteria of Recurrent HCC

Patients after curative treatment for HCC were routinely managed by the sequential follow-up protocol, which consisted of contrast-enhanced computed tomography (CT) or ethoxybenzyl diethylenetriamine pentaacetic acid-enhanced magnetic resonance imaging (EOB-MRI) of the liver within 3 months after the therapy and thereafter every 3 months. Recurrent HCC was diagnosed based on nodules detected by these imaging studies and/or pathologic examinations, such as needle or excisional biopsy, according to the diagnostic algorithm for HCC proposed by the Liver Cancer Study Group of Japan [12].

2.3. Treatment Strategy

The treatment strategy for HCC was mainly according to the Japanese guidelines for HCC [2] and was determined by a cluster conference consisting of gastroenterological physicians, radiologists, pathologists, and hepatobiliary surgeons at Keio University Hospital. The hepatectomy was performed by board-certified hepatobiliary surgeons. RFA was performed by well-experienced gastroenterological physicians using a percutaneous, transhepatic approach guided by ultrasonography. TACE was performed by skilled radiologists.

The indications for salvage hepatectomy were mainly classified into the following categories: technical difficulty of repeated locoregional treatment, tumor thrombus, local recurrence after locoregional therapy, and patient preference. The suitable procedure and approach were selected by experienced hepatobiliary surgeons, taking into account the tumor characteristics and the remnant liver function.

Adjuvant systemic chemotherapy and/or local therapy were not routinely administered, even to patients with recurrent HCC. In cases of extrahepatic recurrence after hepatectomy, multidisciplinary treatment, including systemic chemotherapy, radiation therapy, and hepatic arterial infusion chemotherapy, was chosen depending on the patient and tumor condition.

2.4. Definition of LR-HCC and OR-HCC

Among intrahepatic recurrence of HCC, LR-HCC was microscopically defined by pathologists as follows: viable tumor cells adjacent to necrotic tissue due to locoregional therapy; morphological similarity to coagulated necrotic tumor cells, which were evaluated by silver stain especially focused on structure and nuclear atypia. In the case of viable tumor cells left in the targeted area of locoregional therapy, the transitional area from the coagulated necrotic tissue was also evaluated. On the other hand, other types of recurrent HCC (OR-HCC) were defined as recurrent HCC that did not meet the definition of LR-HCC above.

2.5. Statistical Analysis

Categorical variables were compared using the chi-square test or Fisher's exact test, as appropriate. Continuous variables were compared using the Mann–Whitney U test. Survival was analyzed using Kaplan–Meier curves and the log-rank test. OS, RFS, and disease-specific survival (DSS) were calculated using the date of the first operation for recurrent HCC. In the total cohort study, the expected deviation in the patients' backgrounds between the hepatectomy and locoregional groups was calculated, and DSS was evaluated for their prognoses. The optimum cut-off values of each continuous parameter for RFS were determined using the minimum p-values calculated using the log-rank test. Hazard ratios were estimated by univariate and multivariate survival analyses using the Cox regression model. Variables with $p < 0.10$ in the univariate log-rank test were further explored in the multivariate setting. Differences were considered statistically significant at $p < 0.05$. All analyses were performed using the SPSS software program, version 28.0 (IBM Corp., Chicago, IL, USA).

3. Results

3.1. Patient and Tumor Background

We retrospectively reviewed 273 consecutively resected HCC cases at a single center. After excluding 132 cases that underwent hepatectomy only for the primary HCC and not for the recurrent HCC and 39 cases that underwent repeated liver resections for recurrent HCC, 102 resected recurrent HCC cases were extracted.

The clinicopathological characteristics and comparisons according to the previous treatment modalities are listed in Table 1. A total of 35 cases had recurrent HCC after hepatectomy (17 cases after anatomical resection and 18 cases after non-anatomical resection), and 67 cases had recurrent HCC after locoregional therapy (39 cases after RFA and 28 cases after TACE). There were no differences in liver function and tumor markers between the previous treatment modalities. The number of therapies that had been given before was higher in the locoregional treatment group ($p < 0.001$). Surgical outcomes were not significantly different between the two groups except for postoperative complications. The tumors in the locoregional treatment group were significantly larger ($p = 0.018$). In addition, cirrhosis was observed significantly more frequently in the locoregional treatment group ($p = 0.002$). There were no other differences in pathologic features between the two groups. As for surgical margins, all the tumors considered to be positive were microscopically positive (R1). The median follow-up period was 85 months, and the median OS after surgery for recurrence was 83 months. Both OS and RFS of the locoregional therapy group were significantly worse than those of the hepatectomy group (Figure 1A,B). However, the DSS was not significantly different between the two groups (Figure 1C). At the time of initial recurrence, 19 patients had extrahepatic metastases (Table 1), and those who opted for systemic chemotherapy chose sorafenib or the folinate/uracil/tegafur regimen.

Table 1. Patient characteristics stratified by the previous treatment modalities.

Variables	Recurrence after Hepatectomy ($n = 35$)	Recurrence after Locoregional Therapy ($n = 67$)	p-Value
Age (year, median)	70 (33–82)	71 (50–86)	0.73
Sex			0.58
Female	9	14	
Male	26	53	
Etiology			0.114
HBV	14	16	
HBV + HCV	0	1	
HCV	12	38	
NBNC	9	9	
Child–Pugh classification			0.296
A	35	63	
B	0	4	
Liver damage			0.206
A	32	53	
B	3	13	
C	0	1	
Platelet count ($\times 10^3/\mu L$, median)	13.6 (5.1–28.5)	11.8 (4.1–37.4)	0.347
AFP (ng/mL, median)	6 (2–18,000)	10 (0–80,977)	0.286
AFP-L3 (%, median)	7.2 (0–50.3)	9.2 (0–84.9)	0.304
DCP (mAU/mL, median)	21 (9–5220)	25 (7–23,000)	0.956
Number of pretreatments	1 (1–19)	3 (1–10)	<0.001
Surgical approach			0.883
Open	23	45	
Laparoscopic	12	22	
Procedures			0.13
Partial resection	27	44	
Segmentectomy	1	5	
Sectionectomy	6	8	
Hemihepatectomy	1	10	
Operation time (min, median)	291 (118–780)	359 (84–1500)	0.087
Estimated blood loss (g, median)	300 (1–4560)	300 (1–16,156)	0.915
Morbidities (Clavien–Dindo $\geq$ IIIa)			0.048
No	28	40	
Yes	7	26	

Table 1. Cont.

Variables	Recurrence after Hepatectomy (n = 35)	Recurrence after Locoregional Therapy (n = 67)	p-Value
Postoperative hospital stay (day, median)	13 (6–40)	15 (4–217)	0.313
Tumor multiplicity			0.236
Solitary	20	30	
Multiple	15	37	
Tumor size (mm, median)	18 (6–42)	20 (7–140)	0.018
Histology			0.429
Well	4	7	
Moderate	23	50	
Poor	7	10	
Other	1	0	
Portal venous invasion			0.532
No	19	32	
Yes	16	35	
Hepatic venous invasion			0.658
No	34	63	
Yes	1	4	
Hepatic arterial invasion			1
No	35	66	
Yes	0	1	
Bile duct invasion			0.658
No	34	63	
Yes	1	4	
Surgical margin			0.678
Negative	26	48	
Positive	7	16	
Background liver condition			0.002
Normal	2	0	
Chronic hepatitis	24	30	
Cirrhosis	7	33	
Initial recurrence site			0.136
Liver	19	41	
Extrahepatic	0	5	
Both	3	11	
Recurrence pattern in liver			0.662
Intrahepatic metastasis/Multicentric occurrence	22	47	
Local recurrence	1	5	

Categorical data are expressed as n (%). Continuous variables are presented as the median [range]. AFP, alpha-fetoprotein; AFP-L3, lens culinaris agglutinin-reactive AFP; DCP, des-γ-carboxy prothrombin; HBV, hepatitis B virus; HCV, hepatitis C virus; NBNC, non-HBV non-HCV.

3.2. Clinicopathologic Characteristics of Patients with LR-HCC

The recurrence pattern was assessed by the pathologic review: 30 cases were diagnosed as LR-HCC and 37 cases as OR-HCC in the locoregional therapy group. Table 2 shows the clinicopathologic features of patients with LR-HCC. Compared with the OR-HCC group, the LR-HCC group had higher serum levels of AFP and AFP-L3 ($p = 0.031$ and $p = 0.033$, respectively). The incidence of postoperative complications tended to be higher in patients with LR-HCC. Pathologic assessment showed that the incidence of positive surgical margins tended to be higher in these patients. There were no obvious differences between the initial recurrence site and the recurrence pattern in the liver after curative surgery. The prognosis was not different between the LR-HCC and OR-HCC groups (Figure 2A,B).

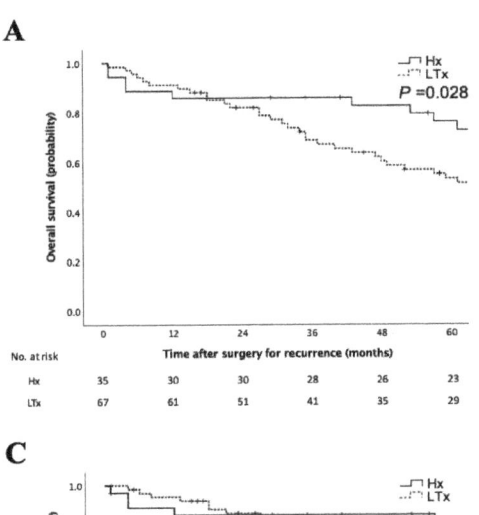
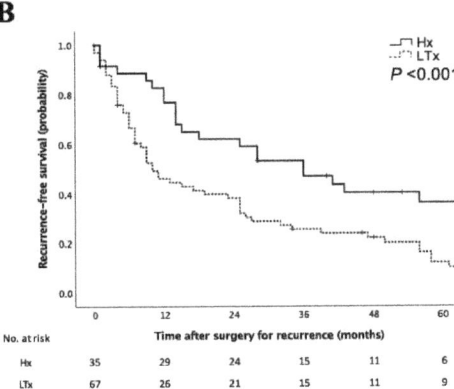
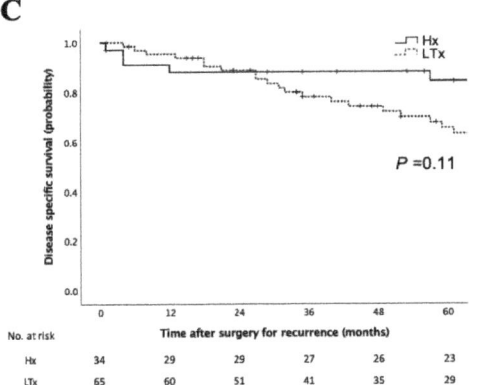

Figure 1. Survival analyses according to the previous treatment modalities. Kaplan–Meier curves for overall survival rates (**A**), recurrence-free survival rates (**B**), and disease-specific survival (**C**) of patients according to the previous treatment modalities. Survival rates in patients with previous locoregional therapy were significantly worse than those in patients with previous hepatectomy in the log–rank test. Hx, recurrence after hepatectomy; LTx, recurrence after locoregional therapy.

Table 2. Patient characteristics stratified by the recurrence pattern after locoregional therapy.

Variables	LR-HCC (n = 30)	OR-HCC (n = 37)	p-Value
Age (year, median)	68 (52–86)	70 (50–80)	0.94
Sex			0.871
Female	6	8	
Male	24	29	
Etiology			0.031
HBV	12	4	
HBV + HCV	0	1	
HCV	14	24	
NBNC	4	8	
Child–Pugh classification			1
A	28	35	
B	2	2	
Liver damage			0.548
A	24	29	
B	6	7	
C	0	1	

Table 2. Cont.

Variables	LR-HCC (n = 30)	OR-HCC (n = 37)	p-Value
Platelet count ($\times 10^3/\mu L$, median)	11.1 (5.1–19.1)	12.8 (5.1–28.5)	0.57
AFP (ng/mL, median)	35 (4–47,598)	7 (0–314)	0.031
AFP-L3 (%, median)	17.3 (0–84.9)	7.3 (0–50.3)	0.033
DCP (mAU/mL, median)	32 (10–10,520)	19 (7–23,000)	0.897
Number of pretreatments	3 (1–7)	3 (1–10)	0.253
Surgical approach			0.938
Open	20	25	
Laparoscopic	10	12	
Procedures			0.297
Partial resection	16	28	
Segmentectomy	3	2	
Sectionectomy	5	3	
Hemihepatectomy	6	4	
Operation time (min, median)	363 (155–650)	310 (84–1500)	0.123
Estimated blood loss (g, median)	475 (1–2537)	275 (1–16,156)	0.197
Morbidities (Clavien–Dindo $\geq$ IIIa)			0.07
No	14	26	
Yes	15	11	
Postoperative hospital stay (day, median)	16 (7–43)	12 (4–217)	0.232
Tumor multiplicity			0.439
Solitary	15	15	
Multiple	15	22	
Tumor size (mm, median)	25 (7–50)	22 (10–80)	0.705
Histology			0.577
Well	3	4	
Moderate	21	29	
Poor	6	4	
Other	0	0	
Portal venous invasion			0.102
No	11	21	
Yes	19	16	
Hepatic venous invasion			0.318
No	27	36	
Yes	3	1	
Hepatic arterial invasion			0.448
No	29	37	
Yes	1	0	
Bile duct invasion			1
No	28	35	
Yes	2	2	
Surgical margin			0.081
Negative	18	30	
Positive	10	6	
Background liver condition			0.268
Normal	0	0	
Chronic hepatitis	16	14	
Cirrhosis	13	20	
Initial recurrence site			0.689
Liver	18	23	
Extrahepatic	3	2	
Both	6	5	
Recurrence pattern in the liver			1
Intrahepatic metastasis/Multicentric occurrence	22	25	
Local recurrence	2	3	

Categorical data are expressed as n (%). Continuous variables are presented as the median [range]. AFP, alpha-fetoprotein; AFP-L3, lens culinaris agglutinin-reactive AFP; DCP, des-γ-carboxy prothrombin; HBV, hepatitis B virus; HCV, hepatitis C virus; LR-HCC, locally recurrent hepatocellular carcinoma after locoregional therapy; NBNC, non-HBV non-HCV; OR-HCC, other types of recurrent hepatocellular carcinoma after locoregional therapy.

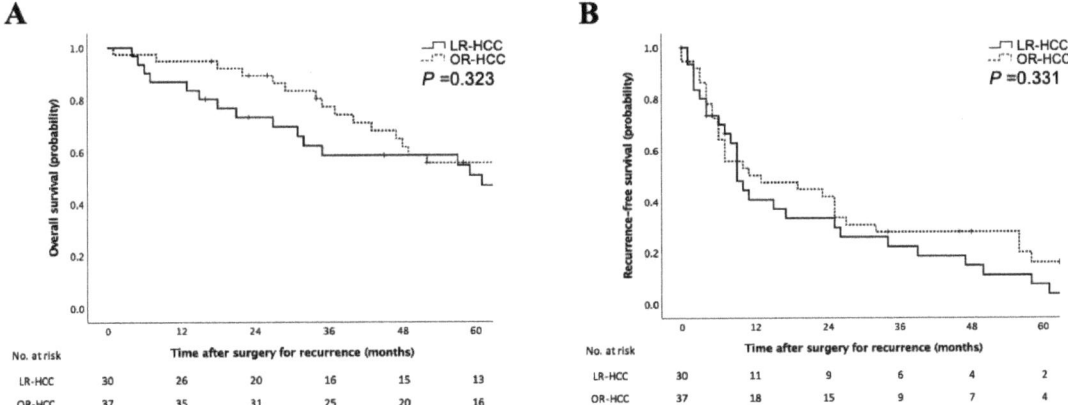

Figure 2. Survival analyses according to recurrence patterns after the locoregional treatment. Kaplan–Meier curves for overall survival rates (**A**) and recurrence-free survival rates (**B**) of patients according to recurrence patterns after the locoregional treatment. Survival rates were comparable between locally recurrent and other types of recurrent hepatocellular carcinoma in the log–rank test. LR-HCC, locally recurrent hepatocellular carcinoma after locoregional therapy; OR-HCC, other types of recurrent hepatocellular carcinoma after locoregional therapy.

3.3. Characteristics and Prognosis of Patients with LR-HCC after RFA and TACE

Table 3 shows the clinicopathologic differences between RFA and TACE stratified by the previous treatment modalities in LR-HCC. LR-HCC after RFA had higher values of des-γ-carboxy prothrombin (DCP) ($p = 0.041$). There were no other differences between the two groups. The prognosis was not different between the two groups (Figure 3A,B).

Table 3. Patient characteristics stratified by the previous locoregional therapies for LR-HCC.

Variables	Local Recurrence after RFA ($n = 15$)	Local Recurrence after TACE ($n = 15$)	p-Value
Age (year, median)	64 (52–86)	73 (54–79)	0.713
Sex			1
Female	3	3	
Male	12	12	
Etiology			0.513
HBV	6	6	
HCV	8	6	
NBNC	1	3	
Child–Pugh classification			0.483
A	13	15	
B	2	0	
Liver damage			0.651
A	11	13	
B	4	2	
Platelet count ($\times 10^3/\mu L$, median)	14.2 (5.1–25.8)	11.6 (7.1–29.0)	0.624
AFP (ng/mL, median)	71 (3–47,598)	9 (1–80,977)	0.367
AFP-L3 (%, median)	14.1 (0–84.9)	22.6 (0–58.0)	0.591
DCP (mAU/mL, median)	45 (10–6060)	15 (9–10,520)	0.041
Number of pretreatments	3 (1–5)	3 (1–11)	0.217
Surgical approach			1
Open	10	10	
Laparoscopic	5	5	
Procedures			0.4

Table 3. Cont.

Variables	Local Recurrence after RFA (n = 15)	Local Recurrence after TACE (n = 15)	p-Value
Partial resection	8	8	
Segmentectomy	1	2	
Sectionectomy	4	1	
Hemihepatectomy	2	4	
Operation time (time, median)	351 (155–691)	403 (246–801)	0.505
Estimated blood loss (g, median)	400 (1–2537)	510 (1–7100)	0.88
Morbidities (Clavien-Dindo ≥IIIa)			0.858
No	7	7	
Yes	8	7	
Postoperative hospital stay (day, median)	21 (7–160)	16 (6–101)	0.935
Tumor multiplicity			0.273
Solitary	9	6	
Multiple	6	9	
Tumor size (mm, median)	20 (7–55)	23 (13–140)	0.806
Histology			
Well	2	1	0.587
Moderate	11	10	
Poor	2	4	
Portal venous invasion			0.256
No	7	4	
Yes	8	11	
Hepatic venous invasion			1
No	14	13	
Yes	1	2	
Hepatic arterial invasion			0.309
No	15	14	
Yes	0	1	
Bile duct invasion			0.483
No	15	13	
Yes	0	2	
Surgical margin			1
Negative	9	9	
Positive	5	5	
Background liver condition			0.34
Normal	0	0	
Chronic hepatitis	7	9	
Cirrhosis	8	5	
Initial recurrence site			0.453
Liver	7	11	
Extrahepatic	1	2	
Both	4	2	
Recurrence pattern in the liver			0.482
Intrahepatic metastasis/ Multicentric occurrence	11	11	
Local recurrence	0	2	

Categorical data are expressed as n (%). Continuous variables are presented as the median [range]. AFP, alpha-fetoprotein; AFP-L3, lens culinaris agglutinin-reactive AFP; DCP, des-γ-carboxy prothrombin; HBV, hepatitis B virus; HCV, hepatitis C virus; NBNC, non-HBV non-HCV.

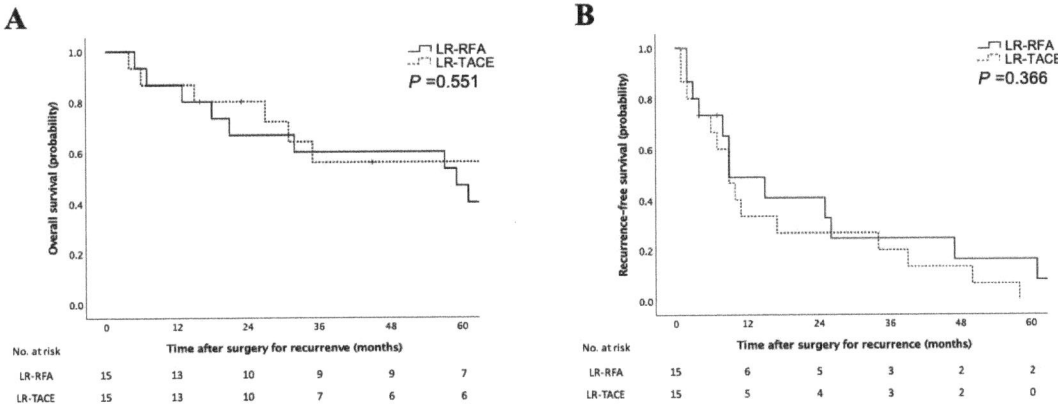

Figure 3. Survival analyses according to the previous locoregional therapy in LR-HCC. Kaplan–Meier curves for overall survival rates (**A**) and recurrence-free survival rates (**B**) of patients according to the previous locoregional therapy in locally recurrent hepatocellular carcinoma. Survival rates were comparable between RFA and TACE before recurrence in the log–rank test. LR-RFA, locally recurrent hepatocellular carcinoma after RFA; LR-TACE, locally recurrent hepatocellular carcinoma after TACE.

3.4. Prognostic Factors for the RFS of Recurrent HCC

The univariate and multivariate analyses of RFS for recurrent HCC are shown in Table 4. The optimal cut-off values of tumor markers to assign the patients into the two groups based on the greatest difference in the RFS were 20 ng/mL for AFP (p = 0.009), 10% for AFP-L3 (p = 0.04), and 40 mAU/mL for DCP (p = 0.076) when the minimum p-value approach was used (Supplementary Figure S1A–C). Multivariate analysis revealed that locoregional therapy as the previous treatment, multiple tumors, and portal venous invasion were the prognostic factors of RFS in recurrent HCC.

Table 4. Univariate and multivariate analyses of recurrence-free survival.

Variables	n	Median RFS	Univariate p-Value	Multivariate HR (95% CI)	p-Value
Etiology			0.208		
HBV	30	26			
HBV + HCV	1	56			
HCV	50	11			
NBNC	21	27			
Child–Pugh classification			0.946		
A	98	17			
B	4	32			
Liver damage			0.404		
A	85	18			
B + C	17	10			
AFP (ng/mL, median)			0.009		0.061
<20	69	25		1 (ref)	
≥20	33	10		1.65 (0.98–2.77)	
AFP-L3 (%, median)			0.04		0.388
<10	81	25		1 (ref)	
≥10	21	10		1.31 (0.71–2.39)	
DCP (mAU/mL, median)			0.076		0.899
<40	67	23		1 (ref)	
≥40	35	13		1.04 (0.60–1.80)	

Table 4. Cont.

Variables	n	Median RFS	Univariate p-Value	Multivariate HR (95% CI)	p-Value
Number of pretreatments			0.018		0.712
1	47	25		1 (ref)	
≥2	55	11		1.10 (0.67–1.79)	
Pretreatment modality			<0.001		0.005
Hepatectomy	35	36		1 (ref)	
Locoregional therapy	67	10		2.04 (1.24–3.39)	
Tumor multiplicity			<0.001		<0.001
Solitary	50	34		1 (ref)	
Multiple	52	8		2.78 (1.71–4.49)	
Tumor size (mm)			0.029		0.577
≤20	56	25		1 (ref)	
>20	46	14		1.20 (0.66–2.19)	
Portal venous invasion			<0.001		0.001
No	51	25		1 (ref)	
Yes	51	10		2.27 (1.39–3.71)	
Hepatic venous invasion			0.281		
No	97	17			
Yes	5	11			
Hepatic arterial invasion			0.495		
No	101	17			
Yes	1	11			
Bile duct invasion			<0.001		0.19
No	97	19		1 (ref)	
Yes	5	2		1.95 (0.72–5.28)	
Surgical margin			0.049		0.521
Negative	74	25		1 (ref)	
Positive	23	7		1.22 (0.67–2.23)	
Background liver condition			0.411		
Normal/Chronic hepatitis	56	25			
Cirrhosis	40	17			
Recurrence pattern			0.014		0.644
Local recurrence	30	9		1.15 (0.64–2.08)	
Other types of recurrence	72	25		1 (ref)	

Categorical data are expressed as n. AFP, alpha-fetoprotein; AFP-L3, lens culinaris agglutinin-reactive AFP; CI, confidence interval; DCP, des-γ-carboxy prothrombin; HBV, hepatitis B virus; HCV, hepatitis C virus; HR, hazard ratio; NBNC, non-HBV non-HCV; ref, reference; RFS, recurrence-free survival.

4. Discussion

The present study was designed to investigate the clinical benefit of salvage hepatectomy for LR-HCC. In this study, the incidence of postoperative complications was significantly high, which implies that salvage hepatectomy for LR-HCC was technically demanding. On the other hand, the prognosis of LR-HCC after RFA was comparable to those in previous studies [7,9–11]. The prognosis of LR-HCC after TACE was shown to be equivalent to that of LR-HCC after RFA. Taken together, these findings suggest that salvage hepatectomy for LR-HCC had favorable OS despite the high incidence of recurrence after curative surgery. In the multivariate analysis, LR-HCC was not a prognostic factor for RFS. Therefore, considering that multidisciplinary sequential therapies are mostly required for LR-HCC because of its highly malignant potential, surgical intervention should be considered as part of treatments if LR-HCC is resectable. It is important to consider hepatectomy and other local treatments as complementary and not exclusive. The dissociation between a low RFS and a rather high OS reflects the slow progression of the disease and the importance of repeating the treatment. Kishi et al. reported that the number rather than the type of treatment for tumor recurrence was associated with prolonged survival [13].

In general, LR-HCC is reported to have a high malignant potential among recurrent HCC [13]. The mechanism of the aggressive behavior remains unclarified. Some studies have concluded that increased intratumoral pressure caused by RFA may favor intravascular tumor spread. Several studies have documented that some recurrent HCC after RFA exhibit aggressive recurrence patterns as reflected in the rate of positive macroscopic tumor thrombus and more extensive tumor distribution. Especially, LR-HCC after RFA tended to be invasive because of lower differentiation grade, capsule invasion, and vascular invasion. However, the present study showed no evident findings rather than high serum levels of tumor markers compared with the other types of recurrent HCC. Immunohistological or genomic assessment of the tumor and tumor microenvironment might reveal reasonable causes of the aggressive behavior of LR-HCC.

Treatments for recurrent HCC are generally selected based on the same criteria as for primary HCC. Therefore, locoregional therapies are easily used again for recurrent HCC after locoregional therapy due to problems such as impaired liver function. Repeating locoregional treatment for intrahepatic recurrence prolongs patient survival and provides a comparable prognosis after RFA to repeat hepatectomy [14–17]. However, repeated locoregional treatment may lead to poor prognosis when liver resection may be preferable to locoregional treatment from an oncological standpoint in the case of LR-HCC. Appropriate timing of surgical intervention and the establishment of indications for salvage hepatectomy are warranted.

Even in cases where local treatment has been selected due to unresectable factors, surgical treatment may become possible by reviewing the timing and planning tailor-made procedures. In some cases, improvement of liver function through viral therapy or abstinence from alcohol could help preserve postoperative liver function. Recently, minimally invasive surgeries (MIS) have reduced the amount of abdominal wall destruction, thereby reducing leakage of ascites and pleural effusions [18]. In addition to the magnified view of MIS, the development of simulation technology has made it possible to perform accurate resection of the liver based on the understanding of the precise anatomy [19], and partial anatomical resection is now performed to ensure oncological cure, taking into account the remnant liver function. Furthermore, the number of postoperative complications has decreased due to the standardization of surgical techniques, the establishment of a board certification system [20], and the advancement of medical instruments relating to liver dissection and hemostasis methods, which may have fewer adverse effects on postoperative liver regeneration. These factors may have contributed to the selection of liver resection at the time of recurrence, even for patients who would previously have been considered more suitable for local treatment due to unresectable factors in the present study.

Liver transplantation, especially salvage liver transplantation, is the most promising treatment option for recurrent HCC. A meta-analysis reported that the 5-year survival rate after salvage liver transplantation was 53.9%, which was comparable to that after primary liver transplantation (56.5%) [21]. However, the shortage of donor organs, high medical costs, and contraindications for older patients limit the standardization of this strategy. Therefore, salvage hepatectomy might be an alternative treatment to liver transplantation for recurrent HCC, especially for LR-HCC.

To date, no adjuvant therapies have been shown to have benefits, but there are ongoing clinical trials. The IMbrave 050 trial revealed that atezolizumab plus bevacizumab as adjuvant chemotherapy showed prolonged RFS for patients at high risk of HCC recurrence who underwent locoregional or surgical therapy [22]. Considering that the treatment principle of recurrent HCC is the same as that of primary HCC, recurrent HCC with recurrence risk factors might be a good target of adjuvant therapies, including immune checkpoint inhibitors. Moreover, these therapies have the potential to improve the prognosis of patients with highly malignant LR-HCC.

Cytokeratin 19 (CK19) and epithelial cell adhesion molecule (EpCAM) have been known as prognostic biomarkers for HCC [23–25]. They might be useful in considering treatment strategies for resectable recurrent HCC. Neoadjuvant or adjuvant therapies might improve CK19- or EpCAM-positive recurrent HCC.

Our study has several limitations. First, it is a retrospective, single-center, small case-series study conducted by expert hepatobiliary surgeons. In addition, it has potential selection bias because the patients in this study had all undergone hepatectomy. We might have chosen patients with better background liver function and fewer multinodular tumors. In particular, the prognosis of the patients with LR-HCC who were treated using non-surgical therapies was unknown. Second, the starting point for prognostic evaluation was the date of resection of recurrent HCC, and previous therapies were not detailed, resulting in potentially varied patient and tumor characteristics. As a result, the prognosis of LR-HCC could not have been fully evaluated. Therefore, the indications and clinical benefit of salvage hepatectomy for LR-HCC were not directly generalized. Multi-institutional prospective cohort studies are warranted to decrease the influence of the potential bias in this study. However, we believe that the results of this study will support the validity of salvage hepatectomy for LR-HCC in selected patients.

5. Conclusions

Our study showed that salvage hepatectomy for LR-HCC after locoregional therapies has potentially favorable oncologic outcomes despite being technically demanding. Surgical treatment should be considered for LR-HCC in selected patients.

Supplementary Materials: The following supporting information can be downloaded at: https://www.mdpi.com/article/10.3390/cancers15082320/s1, Figure S1: Optimal cut-off values of tumor markers based on the prognostic differences in the recurrence-free survival of the patients; 20 ng/mL for AFP ($p = 0.009$) (**A**), 10% for AFP-L3 ($p = 0.04$) (**B**), and 40 mAU/mL for DCP ($p = 0.076$) (**C**).

Author Contributions: Conceptualization, T.M. and O.I.; methodology, T.M.; acquisition of data, M.K., Y.A., H.Y. and T.H.; analysis and interpretation of data, T.M., H.O. and M.S. (Masahiro Shinoda); writing—original draft preparation, T.M.; writing—review and editing, O.I. and M.S. (Michiie Sakamoto); supervision, Y.K.; project administration, O.I. All authors have read and agreed to the published version of the manuscript.

Funding: This research received no external funding.

Institutional Review Board Statement: The study was conducted in accordance with the Declaration of Helsinki and approved by the Institutional Review Board of Keio University School of Medicine (unique number: 20120280).

Informed Consent Statement: Informed consent was waived due to it's a retrospective study.

Data Availability Statement: Not applicable.

Conflicts of Interest: Y.K. received grants and personal fees from Chugai Pharmaceutical Co., Ltd., grants from Eisai Co., Ltd., and grants and personal fees from Takeda Pharmaceutical Company Limited, outside the submitted work. The other authors declare no conflict of interest.

References

1. Sung, H.; Ferlay, J.; Siegel, R.L.; Laversanne, M.; Soerjomataram, I.; Jemal, A.; Bray, F. Global Cancer Statistics 2020: GLOBOCAN Estimates of Incidence and Mortality Worldwide for 36 Cancers in 185 Countries. *CA Cancer J. Clin.* **2021**, *71*, 209–249. [CrossRef]
2. Arii, S.; Teramoto, K.; Kawamura, T.; Okamoto, H.; Kaido, T.; Mori, A.; Imamura, M. Characteristics of recurrent hepatocellular carcinoma in Japan and our surgical experience. *J. Hepatobiliary Pancreat. Surg.* **2001**, *8*, 397–403. [CrossRef]
3. European Association for the Study of the Liver. Electronic address: Easloffice@easloffice.eu; European Association for the Study of the Liver: EASL Clinical Practice Guidelines: Management of hepatocellular carcinoma. *J. Hepatol.* **2018**, *69*, 182–236. [CrossRef]
4. Kudo, M.; Kawamura, Y.; Hasegawa, K.; Tateishi, R.; Kariyama, K.; Shiina, S.; Toyoda, H.; Imai, Y.; Hiraoka, A.; Ikeda, M.; et al. Management of Hepatocellular Carcinoma in Japan: JSH Consensus Statements and Recommendations 2021 Update. *Liver Cancer* **2021**, *10*, 181–223. [CrossRef] [PubMed]
5. Heimbach, J.K.; Kulik, L.M.; Finn, R.S.; Sirlin, C.B.; Abecassis, M.M.; Roberts, L.R.; Zhu, A.X.; Murad, M.H.; Marrero, J.A. AASLD guidelines for the treatment of hepatocellular carcinoma. *Hepatology* **2018**, *67*, 358–380. [CrossRef] [PubMed]

6. The NCCN Clinical Practice Guidelines in Oncology (NCCN Guidelines®) Hepatobiliary Cancers (Version 5.2022). Available online: https://www.nccn.org/professionals/physician_gls/pdf/hepatobiliary.pdf (accessed on 13 January 2023).
7. Torzilli, G.; Del Fabbro, D.; Palmisano, A.; Marconi, M.; Makuuchi, M.; Montorsi, M. Salvage hepatic resection after incomplete interstitial therapy for primary and secondary liver tumours. *Br. J. Surg.* 2007, *94*, 208–213. [CrossRef]
8. Masuda, T.; Beppu, T.; Ishiko, T.; Horino, K.; Baba, Y.; Mizumoto, T.; Hayashi, H.; Okabe, H.; Horlad, H.; Doi, K.; et al. Intrahepatic dissemination of hepatocellular carcinoma after local ablation therapy. *J. Hepatobiliary Pancreat. Surg.* 2008, *15*, 589–595. [CrossRef] [PubMed]
9. Portolani, N.; Baiocchi, G.L.; Coniglio, A.; Grazioli, L.; Frassi, E.; Gheza, F.; Giulini, S.M. Sequential multidisciplinary treatment of hepatocellular carcinoma: The role of surgery as rescue therapy for failure of percutaneous ablation therapies. *J. Surg. Oncol.* 2009, *100*, 580–584. [CrossRef]
10. Sugo, H.; Ishizaki, Y.; Yoshimoto, J.; Imamura, H.; Kawasaki, S. Salvage hepatectomy for local recurrent hepatocellular carcinoma after ablation therapy. *Ann. Surg. Oncol.* 2012, *19*, 2238–2245. [CrossRef]
11. Imai, K.; Beppu, T.; Chikamoto, A.; Mima, K.; Okabe, H.; Hayashi, H.; Nitta, H.; Ishiko, T.; Baba, H. Salvage treatment for local recurrence of hepatocellular carcinoma after local ablation therapy. *Hepatol. Res.* 2014, *44*, E335–E345. [CrossRef]
12. Kudo, M.; Matsui, O.; Izumi, N.; Iijima, H.; Kadoya, M.; Imai, Y.; Okusaka, T.; Miyayama, S.; Tsuchiya, K.; Ueshima, K.; et al. JSH consensus-based clinical practice guidelines for the management of hepatocellular carcinoma: 2014 updates by the Liver Cancer Study Group of Japan. *Liver Cancer* 2014, *3*, 458–468. [CrossRef]
13. Kishi, Y.; Shimada, K.; Nara, S.; Esaki, M.; Kosuge, T. Role of hepatectomy for recurrent or initially unresectable hepatocellular carcinoma. *World J. Hepatol.* 2014, *6*, 836–843. [CrossRef] [PubMed]
14. Taura, K.; Ikai, I.; Hatano, E.; Fujii, H.; Uyama, N.; Shimahara, Y. Implication of frequent local ablation therapy for intrahepatic recurrence in prolonged survival of patients with hepatocellular carcinoma undergoing hepatic resection: An analysis of 610 patients over 16 years old. *Ann. Surg.* 2006, *244*, 265–273. [CrossRef]
15. Poon, R.T.P.; Ngan, H.; Lo, C.M.; Liu, C.L.; Fan, S.T.; Wong, J. Transarterial chemoembolization for inoperable hepatocellular carcinoma and postresection intrahepatic recurrence. *J. Surg. Oncol.* 2000, *73*, 109–114. [CrossRef]
16. Choi, D.; Lim, H.K.; Rhim, H.; Kim, Y.S.; Yoo, B.C.; Paik, S.W.; Joh, J.W.; Park, C.K. Percutaneous radiofrequency ablation for recurrent hepatocellular carcinoma after hepatectomy: Long-term results and prognostic factors. *Ann. Surg. Oncol.* 2007, *14*, 2319–2329. [CrossRef]
17. Okuwaki, Y.; Nakazawa, T.; Kokubu, S.; Hidaka, H.; Tanaka, Y.; Takada, J.; Watanabe, M.; Shibuya, A.; Minamino, T.; Saigenji, K. Repeat radiofrequency ablation provides survival benefit in patients with intrahepatic distant recurrence of hepatocellular carcinoma. *Am. J. Gastroenterol.* 2009, *104*, 2747–2753. [CrossRef] [PubMed]
18. Cipriani, F.; Fantini, C.; Ratti, F.; Lauro, R.; Tranchart, H.; Halls, M.; Scuderi, V.; Barkhatov, L.; Edwin, B.; Troisi, R.I.; et al. Laparoscopic liver resections for hepatocellular carcinoma. Can we extend the surgical indication in cirrhotic patients? *Surg. Endosc.* 2018, *32*, 617–626. [CrossRef]
19. Wakabayashi, G.; Cherqui, D.; Geller, D.A.; Hilal, M.A.; Berardi, G.; Ciria, R.; Abe, Y.; Aoki, T.; Asbun, H.J.; Chan, A.C.Y.; et al. The Tokyo 2020 terminology of liver anatomy and resections: Updates of the Brisbane 2000 system. *J. Hepatobiliary Pancreat. Sci.* 2022, *29*, 6–15. [CrossRef]
20. Arita, J.; Yamamoto, H.; Kokudo, T.; Hasegawa, K.; Miyata, H.; Toh, Y.; Gotoh, M.; Kokudo, N.; Kakeji, Y.; Seto, Y. Impact of board certification system and adherence to the clinical practice guidelines for liver cancer on post-hepatectomy risk-adjusted mortality rate in Japan: A questionnaire survey of departments registered with the National Clinical Database. *J. Hepatobiliary Pancreat. Sci.* 2021, *28*, 801–811. [CrossRef]
21. Guerrini, G.P.; Esposito, G.; Olivieri, T.; Magistri, P.; Ballarin, R.; Di Sandro, S.; Di Benedetto, F. Salvage versus primary liver transplantation for hepatocellular carcinoma: A twenty-year experience meta-analysis. *Cancers* 2022, *14*, 3465. [CrossRef]
22. Hack, S.P.; Spahn, J.; Chen, M.; Cheng, A.L.; Kaseb, A.; Kudo, M.; Lee, H.C.; Yopp, A.; Chow, P.; Qin, S. IMbrave 050: A Phase III trial of atezolizumab plus bevacizumab in high-risk hepatocellular carcinoma after curative resection or ablation. *Future Oncol.* 2020, *16*, 975–989. [CrossRef] [PubMed]
23. Kim, H.; Choi, G.H.; Na, D.C.; Ahn, E.Y.; Kim, G.I.; Lee, J.E.; Cho, J.Y.; Yoo, J.E.; Choi, J.S.; Park, Y.N. Human hepatocellular carcinomas with "Stemness"-related marker expression: Keratin 19 expression and a poor prognosis. *Hepatology* 2011, *54*, 1707–1717. [CrossRef] [PubMed]
24. Yamashita, T.; Ji, J.; Budhu, A.; Forgues, M.; Yang, W.; Wang, H.Y.; Jia, H.; Ye, Q.; Wauthier, E.; Reid, L.M.; et al. EpCAM-positive hepatocellular carcinoma cells are tumor-initiating cells with stem/progenitor cell features. *Gastroenterology* 2009, *136*, 1012–1024. [CrossRef] [PubMed]
25. Tsujikawa, H.; Masugi, Y.; Yamazaki, K.; Itano, O.; Kitagawa, Y.; Sakamoto, M. Immunohistochemical molecular analysis indicates hepatocellular carcinoma subgroups that reflect tumor aggressiveness. *Hum. Pathol.* 2016, *50*, 24–33. [CrossRef]

Disclaimer/Publisher's Note: The statements, opinions and data contained in all publications are solely those of the individual author(s) and contributor(s) and not of MDPI and/or the editor(s). MDPI and/or the editor(s) disclaim responsibility for any injury to people or property resulting from any ideas, methods, instructions or products referred to in the content.

MDPI
St. Alban-Anlage 66
4052 Basel
Switzerland
www.mdpi.com

Cancers Editorial Office
E-mail: cancers@mdpi.com
www.mdpi.com/journal/cancers

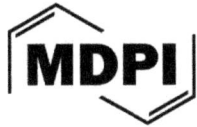

Disclaimer/Publisher's Note: The statements, opinions and data contained in all publications are solely those of the individual author(s) and contributor(s) and not of MDPI and/or the editor(s). MDPI and/or the editor(s) disclaim responsibility for any injury to people or property resulting from any ideas, methods, instructions or products referred to in the content.

www.ingramcontent.com/pod-product-compliance
Lightning Source LLC
LaVergne TN
LVHW070713100526
838202LV00013B/1083